T0263717

Central Nervous System Infections

Editor

TCHOYOSON LIM

NEUROIMAGING CLINICS OF NORTH AMERICA

www.neuroimaging.theclinics.com

Consulting Editor
SURESH K. MUKHERJI

February 2023 • Volume 33 • Number 1

ELSEVIER

1600 John F. Kennedy Boulevard • Suite 1800 • Philadelphia, Pennsylvania, 19103-2899

http://www.neuroimaging.theclinics.com

NEUROIMAGING CLINICS OF NORTH AMERICA Volume 33, Number 1
February 2023 ISSN 1052-5149, ISBN 13: 978-0-323-84950-0

Editor: John Vassallo (j.vassallo@elsevier.com)
Developmental Editor: Karen Solomon

© **2023 Elsevier Inc. All rights reserved.**

This publication and the individual contributions contained in it are protected under copyright by Elsevier, and the following terms and conditions apply to their use:

Photocopying
Single photocopies of single articles may be made for personal use as allowed by national copyright laws. Permission of the Publisher and payment of a fee is required for all other photocopying, including multiple or systematic copying, copying for advertising or promotional purposes, resale, and all forms of document delivery. Special rates are available for educational institutions that wish to make photocopies for non-profit educational classroom use. For information on how to seek permission visit www.elsevier.com/permissions or call: (+44) 1865 843830 (UK)/(+1) 215 239 3804 (USA).

Derivative Works
Subscribers may reproduce tables of contents or prepare lists of articles including abstracts for internal circulation within their institutions. Permission of the Publisher is required for resale or distribution outside the institution. Permission of the Publisher is required for all other derivative works, including compilations and translations (please consult www.elsevier.com/permissions).

Electronic Storage or Usage
Permission of the Publisher is required to store or use electronically any material contained in this periodical, including any article or part of an article (please consult www.elsevier.com/permissions). Except as outlined above, no part of this publication may be reproduced, stored in a retrieval system or transmitted in any form or by any means, electronic, mechanical, photocopying, recording or otherwise, without prior written permission of the Publisher.

Notice
No responsibility is assumed by the Publisher for any injury and/or damage to persons or property as a matter of products liability, negligence or otherwise, or from any use or operation of any methods, products, instructions or ideas contained in the material herein. Because of rapid advances in the medical sciences, in particular, independent verification of diagnoses and drug dosages should be made.

Although all advertising material is expected to conform to ethical (medical) standards, inclusion in this publication does not constitute a guarantee or endorsement of the quality or value of such product or of the claims made of it by its manufacturer.

Neuroimaging Clinics of North America (ISSN 1052-5149) is published quarterly by Elsevier Inc., 360 Park Avenue South, New York, NY 10010-1710. Months of issue are February, May, August, and November. Business and editorial offices: 1600 John F. Kennedy Blvd., Suite 1800, Philadelphia, PA 19103-2899. Business and editorial offices: 6277 Sea Harbor Drive, Orlando, FL 32887-4800. Periodicals postage paid at New York, NY, and additional mailing offices. Subscription prices are USD 413 per year for US individuals, USD 745 per year for US institutions, USD 100 per year for US students and residents, USD 483 per year for Canadian individuals, USD 949 per year for Canadian institutions, USD 562 per year for international individuals, USD 949 per year for international institutions, USD 100 per year for Canadian students and residents and USD 260 per year for foreign students and residents. To receive student/resident rate, orders must be accompanied by name of affiliated institution, date of term, and the *signature* of program/residency coordinator on institution letterhead. Orders will be billed at individual rate until proof of status is received. Foreign air speed delivery is included in all *Clinics* subscription prices. All prices are subject to change without notice. POSTMASTER: Send address changes to *Neuroimaging Clinics of North America*, Elsevier Health Sciences Division, Subscription **Customer Service, 3251 Riverport Lane, Maryland Heights, MO 63043. Telephone: 1-800-654-2452 (U.S. and Canada); 314-447-8871 (outside U.S. and Canada). Fax: 314-447-8029. E-mail: journalscustomerservice-usa@elsevier.com (for print support); journals onlinesupport-usa@elsevier.com (for online support).**

Reprints. For copies of 100 or more of articles in this publication, please contact the Commercial Reprints Department, Elsevier Inc., 360 Park Avenue South, New York, NY 10010-1710. Tel.: 212-633-3874; Fax: 212-633-3820; E-mail: reprints@elsevier.com.

Neuroimaging Clinics of North America is covered by *Excerpta Medical/EMBASE,* the RSNA Index of Imaging Literature, *MEDLINE/PubMed (Index Medicus),* MEDLINE/MEDLARS, SciSearch, Research Alert, and Neuroscience Citation Index.

PROGRAM OBJECTIVE
The goal of *Neuroimaging Clinics of North America* is to keep practicing radiologists and radiology residents up to date with current clinical practice in radiology by providing timely articles reviewing the state of the art in patient care.

TARGET AUDIENCE
Practicing radiologists, radiology residents, and other healthcare professionals who utilize neuroimaging findings to provide patient care.

LEARNING OBJECTIVES
Upon completion of this activity, participants will be able to:
1. Review typical and atypical neuroimaging findings in order to promote early diagnosis and monitoring of CNS infections.
2. Discuss the advantages of using neuroimaging into CNS infection diagnosis and treatment planning.
3. Recognize the value of using neuroimaging in multidisciplinary teams to rapidly develop, precisely diagnose, and treat CNS infections.

ACCREDITATION
The Elsevier Office of Continuing Medical Education (EOCME) is accredited by the Accreditation Council for Continuing Medical Education (ACCME) to provide continuing medical education for physicians.

The EOCME designates this journal-based CME activity for a maximum of 13 *AMA PRA Category 1 Credit*(s)™.Physicians should claim only the credit commensurate with the extent of their participation in the activity.

All other healthcare professionals requesting continuing education credit for this enduring material will be issued a certificate of participation.

DISCLOSURE OF CONFLICTS OF INTEREST
The EOCME assesses conflict of interest with its instructors, faculty, planners, and other individuals who are in a position to control the content of CME activities. All relevant conflicts of interest that are identified are thoroughly vetted by EOCME for fair balance, scientific objectivity, and patient care recommendations. EOCME is committed to providing its learners with CME activities that promote improvements or quality in healthcare and not a specific proprietary business or a commercial interest.

The planning committee, staff, authors, and editors listed below have identified no financial relationships or relationships to products or devices they or their spouse/life partner have with commercial interest related to the content of this CME activity:
Brenda Sze Peng Ang, MBBS, M Med, MPH; Yun Jung Bae, MD; Puneet Belani, MD; Sanders Chang, MD; Tchoyoson Lim Choie Cheio, MBBS, MMed; Thoon Koh Cheng, MBBS, MRCPCH, MMed; Michael Tran Duong, PhD; Christopher G. Filippi, MD; Rakesh Gupta, MD; Rajan Jain, MD; Pradeep Kuttysankaran; Aleum Lee, MD, PhD; Leandro Tavares Lucato, MD, PhD; Thiago Augusto Vasconcelos Miranda, MD; Monique A. Mogensen, MD; Suyash Mohan, MD,PDCC; Yoshiaki Ota, MD; Mina Park, MD, PhD; Norlisah Mohd Ramli, MBBS, FRCR,FAMM; Jeffrey D. Rudie, MD, PhD; Jitender Saini, MBBS, MD; Shilpa Sankhe, MBBS, MD; Michael Schecht, MD; Rekha Siripurapu, MBBS, MRCP, FRCR; E. Turgut Tali, MD; Chong Tin Tan, MBBS, FRCP, MD; Phua Hwee Tang, MBBS, MMed, FRCR; Umapathi Thirugnanam, MBBS; Doreen Thomas-Payne, MSN, BSN, RN, PMHNP-BC; Kazuhiro Tsuchiya; Kum Thong Wong, MBBS, MPath, FRCPath, MD; Jun Fang Xian, MD, PhD; Hajime Yokota, MD, PhD

The planning committee, staff, authors and editors listed below have identified financial relationships or relationships to products or devices they or their spouse/life partner have with commercial interest related to the content of this CME activity:
Joel M. Stein, MD, PhD: Researcher: Hyperfine, Inc; Consultant: Centaur Labs

UNAPPROVED / OFF-LABEL USE DISCLOSURE
The EOCME requires CME faculty to disclose to the participants:
1. When products or procedures being discussed are off-label, unlabelled, experimental, and/or investigational (not US Food and Drug Administration [FDA] approved); and
2. Any limitations on the information presented, such as data that are preliminary or that represent ongoing research, interim analyses, and/or unsupported opinions. Faculty may discuss information about pharmaceutical agents that is outside of FDA-approved labelling. This information is intended solely for CME and is not intended to promote off-label use of these medications. If you have any questions, contact the medical affairs department of the manufacturer for the most recent prescribing information.

TO ENROLL
To enroll in the *Neuroimaging Clinics of North America* Continuing Medical Education program, call customer service at 1-800-654-2452 or sign up online at http://www.theclinics.com/home/cme. The CME program is available to subscribers for an additional annual fee of USD 265.00.

METHOD OF PARTICIPATION

In order to claim credit, participants must complete the following:
1. Complete enrolment as indicated above.
2. Read the activity.
3. Complete the CME Test and Evaluation. Participants must achieve a score of 70% on the test. All CME Tests and Evaluations must be completed online.

CME INQUIRIES/SPECIAL NEEDS

For all CME inquiries or special needs, please contact elsevierCME@elsevier.com.

NEUROIMAGING CLINICS OF NORTH AMERICA

FORTHCOMING ISSUES

May 2023
MRI and Brain Trauma
Pejman Jabehdar Maralani and Sean Symons,
Editors

August 2023
Spine Tumors
Carlos Torres, *Editor*

November 2023
Pediatric Head and Neck Imaging
William T. O'Brien, Sr., *Editor*

RECENT ISSUES

November 2022
Neuroimaging Anatomy, Part 2: Head, Neck, and Spine
Tarik F. Massoud, *Editor*

August 2022
Neuroimaging Anatomy, Part 1: Brain and Skull
Tarik F. Massoud, *Editor*

May 2022
Mimics, Pearls, and Pitfalls of Head and Neck Imaging
Gul Moonis and Daniel T. Ginat, *Editors*

SERIES OF RELATED INTEREST

Advances in Clinical Radiology
Available at: Advancesinclinicalradiology.com
MRI Clinics of North America
Available at: MRI.theclinics.com
PET Clinics
Available at: https://www.pet.theclinics.com/
Radiologic Clinics of North America
Available at: Radiologic.theclinics.com

THE CLINICS ARE AVAILABLE ONLINE!
Access your subscription at:
www.theclinics.com

NEUROIMAGING CLINICS OF NORTH AMERICA

FORTHCOMING ISSUES

May 2022
MRI and Brain Trauma
Pejman Jabehdar Maralani and Sean Symons,
Editors

August 2022
Spine Tumors
Carlos Torres, Editor

November 2022
Pediatric Head and Neck Imaging
William T. O'Brien, Sr., Editor

RECENT ISSUES

February 2022
Neuroimaging Anatomy, Part 2: Head, Neck, and Spine
Tarik F. Massoud, Editor

November 2021
Neuroimaging Anatomy, Part 1: Brain and Skull
Tarik F. Massoud, Editor

May 2021
Mimics, Pearls, and Pitfalls of Head and Neck Imaging
Gul Moonis and Daniel T. Ginat, Editors

SERIES OF RELATED INTEREST

Radiologic Clinics of North America
https://www.radiologic.theclinics.com

THE CLINICS ARE AVAILABLE ONLINE!
Access your subscription at:
www.theclinics.com

Contributors

CONSULTING EDITOR

SURESH K. MUKHERJI, MD, MBA, FACR
Clinical Professor of Radiology and Radiation
Oncology, University of Illinois, Peoria, Illinois,
USA; Robert Wood Johnson Medical School,
Rutgers University, New Brunswick, New
Jersey, USA; Faculty, Otolaryngology Head
Neck Surgery, Michigan State University,
Farmington Hills, Michiga, USAn; National
Director of Head and Neck Radiology, ProScan
Imaging, Carmel, Indiana, USA

EDITOR

TCHOYOSON LIM, MBBS, MMed
Clinical Professor, Neuroradiology, National
Neuroscience Institute, Singapore

AUTHORS

**BRENDA SZE PENG ANG, MBBS, MMed,
MPH**
Senior Consultant, Department of Infectious
Diseases, Clinical Director, Department of
Infection Prevention and Control, Adjunct
Associate Professor, LKC School of Medicine,
Singapore

YUN JUNG BAE, MD, PhD
Department of Radiology, Seoul National
University Bundang Hospital, Seoul National
University College of Medicine, Seoul,
Republic of Korea

PUNEET BELANI, MD
Departments of Diagnostic, Molecular and
Interventional Radiology, and Neurosurgery,
Icahn School of Medicine at Mount Sinai, New
York, New York, USA

SANDERS CHANG, MD
Department of Diagnostic, Molecular and
Interventional Radiology, Icahn School of
Medicine at Mount Sinai, New York, New York,
USA

MICHAEL TRAN DUONG, PhD
Division of Neuroradiology, Department
of Radiology, Perelman School of
Medicine at the University of
Pennsylvania, Philadelphia, Pennsylvania,
USA

CHRISTOPHER G. FILIPPI, MD
Professor and Chairman, Department of
Radiology, Tufts University School of Medicine,
Boston, Massachusetts, USA

RAKESH K. GUPTA, MD
Department of Radiology, Fortis Memorial
Research Institute, Gurugram, Haryana,
India

**TANG PHUA HWEE, MBBS (SINGAPORE),
MMED (DIAGNOSTIC RADIOLOGY), FRCR
(UK)**
Senior Consultant Radiologist, Department of
Diagnostic and Interventional Imaging, KK
Women's and Children's Hospital, Singapore,
Singapore

RAJAN JAIN, MD
Departments of Radiology and Neurosurgery, NYU Grossman School of Medicine, New York, New York, USA

THOON KOH CHENG, MBBS, MRCPCH, MMED (PAEDS)
Department of Paediatrics, Head and Senior Consultant, Infectious Disease, KK Women's and Children's Hospital, Singapore, Singapore

ALEUM LEE, MD, PhD
Associate Professor, Department of Radiology, Soon Chun Hyang University Hospital, Bucheon, Republic of Korea

TCHOYOSON LIM, MBBS, MMed
Clinical Professor, Neuroradiology, National Neuroscience Institute, Singapore

LEANDRO TAVARES LUCATO, MD, PhD
Chief of Diagnostic Neuroradiology Section, Hospital das Clínicas da Faculdade de Medicina da Universidade de São Paulo, Grupo Fleury, São Paulo, São Paulo, Brazil

MONIQUE A. MOGENSEN, MD
Assistant Professor, Department of Radiology, University of Washington School of Medicine, Seattle, Washington, USA

SUYASH MOHAN, MD, PDCC
Division of Neuroradiology, Department of Radiology, Perelman School of Medicine at the University of Pennsylvania, Philadelphia, Pennsylvania, USA

YOSHIAKI OTA, MD
Division of Neuroradiology, Department of Radiology, University of Michigan, Ann Arbor, Michigan, USA

MINA PARK, MD, PhD
Department of Radiology, Gangnam Severance Hospital, Yonsei University College of Medicine, Gangnam-gu, Seoul, South Korea

NORLISAH MOHD RAMLI, MBBS, FRCR
Department of Biomedical Imaging, Faculty of Medicine, University of Malaya, Kuala Lumper, Malaysia

JEFFREY D. RUDIE, MD, PhD
Department of Radiology, Scripps Clinic, La Jolla, California, USA

JITENDER SAINI, MBBS, MD
Professor, Department of Neuroimaging & Interventional Radiology, National institute of Mental Health and Neurosciences, Bangalore, India

SHILPA S. SANKHE, MD, DNB
Associate Professor of Radiology, King Edward Memorial Hospital, Parel, Mumbai, India

MICHAEL SCHECHT, MD
Department of Diagnostic, Molecular and Interventional Radiology, Icahn School of Medicine at Mount Sinai, New York, New York, USA

REKHA SIRIPURAPU, MBBS, MRCP, FRCR
Consultant Neuroradiologist, Department of Neuroradiology, Manchester Centre for Clinical Neurosciences, Salford Royal Hospital, Northern Care Alliance NHS Foundation Trust, Salford, United Kingdom

JOEL M. STEIN, MD, PhD
Assistant Professor of Radiology, Division of Neuroradiology, Department of Radiology, Hospital of the University of Pennsylvania, Philadelphia, Pennsylvania, USA

E. TURGUT TALI, MD
Professor of Radiology and Neuroradiology, Director, Section of Neuroradiology Lokman Hekim University School of Medicine, Sogutozu, Ankara, Turkey

CHONG TIN TAN, MBBS, FRCP, MD
Professor, Department of Medicine, University of Malaya, Kuala Lumpur, Malaysia

KAZUHIRO TSUCHIYA, MD, PhD
JR Tokyo General Hospital, Shibuya City, Tokyo, Japan

THIRUGNANAM UMAPATHI, MBBS
Associate Professor, Neurology, National Neuroscience Institute, Singapore

THIAGO AUGUSTO VASCONCELOS MIRANDA, MD
Emergency Radiology Section, Hospital das Clínicas da Faculdade de Medicina da Universidade de São Paulo, São Paulo, Brazil

KUM THONG WONG, MBBS, MPath, FRACPath
Department of Medicine, University of Malaya, Kuala Lumpur, Malaysia

JUNFANG XIAN, MD, PhD
Professor and Chair, Department of Radiology, Capital Medical University, Beijing, China

HAJIME YOKOTA, MD, PhD
Department of Diagnostic Radiology and Radiation Oncology, Graduate School of Medicine, Chiba University, Chuo-ku, Chiba, Japan

Contents

Foreword: Central Nervous System Infections   xv

Suresh K. Mukherji

Preface: Imaging CNS Infection: Now more relevant than ever   xvii

Tchoyoson Lim

The Changing Epidemiology of Central Nervous System Infection: Can Radiologists Keep
Up?   1

Brenda Sze Peng Ang, Thirugnanam Umapathi, and Tchoyoson Lim

Diagnostic radiologists can increase their clinical value by supplementing image pattern recognition with knowledge of epidemiology and geographic distribution of central nervous system (CNS) infections and their causative organisms. This article reviews the changing global disease patterns, as well as zoonotic outbreaks of henipaviruses, coronaviruses, and other emerging, reemerging, and vector-borne organisms; case examples highlight typical imaging features of CNS infections and their mimics. Technical advances in neuroimaging help to enhance the value of radiologists to the multidisciplinary team and the responses to future pandemic preparation.

Neuroimaging Patterns of Intracranial Infections: Meningitis, Cerebritis, and Their
Complications   11

Michael Tran Duong, Jeffrey D. Rudie, and Suyash Mohan

Neuroimaging provides rapid, noninvasive visualization of central nervous system infections for optimal diagnosis and management. Generalizable and characteristic imaging patterns help radiologists distinguish different types of intracranial infections including meningitis and cerebritis from a variety of bacterial, viral, fungal, and/or parasitic causes. Here, we describe key radiologic patterns of meningeal enhancement and diffusion restriction through profiles of meningitis, cerebritis, abscess, and ventriculitis. We discuss various imaging modalities and recent diagnostic advances such as deep learning through a survey of intracranial pathogens and their radiographic findings. Moreover, we explore critical complications and differential diagnoses of intracranial infections.

Structured Imaging Approach for Viral Encephalitis   43

Norlisah Mohd Ramli and Yun Jung Bae

MR imaging is essential in diagnosing viral encephalitis. Clinical features, cerebrospinal fluid analysis and pathogen confirmation by polymerase chain reaction can be supported by assessing imaging features. MR imaging patterns with typical locations can identify pathogens such as temporal lobe for herpes simplex virus type 1; bilateral thalami for Japanese encephalitis and influenza virus; and brainstem for enterovirus and rabies. In this article, we have reviewed representative viral encephalitis and its MR imaging patterns. In addition, we also presented acute viral encephalitis without typical MR imaging patterns, such as dengue and varicella-zoster virus encephalitis.

Acute Neurological Complications of Coronavirus Disease   57

Sanders Chang, Michael Schecht, Rajan Jain, and Puneet Belani

> The coronavirus disease (COVID-19) pandemic has impacted many lives globally. Neurologic manifestations have been observed among individuals at various stages and severity of the disease, the most common being stroke. Prompt identification of these neurologic diagnoses can affect patient management and prognosis. This article discusses the acute neuroradiological features typical of COVID-19, including cerebrovascular disease, intracerebral hemorrhage, leukoencephalopathy, and sensory neuropathies.

Coronavirus Disease: Subacute to Chronic Neuroimaging Findings   69

Monique A. Mogensen and Christopher G. Filippi

> Several neurologic disorders are associated with coronavirus disease 2019 (COVID-19). In this article, clinical syndromes typically occurring in the subacute to chronic phase of illness and their neuroimaging findings are described with discussion of their COVID-19 specific features and prognosis. Proposed pathogenic mechanisms of these neuroimaging findings and challenges in determining etiology are reviewed.

Imaging of Uncommon Bacterial, Rickettsia, Spirochete, and Fungal Infections   83

Jitender Saini, Shilpa S. Sankhe, and Aleum Lee

> This article reviews uncommon bacterial (brucellosis, actinomycosis, neuromelioidosis, nocardiosis, whipple disease, and listeriosis), Rickettsia, spirochete (neurosyphilis and Lyme disease), and fungal (mucormycosis, aspergillosis, candidiasis, cryptococcosis, and Cladophialophora bantiana) diseases affecting central nervous system (CNS), focusing primarily on their cranial manifestations. These infections often show a variety of neuroimaging features that may be similar or differ from typical pyogenic bacterial meningitis and abscess. Familiarity with these patterns is essential for timely recognition and initiation of appropriate management. Neuroimaging is also useful for identifying complications of CNS infections and follow-up evaluation after initiation of treatment.

Central Nervous System Mycobacterium Infection: Tuberculosis and Beyond   105

Mina Park and Rakesh K. Gupta

> Tuberculosis is a contagious infectious disease caused by Mycobacterium tuberculosis, and is the leading cause of death from a single infectious agent worldwide. Imaging plays an important role in the early diagnosis of central nervous system tuberculosis and may prevent unnecessary morbidity and mortality. This article presents an extensive review of pathogenesis, clinical symptoms, typical and atypical imaging appearances of intracranial and spinal tuberculosis, and advanced imaging of intracranial tuberculosis. Furthermore, we explore central nervous system infection of nontuberculous mycobacteria and leprosy and their imaging findings.

Imaging of Central Nervous System Parasitic Infections   125

Thiago Augusto Vasconcelos Miranda, Kazuhiro Tsuchiya, and Leandro Tavares Lucato

> Parasitic infections of the central nervous system (CNS) constitute a wide range of diseases, some quite prevalent across the world, some exceedingly rare. Causative parasites can be divided into two groups: unicellular protozoa and multicellular

helminthic worms. This includes diseases such as neurotoxoplasmosis and neuro-cysticercosis, which represent a major cause of pathology among certain popula-tions, and some more uncommon diseases, as primary amebic meningoencephalitis and neuroschistosomiasis. In this review, we focus on imaging manifestation and some helpful clinical and epidemiologic features of such condi-tions, providing radiologists with helpful information to identify and correctly diag-nose the most common of those pathologies.

Human Immunodeficiency Virus: Opportunistic Infections and Beyond   147

Rekha Siripurapu and Yoshiaki Ota

Human immunodeficiency virus (HIV) infection causes substantial morbidity and mortality worldwide. Although antiretroviral therapy (ART) has changed the epidemi-ology of HIV in the last 20 years with increased survival and decreasing incidence of opportunistic infections (OI), CNS OI remain a major cause of morbidity. Improved survival has also increased neurological presentations due to co morbid conditions, treatment related side effects and inflammatory syndromes. Being familiar with the imaging findings, the impact of ART and interpretation of imaging in the context of clinical and laboratory findings is important for radiologists as well as clinicians in the management of HIV-infected patients.

Spinal Infections   167

Hajime Yokota and E. Turgut Tali

Spinal cord infections can present with a wide variety of imaging findings, depending on the pathogen and the host's immune status. Infectious myelitis can have a char-acteristic distribution of lesions within the spinal cord, which refine the differential disease. Some spinal infections do not show typical imaging features, and many noninfectious may mimic spinal infections with similar MR imaging findings. Infec-tious arachnoiditis and meningitis must be differentiated from neoplasms. Spondy-litis has many mimickers and requires careful interpretations of images, clinical findings, and follow-up information.

Imaging of Head and Neck Infections   185

Joel M. Stein and Junfang Xian

The complex anatomy and deep spaces of the head and neck limit physical exam-ination while also offering many points for entry and spread of infection. Radiologic imaging plays a crucial role in managing head and neck infections by defining the location and extent of disease, facilitating abscess drainage, and identifying compli-cations. This review provides essential background and examples for imaging infec-tion throughout the head and neck region.

Imaging of Congenital/Childhood Central Nervous System Infections   207

TANG Phua Hwee and THOON Koh Cheng

This article highlights the changing profile of the pediatric patient with central ner-vous system infection as countries develop and the roles of different imaging modal-ities such as cranial ultrasound, MR imaging, and computed tomography. It discusses the commonly encountered congenital toxoplasmosis, rubella, cytomeg-alovirus, herpes simplex (TORCH) infections, Group B Streptococcal and Escheri-chia coli infections in the neonatal period, and disease outbreaks affecting children. Iatrogenic, opportunistic, and immune-mediated changes as well as long-term effects of infection and mimics of infection are also discussed. Variety of images is provided to show the range of neuroimaging findings encountered, particularly on cranial ultrasound and MR imaging.

Beyond Pattern Recognition: Radiology-Pathology-Clinical Correlation   225

Kum Thong Wong, Chong Tin Tan, and Tchoyoson Lim

Radiology-pathology correlation is essential for multidisciplinary collaboration in diagnosis and understanding the mechanism of CNS damage in infectious processes. The microscopic acute inflammatory processes are well established and are supplemented by a variety of less-invasive microbial and immunohistochemical investigations. Understanding the pathogenesis of pathogen spread and neuroinvasion, vascular and immune-mediated brain, and spinal cord damage are essential for interpreting radiological images.

Foreword
Central Nervous System Infections

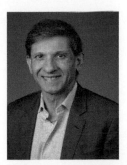

Suresh K. Mukherji, MD, MBA, FACR
Consulting Editor

I could not help but notice the unfortunate irony that Dr Tchoyoson C.C. Lim has been working on his issue of *Neuroimaging Clinics* devoted to Central Nervous System Infections as we were all struggling with the COVID pandemic. This issue is certainly timely and topical, and I thank Dr Lim, who persevered during this difficult time to produce such an outstanding issue.

This issue beautifully covers the spectrum of central nervous system (CNS) infections with unique articles devoted to infections we rarely see in the western hemisphere, such as rickettsia, spirochete, and parasitic infections. There are also specific articles devoted to spine, head and neck, and pediatric CNS infections, with an especially interesting article on the radiology-pathology correlation.

Thank you to all the article authors for your exquisite efforts during these challenging times. The authors are world renowned for their expertise, and the contributions are superb. Finally, a very special thanks to Dr Tchoyoson Lim for accepting our invitation to guest edit this unique issue. This is a wonderful contribution that will have a lasting impact for many years to come!

Suresh K. Mukherji, MD, MBA, FACR
Marian University, Head and Neck Radiology,
ProScan Imaging, Carmel, IN 46032, USA

E-mail address:
sureshmukherji@hotmail.com

Neuroimag Clin N Am 33 (2023) xv
https://doi.org/10.1016/j.nic.2022.08.002
1052-5149/23/© 2022 Published by Elsevier Inc.

Preface
Imaging CNS Infection: Now more relevant than ever

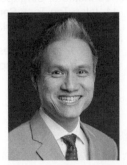

Tchoyoson Lim, MBBS, MMed
Editor

As the authors were preparing and writing the 2023 issue of central nervous system (CNS) infections, they did so in the midst of the COVID-19 pandemic. Sickness, uncertainty, and fear affected us radiologists and other health care professionals just as they did all humanity; however, this difficult time can also represent an opportunity to increase our awareness of the importance of infectious diseases. For too long, these diseases have been neglected and underserved, with an unequal burden of human suffering falling on low- and middle-income countries: what might appear to be an "exotic" case to radiologists in the developed world can actually be far too common, and we don't know about it because of our ignorance and inadequate access to advanced imaging technology.

At the same time, the COVID-19 pandemic has exposed shortcoming in practice and the widespread lack of robust primary scientific data from rigorous hypothesis-driven research in CNS infections, compared with neoplasia or stroke. Better disease registries and clinical trials are needed, so that scientific rigor in sensitivity, specificity, and generalizability of imaging features can accurately inform our radiology practice.

There are multiple possible classifications of neuroimaging in CNS infections, and this issue takes a mixed approach, by taxonomy of pathogen (bacteria, virus, parasite), anatomical location (spine, head, and neck), and special situations (pediatrics, tuberculosis, HIV, acute COVID-19, and subacute/chronic COVID-19). Bookended by epidemiology and radiology-pathology correlation, the longest overview is the article entitled, "Imaging Patterns of Meningitis, Ventriculitis, Cerebritis and Abscess," which serves as an anchor that links all articles. Readers are encouraged to digest the entire issue as a whole, knowing that there will be substantive overlap and oversimplification.

Clinical problem-solving based on pattern recognition has long been a core pillar of diagnostic imaging. Our knowledge of "classic" CT and MRI features and their typical anatomical distribution has enabled us to process new data in new diseases, in light of past differential diagnosis algorithms. There is also tremendous untapped potential in machine learning and the physiologic information that can be extracted from advanced imaging techniques. It is hoped that future iterations of our work will tease out the mechanisms of neuronal damage and immune response in CNS infections.

I would like to thank Suresh Mukherji, the consulting editor, for inviting me to be the guest editor, and Karen Solomon and John Vassallo from Elsevier, for their patience and professionalism. I am very grateful to this diverse group of authors (who had to endure my incessant nagging)

Neuroimag Clin N Am 33 (2023) xvii–xviii
https://doi.org/10.1016/j.nic.2022.08.001
1052-5149/23/© 2022 Published by Elsevier Inc.

from Asia, Europe, and North and South America; they represent teamwork between different disciplines, hospitals, nations, and practices. This issue is dedicated to my wife, parents, and children (who have to endure all my other faults), to our health care professional colleagues who labored alongside us in the "trenches" during the pandemic, and finally, to our patients, who teach us to learn from our past. May we, with better education and research, face future pandemics with stronger preparedness, multidisciplinary collaboration, and compassion for our patients.

Tchoyoson Lim, MBBS, MMed
Department of Neuroradiology
National Neuroscience Institute, Singapore
11 Jalan Tan Tock Seng
Singapore 308433

E-mail address:
tchoyoson@gmail.com

The Changing Epidemiology of Central Nervous System Infection
Can Radiologists Keep Up?

Brenda Sze Peng Ang, MBBS, M Med, MPH[a], Thirugnanam Umapathi, MBBS[b], Tchoyoson Lim, MBBS, MMed[c],*

KEYWORDS

- Epidemiology • Multidisciplinary teams (MDT) • Emerging infection • Zoonotic outbreak • Mimics

KEY POINTS

- Radiologists should be aware of disease outbreaks, typical imaging features of central nervous system (CNS) infections, and their mimics.
- The epidemiology of CNS infections is constantly changing, and vaccines improve the meningitis outlook in both developed and low- and middle-income countries.
- Human factors and genetic adaptation by pathogens increase the extent, severity, and likelihood of outbreaks of emerging and reemerging diseases.
- Radiologists add value to the multidisciplinary team (MDT), and flexible systems responses are required for future pandemic preparation.

INTRODUCTION

Although noncommunicable chronic diseases, such as heart disease and cancer, dominate in many developed nations, the ongoing COVID-19 pandemic has shown that infectious diseases are not limited to low- and middle-income countries (LMIC), but have the potential to pose a public health threat worldwide.[1,2] Many pathogens can cause central nervous system (CNS) infection, including bacteria, viruses, fungi, mycobacteria, and parasites; transmissible prion disease in bovine spongiform encephalopathy and variant Creutzfeldt-Jakob disease will not be reviewed.

Although the radiologist is not expected to be able to identify a specific microbial cause from radiologic pattern recognition alone, some knowledge of epidemiology, neurology, and pathology of the causative organisms is important to understand pretest probability and relative risk.[3]

Radiologists assessing images in infectious disease need to take into account information such as the patient's age, background, immune status, exposures, vaccination status, surgical interventions, and epidemiology and geographic distribution of infectious diseases. Multidisciplinary discussions between the managing team, neuroradiologist, and an infectious disease physician will facilitate rapid recognition and diagnosis, leading to prompt appropriate antimicrobial treatment to achieve favorable clinical outcomes.

EMERGING CENTRAL NERVOUS SYSTEM INFECTIONS AND ZOONOTIC OUTBREAKS

Emerging diseases are those infecting human hosts for the first time; reemerging diseases are either infections that become drug-resistant, reappear after being controlled, present with new unusual manifestations, or emerge in locations where they were

[a] Department of Infectious Diseases, Tan Tock Seng Hospital, 11 Jalan Tan Tock Seng, Singapore 308433;
[b] Department of Neurology, National Neuroscience Institute, 11 Jalan Tan Tock Seng, Singapore 308433;
[c] Department of Neuroradiology, National Neuroscience Institute, Singapore, 11 Jalan Tan Tock Seng, Singapore 308433
* Corresponding author.
E-mail address: tchoyoson@gmail.com

Neuroimag Clin N Am 33 (2023) 1–10
https://doi.org/10.1016/j.nic.2022.03.002
1052-5149/23/© 2022 Elsevier Inc. All rights reserved.

previously not seen.[4] Factors that favor emergence and reemergence from the human perspective include occupational exposure, travel and migration, and conflict and warfare, although misuse of antibiotics, genetic mutation, habitat, ecosystem, and climate changes have impact on microbes.[5,6]

Increasing contact with wild animal reservoirs (notably bats) has meant that up to 76% of emerging diseases (especially viruses) are zoonotic: Zoonoses are infectious agents that spill over from animal reservoirs to novel human hosts; examples are the 2009 pandemic "swine flu" influenza H1N1 and avian influenza H5N1, H9N2 subtypes.[3,7] Other pathogens need intermediate arthropod vectors (typically mosquitos, ticks, sand flies) to indirectly spread from either humans or animals. Table 1 shows examples of zoonotic diseases that have been associated with CNS manifestations that radiologists should be familiar with, to better understand past and future zoonotic disease outbreaks.[3]

Henipaviruses: Hendra and Nipah Virus Outbreaks

One of the first large outbreaks of an emerging disease with significant involvement of CNS was seen with Hendra (HeV) and Nipah (NiV) viruses, which caused fatal encephalitis and pneumonia outbreaks in 1994 and 1998, associated with horses in Australia and pigs in Malaysia and Singapore, respectively.[8–12] On brain MR imaging, both were associated with widespread cortical lesions; some

patients with NiV manifested a different pattern of multifocal, bilateral tiny abnormalities, especially within the subcortical deep white matter, attributed to virus-associated microangiopathy and ischemic microinfarction with subacute laminar necrosis.[13,14] Follow-up MR imaging studies in seropositive but asymptomatic Singapore pig slaughterhouse workers revealed similar abnormalities, and in a possible harbinger of long COVID, 8 out of 9 recovering patients developed psychiatric sequelae, including depression, personality changes, deficits in attention, and memory.[15,16] On the other hand, 12 Malaysian NiV survivors suffered relapses, with 3 showing different MR imaging features of late-onset encephalitis.[17,18]

Although the initial NiV outbreak in Malaysia was ended by drastic pig culling, localized NiV outbreaks have been reported in multiple locations in India and Bangladesh, caused by direct transmission from the wide-ranging fruit bat (genus *Pteropus*) reservoir by consumption of contaminated fruit or date palm sap, contact with infected animals, or human-to-human spread.[19] Sporadic HeV cases have also been reported as recently as 2015.[20]

Coronaviruses: SARS-CoV-1, Middle East respiratory syndrome coronavirus, SARS-CoV-2 Outbreaks

Before SARS-CoV-2 emerged in 2019, 2 newly discovered, aggressive β-coronaviruses with respective animal hosts were SARS-CoV-1

Table 1
Zoonotic diseases with central nervous system manifestations

Pathogen Type	Animal Reservoir	Zoonotic Species/Agent
Viral	Bats	Rabies virus, Australian bat lyssavirus, Hendra virus (HeV), Nipah virus (NiV), SARS-CoV, MERS-CoV, SARS-CoV-2
	Bats, primates, duikers	Ebola virus, Marburg virus
	Poultry, swine	Influenza A virus (H1N1, H1N2, H3N2, H5N1, H7N9)
	Rodents	Hantavirus
	Primates	Herpes B virus
Bacteria	Ruminants	*Brucella* spp, *Leptospira interrogans*, *Coxiella burnetii*
	Rabbits, rodents	*Francisella tularensis*
	Poultry	*Chlamydia psittaci*
	Fish	*Streptococcus iniae*
Parasitic	Felines	*Toxoplasma gondii*
	Swine	*Taenia solium*
	Sheep, cattle	*Echinococcus* spp
Fungal	Bats, birds, various mammals	*Histoplasma capsulatum*, *Cryptococcus neoformans*, *C gattii*

G.X. Goh, K. Tan, B.S.P. Ang, L.-F. Wang, Tchoyoson Lim, Neuroimaging in Zoonotic Outbreaks Affecting the Central Nervous System: Are We Fighting the Last War?, American Journal of Neuroradiology Oct 2020, 41 (10) 1760-1767; DOI: 10.3174/ajnr.A6727.

(2002, civet cats and other small mammals) and MERS-CoV (2012, camels).[3] Human-to-human transmission and global travel spread SARS-CoV-1 from China to 33 nations, causing severe acute respiratory syndrome (SARS) in 8096 people with 774 deaths.[21] Although SARS manifested primarily as an atypical pneumonia, in one series, 5 seriously ill patients developed large-artery territory cerebral infarction, some with hemorrhagic conversion; 3 died.[22] The increased incidence of associated pulmonary embolism and deep venous thrombosis in SARS perhaps foreshadowed the complex CNS manifestations associated with COVID-19 that includes what appears to be dysimmune acute necrotizing encephalopathy (ANE) and acute disseminated encephalomyelitis (ADEM)-like presentations.[22–25] The SARS outbreak ended after several months in October 2003, and subsequently, there had only been a few cases involving laboratory accidents or animal-to-human transmission.[26,27]

Similarly, the coronavirus MERS-CoV, causing Middle East respiratory syndrome (MERS), spread from Saudi Arabia to 26 other nations, affecting 2519 patients with 866 deaths (35% case fatality ratio).[3,28] MR imaging case reports in 3 patients with multiple organ dysfunction and CNS manifestations described widespread, bilateral abnormalities within the subcortical white matter, corpus callosum, and basal ganglia.[29]

Other Emerging Pathogens and Outbreaks (Enterovirus 71, H1N1 Influenza, Measles)

Enterovirus (EV) 71 causes hand, foot, and mouth disease, a febrile rash, with respiratory and gastrointestinal symptoms. Since the initial epidemic described in 1969,[30] this highly contagious virus has caused seasonal outbreaks, often necessitating school and childcare center closures. CNS involvement in 10% to 20% of patients is associated with severe and fatal outcomes, including rhombencephalitis and acute flaccid paralysis that can be indistinguishable from poliomyelitis. MR imaging features include abnormalities in the cervical cord anterior horn, brainstem, and cerebellum.[31]

Influenza is known to be associated with various fatal neurologic complications, including Reye syndrome, Guillain-Barré syndrome (GBS), transverse myelitis, seizures, and encephalopathy, mainly in pediatric populations. In 2009, a new H1N1 influenza virus emerged, causing the first global flu pandemic in 40 years. A few reports described ANE on neuroimaging.[32,33]

Ebola virus has caused multiple epidemics of severe hemorrhagic fever, but in the recent West African outbreak, it was recognized to infrequently cause encephalitis, in some cases with positive viral polymerase chain reaction in cerebrospinal fluid (CSF). Neuroimaging revealed a variety of features, including stroke, meningoencephalitis, and multiple punctate areas of restriction diffusion suggestive of ischemia in the corpus callosum, cerebral white matter, and spinal cord.[34–36]

Outbreaks of measles, one of the most contagious diseases, have been happening all over the world. Although a vaccine became available in the 1960s, the incidence has been increasing even in countries that previously had it under control. This has been attributed to poor health services, civil strife, complacency, and antivaccination movements. Although neuroimaging patterns range from primary measles encephalitis, ADEM, measles inclusion body encephalitis, and subacute sclerosing panencephalitis, MR imaging is not well described in outbreaks.[4]

Vector-Borne Viruses: Japanese Encephalitis, Dengue, Chikungunya, and Zika Viruses

Arthropod-borne, or arboviruses, include Japanese encephalitis (JE), dengue (DENV), Chikungunya (CHIKV), Zika (ZIKV), West Nile, and numerous tick-borne viruses. JE is a common, serious vector-borne viral encephalitis found worldwide, especially in the Western Pacific and in northern Australia: more than 3 billion individuals live in JE epidemic and/or endemic countries. The fatality rate in JE cases ranges from 20% to 30%, with neurologic or psychiatric sequelae observed in 30% to 50% of survivors.[37]

As DENV is already one of the most common mosquito-borne viruses globally, the incidence of DENV is increasing explosively owing to rapid genetic adaptation and human activity, expanding its geographic range in tropical and subtropical Asia and the Americas. The existence of 4 distinct serotypes that preclude lifelong immunity also makes vaccine development and Aedes species mosquito control extremely challenging. Most patients suffer dengue fever with generalized myalgia and arthralgia, but hemorrhagic fever, shock syndrome, and CNS involvement can occur.[38] Brain imaging patterns are variable, including abnormalities in the bilateral thalamus, pons, cerebellum, corpus callosum, or features similar to posterior reversible encephalopathy syndrome (PRES), ADEM, and acute necrotizing encephalitis.[39,40] There may be cerebral edema, hemorrhage, diffusion restriction, and leptomeningeal enhancement.[41]

Although CHIKV has long been circulating in tropical and subtropical Africa, recent outbreaks emerged in both Africa and Asia, spreading worldwide, causing a febrile, painful arthritic syndrome that is clinically very similar to, but more severe than DENV infection. CNS manifestations include encephalitis and encephalomyelitis, and white matter disease.[42,43]

The ZIKV was discovered in 1947 in East Africa, isolated from *Aedes aegypti* mosquitoes in 1966 in Malaysia and associated with human infections in 1977 in Indonesia; it had most likely been silently circulating among humans, animals, and mosquitoes throughout tropical Africa and Asia, misdiagnosed as other endemic arboviruses like JE or dengue. Genetic changes in virus strains, combined with human factors, were probably responsible for the dramatic South American ZIKV outbreaks in 2015 to 2016 causing microcephaly and severe fetal CNS changes.[44]

Iatrogenic Central Nervous System Infection Outbreaks

In September 2012, a multistate outbreak in the US affected 751 patients who suffered fungal meningitis, stroke, peripheral osteoarticular infection, spinal or paraspinal infection, with 64 deaths. The source was traced to epidural or osteoarticular injection using preservative-free steroid injection contaminated by *Exserohilum rostratum*, a soil organism that previously was an uncommon cause of human infection.[45] This was a large and completely unexpected outbreak. Even a first case of an unusual organisms not previously known to infect humans should alert physicians to potential public health threats and be investigated. Eventual resolution of this outbreak was achieved by vigilance, epidemiologic surveillance, and multidisciplinary collaboration.[46]

CHANGING EPIDEMIOLOGY OF CENTRAL NERVOUS SYSTEM INFECTIONS

Nonzoonotic outbreaks include reemergence of rare transmissible and neurovirulent circulating vaccine-derived poliovirus strains associated with live-attenuated polio vaccines and measles clusters associated with "anti-vaxxer" social movements recently amplified by social media.[47–49] Other nonoutbreak changes in epidemiology that result in changes in relative frequency of species/serotype incidence and mutations arise as a result of selection pressure. For example, among people living with HIV infection, the MR imaging patterns may diverge between the developed countries and LMIC on account of access to highly active antiretroviral therapy (HAART).[50] Some common causes of bacterial, viral, and other CNS infections are shown in **Table 2.**

Bacterial Meningitis

Three bacteria: *Hemophilus influenzae*, *Streptococcus pneumoniae*, and *Neisseria meningitidis*, account for most cases of acute bacterial meningitis. Widespread introduction of Haemophilus influenzae type b polysaccharide-protein conjugate vaccine into national immunization programs of many nations has decreased the incidence of *Hemophilus influenzae B*, with shift to other serotypes, whereas introduction of 7-valent pneumococcal conjugate vaccine (PCV7) conjugate vaccines has not consistently decreased overall pneumococcal meningitis incidence because of the phenomenon of serotype replacement by non-PCV7 serotypes.[51] Several countries have added meningococcal vaccines to national immunization programs, with resulting decrease in incidence of invasive meningococcal disease. However, it continues to be an important cause of morbidity and mortality in both adults and children, and a humanitarian crisis especially in Africa's meningitis belt (**Fig. 1**).[52]

Group B *Streptococcus agalactiae* is the most common cause of neonatal meningitis and sepsis, but intrapartum antibiotic prophylaxis directed at high-risk women for maternal-fetal transmission has resulted in an initial sharp decrease with stability.[53] An unusual adult outbreak of invasive Group B *Streptococcus agalactiae* CNS infections was reported from Singapore, ascribed to consumption of raw farmed freshwater fish infected with invasive serotype III sequence type 283 (ST283).[54,55] In that outbreak, diffusion-weighted imaging (DWI) was sensitive in detecting small collections of subarachnoid and ventricular pus, as well as lesions in the cerebellum and subcortical structures.

Listeria monocytogenes is a food-borne pathogen that may be the third most common cause of bacterial meningitis, with mortalities as high as 30%, especially in the elderly, the immunocompromised, pregnant women, and neonates. The organism is hardy, can survive in refrigerated food with low moisture and high salt concentration, and hence usually is associated with unpasteurized milk and dairy products. However, with globalized food supply chains, new food items, including various fresh, precut, or frozen fruit, like melons, leafy vegetables, sandwiches, and wraps, have been linked to recent outbreaks and food recalls.[56]

Tuberculosis, Fungal, and Parasite Infections

The World Health Organization estimates that one-third of the world's population is infected by *Mycobacterium tuberculosis*, and CNS accounts for 5% to 10% of extrapulmonary tuberculosis (TB); hence, the number of cases of CNS TB could be staggering. Tuberculous meningitis, intracranial

Table 2
Common organisms causing central nervous system infections

Organism	Epidemiologic Characteristics	Remarks
Group B *Streptococcus* spp, *Escherichia coli*, L *monocytogenes*	Common causes of neonatal bacterial meningitis	Neonatal screening has decreased the incidence of meningitis Listeria often causes food-related outbreaks among adult populations, can be deadly to elderly, immunocompromised
Haemophilus influenzae, S *pneumoniae*	Common cause of childhood bacterial meningitis	Vaccination can dramatically decrease the incidence of *Haemophilus influenzae* disease, less so for other organisms
N meningitidis	Common cause of adolescent/adult bacterial meningitis	Outbreaks often in crowded conditions, vaccination may be helpful
Staphylococcus spp, *Streptococcus* spp	Common cause of adult bacterial meningitis & abscess	Commonest Gram+ organisms causing cerebral abscesses in adults, especially in patients with endocarditis and traumatic injury
Anaerobic bacteria	Commonest cause of adult cerebral abscess	Typically, from contiguous oral or ENT source of infection
Enterovirus	Commonest cause of viral meningitis	EV 71 and other serotype outbreaks among preschool children may result in school/childcare closures
Cryptococcus neoformans	Commonest cause of meningitis in HIV patients	
M tuberculosis	Deadly meningitis and complications	TB remains a stubborn disease to eradicate
Vector-borne arboviruses: ZIKV, DENV, CHIKV, and others	Regional/international outbreaks	Increasing range and severity of public health threat

tuberculoma, and spinal tuberculous arachnoiditis, especially affect children, alcoholics, the malnourished, and immunosuppressed, especially HIV patients in LMIC.[57] Lack of public health infrastructure, poverty, and multidrug resistance make TB one of the most devastating and intractable public health problems.

Fungal CNS infections have increased over the past decades, related to an increase in cases of immune suppression, such as HIV, transplantation, and newer cancer chemotherapy; invasion is dependent on both host immune status and fungal virulence. MR imaging interpretation is often complicated by variable clinical presentations, including meningitis, encephalitis, hydrocephalus, cerebral abscesses, and stroke syndromes. Cryptococcus, Coccidioides, and Histoplasma can also cause infection in immunocompetent patients.[2]

Despite several successful eradication campaigns, parasites with complex life cycles and endemicity in resource-limited geographic locations are still responsible for significant mortality and seizure morbidity. Thus, radiologists must have a high index of suspicion for exposure among patients originating from or traveling to endemic areas for work and leisure, as parasites can remain dormant in the host for years until there is immunosuppression or immunosenescence.[4]

ADVANCES IN CLINICAL AND IMAGING METHODS
Neuroimaging Advances

Dedicated negative pressure air-circulation rooms to house computed tomographic (CT) scanners/interventional suites are possible to decrease the

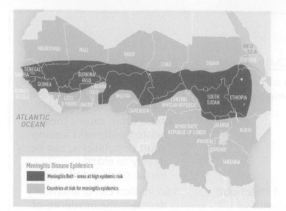

Fig. 1. The "meningitis belt": countries with high-epidemic risk of meningitis. (*From* Sarah A. Mbaeyi, Lucy A. McNamara. Meningococcal Disease. Chapter 4, Travelers Health, CDC https://wwwnc.cdc.gov/travel/yellowbook/2020/travel-related-infectious-diseases/meningococcal-disease#4670.)

risk of airborne cross-infection, not just for sporadic cases of TB, measles, and other highly contagious organisms, but also during times of outbreak and pandemic.[58] Although providing dedicated isolated imaging and interventional facilities may be an impractical luxury for any facility but the most dedicated infectious disease hospitals, the ability of radiology administration to enhance infection control protocols during an outbreak emergency should be a contingency plan for all radiology departments, including mass casualty, terrorism, and climate emergency. Coping with pandemics requires mental agility, fortitude, and responsiveness, coupled with international collaboration that allows learning from global first responders; radiology services need to adjust to prevailing conditions (as well as addressing inherent social/racial inequalities) in each health system.[59]

Continual hardware and software advances in imaging technology benefit patients by providing faster, safer, and more informative biomarkers, such as cytotoxic edema in DWI and microhemorrhage in susceptibility-weighted imaging.[3] Increased accuracy and improved point-of-care access (especially bedside ultrasonography) or at least not denying access to life-saving neurointerventional procedures, such as stroke thrombectomy, are also important.[60] Portable CT scanners and more recently portable low-field MR imaging scanners may improve confidence and access during disease outbreaks, although the limited coverage and other challenges are being revealed and overcome in the current COVID pandemic.[61,62]

Neuroradiologist's Role in Central Nervous System Infections and Outbreaks

Radiologists should recognize typical CT, MR imaging, and angiographic imaging features based on the published literature of CNS infection and past outbreaks.[3] A broad knowledge of pathogenesis would be helpful in interpretation, including direct viral invasion of nervous tissue (when the causative organism is isolated from the CSF or brain), immune-mediated changes ("cytokine storm," ADEM, and GBS), cerebrovascular complications, preexisting comorbidities, or iatrogenic effects in critically ill patients. Often, however, imaging findings may overlap with noninfectious diseases, such as neoplasia or autoimmune encephalitis, and differential diagnosis may be difficult in individual patients. Radiologists can benefit from an awareness of changing epidemiologic trends, active participation at infectious diseases multidisciplinary team conferences, research, and education.[46,54] Although artificial intelligence is in its infancy in radiology and health care applications, sentinel event reporting and caseload surveillance algorithms may help us detect localized case clusters above the baseline disease prevalence in future outbreaks and global pandemics.[63,64] The 2 case examples in later discussion illustrate the value of neuroimaging and clinical radiologists.

ILLUSTRATIVE CASE EXAMPLES
Central Nervous System Parasite Mimicking Brain Tumor

A 32-year-old Singaporean man presented with chronic-onset right hemiplegia and no other significant history. On MR imaging, a single, rounded mass, hyperintense on T2-weighted, hypointense on T1-weighted images with thin rim enhancement was noted at the gray-white matter junction of the parietal lobe, with surrounding white matter vasogenic edema. DWI did not show hyperintensity, and apparent diffusion coefficient (ADC) was unrestricted (Fig. 2). These features did not favor cerebral abscess. At surgical resection for suspected tumor, histology revealed part of a tapeworm consistent with neurocysticercosis. This case illustrates clinical presentation of neurocysticercosis without typical seizures or travel to endemic areas, and that noninvasive differentiation from tumor can be difficult even if pyogenic abscess can be confidently excluded by lack of DWI hyperintensity. A high index of suspicion, direct scolex visualization, advanced imaging such as perfusion or spectroscopy, and a trial of therapy could have been helpful in this case.[65]

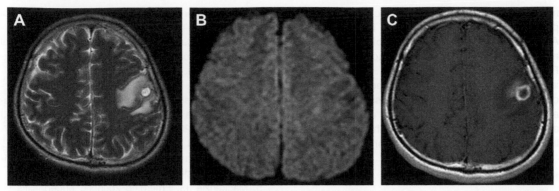

Fig. 2. MR imaging brain in a 32-year-old Singaporean man presenting with chronic-onset right hemiplegia showing a small, rounded mass, hyperintense on T2-weighted (*A*), hypointense on DWI (*B*), thin rim enhancement after contrast injection (*C*) surrounding vasogenic edema in the left frontal lobe. This was interpreted as neoplastic, ruling out pyogenic abscess, and patient proceeded to surgery, which revealed neurocysticercosis.

Inflammatory Disease Mimicking Central Nervous System Infections

A 68-year-old woman presented with fever, headache, and altered mental state. Clinical examination was suggestive of acute meningoencephalomyelitis, supported by diffuse generalized leptomeningeal enhancement on initial MR imaging. Spinal fluid lymphocytic pleocytosis, elevated protein, and low glucose were also consistent, but standard bacteriologic and virologic evaluation was negative. She deteriorated despite antibiotics but improved when antituberculous treatment was initiated together with high-dose dexamethasone. Within 2 weeks of weaning off dexamethasone, she deteriorated again.

Second MR imaging revealed a striking change in the enhancement pattern, with extensive dotlike and linear patterns of perivascular enhancement within the cerebral white matter, oriented radially to the ventricles (**Fig. 3**). In the spinal cord, extensive leptomeningeal enhancement was accompanied by multisegmental intramedullary T2 hyperintensity with patchy enhancement. Spinal fluid TB and bacterial cultures were persistently negative. Because of the characteristic radial MR imaging enhancement pattern, the suspicion of anti-glial fibrillary acidic protein (GFAP) antibody-associated astrocytopathy was investigated and confirmed by high GFAP antibody titers in the spinal fluid. PET scan did not indicate an underlying neoplasm, and patient responded to high-dose corticosteroids.

GFAP autoimmune astrocytopathy is a rare, novel immune-mediated disease characterized by relapse and responsiveness to corticosteroid with a specific GFAP-immunoglobulin G marker; it is sometimes associated with occult

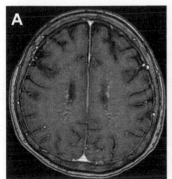
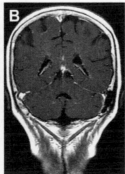
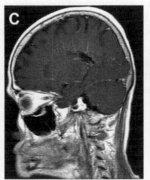
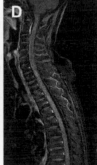

Fig. 3. Second MR imaging brain in a 68-year-old woman presenting with fever, headache, and altered mental state showing extensive bilateral, symmetric dotlike, and linear radiating outwards perpendicular to the lateral ventricles corresponding to the intramedullary veins; similar tiny dotlike enhancement is also seen in the pons and elsewhere (*A–C*). Spinal MR imaging showed leptomeningeal enhancement coating the surface of the cord with multiple, short segmental, intramedullary T2 hyperintensity with patchy enhancement (*D*). Final diagnosis was GFAP-autoimmune astrocytopathy. Courtesy of Sumeet Kumar, Singapore.

malignancy.[66] The characteristic enhancement pattern on MR imaging can mimic TB, sarcoidosis, ADEM, primary progressive multiple sclerosis, primary CNS or intravascular lymphoma, and CLIPPERS syndrome.[67] This case illustrates the importance of radiologists recognizing and considering rare but characteristic patterns of abnormal contrast enhancement and suggesting a differential diagnosis, even if the initial clinical impression supports CNS infection.

SUMMARY

Neuroradiologists should recognize the MR imaging and CT features of past zoonotic outbreaks but be prepared to recognize changes or new imaging manifestations as new data emerge and imaging technology improves. Although challenges continue in vector control, vaccination program rollout, cross-border travel, climate change, and inequalities of access to health care, radiologists continue to play a vital role in future pandemic preparation. The importance of awareness of epidemiologic trends, MDT collaboration, and a vibrant community of practice should be emphasized.

CLINICS CARE POINTS

- Clinicians should be aware of changing epidemiology of CNS infections, and apply the trends to understand locally prevalent and rare, but important organisms.

- Understanding globalization, climate change, genetic adaptation and past outbreaks, helps us stay vigilant against non-endemic and emerging diseases.

- Though vaccines have improved the meningitis outlook in both developed and LMIC, there is some increase in strains not covered by vaccines.

- MDT discussions benefit from radiologists' knowledge of the typical imaging features of CNS infections and their mimics.

DISCLOSURE

The authors have nothing to disclose.

REFERENCES

1. Munoz LS, Garcia MA, Gordon-Lipkin E, et al. Emerging viral infections and their impact on the global burden of neurological disease. Semin Neurol 2018;38:163–75.
2. John CC, Carabin H, Montano SM, et al. Global research priorities for infections that affect the nervous system. Nature 2015;527(7578):S178–86.
3. Goh GX, Tan K, Ang BSP, et al. Neuroimaging in zoonotic outbreaks affecting the central nervous system: are we fighting the last war? AJNR Am J Neuroradiol 2020. https://doi.org/10.3174/ajnr.A6727.
4. do Carmo RL, Alves Simão AK, Faria do Amaral LL, et al. Neuroimaging of emergent and reemergent infections. RadioGraphics 2019;39(6):1649–71.
5. Mackenzie JS. Emerging zoonotic encephalitis viruses: lessons from Southeast Asia and Oceania. J Neurovirol 2005;11:434–40.
6. Parrish CR, Holmes EC, Morens DM, et al. Cross-species virus transmission and the emergence of new epidemic diseases. Microbiol Mol Biol Rev 2008;72:457–70.
7. Wang, L. F. & Cowled, C. Bats and viruses: a new frontier of emerging infectious diseases. Bats and viruses: a new frontier of emerging infectious diseases (2015). doi:10.1002/9781118818824.
8. Murray K, Rogers R, Selvey L, et al. A novel morbillivirus pneumonia of horses and its transmission to humans. Emerg Infect Dis 1995. https://doi.org/10.3201/eid0101.950107.
9. Chua KB, Goh KJ, Wong KT, et al. Fatal encephalitis due to Nipah virus among pig-farmers in Malaysia. Lancet 1999. https://doi.org/10.1016/S0140-6736(99)04299-3.
10. Lee KE, Umapathi T, Tan CB, et al. Neurological manifestations of the Nipah virus. Ann Neurol 1999;46:428–32.
11. Goh KJ, Tan CT, Chew NK, et al. Clinical features of Nipah virus encephalitis among pig farmers in Malaysia. N Engl J Med 2000. https://doi.org/10.1056/NEJM200004273421701.
12. Ang BSP, Lim TCC, Wang L. Nipah virus infection. J Clin Microbiol 2018;56. e01875-17.
13. Lim CCT, Sitoh YY, Hui F, et al. Nipah viral encephalitis or Japanese encephalitis? MR findings in a new zoonotic disease. AJNR Am J Neuroradiol 2000;21:455–61.
14. Lim CCT, Lee KE, Lee WL, et al. Nipah virus encephalitis: serial MR study of an emerging disease. Radiology 2002;222(1):219–26.
15. Lim CCT, Lee WL, Leo YS, et al. Late clinical and magnetic resonance imaging follow up of Nipah virus infection. J Neurol Neurosurg Psychiatry 2003. https://doi.org/10.1136/jnnp.74.1.131.
16. Ng B-Y, Lim CCT, Yeoh A, et al. Neuropsychiatric sequelae of Nipah virus encephalitis. J Neuropsychiatry Clin Neurosci 2004;16(4):500–4.
17. Sarji SA, Abdullah BJJ, Goh KJ, et al. MR imaging features of Nipah encephalitis. Am J Roentgenol 2000;175:437–42.

18. Sejvar JJ, Hossain J, Saha SK, et al. Long-term neurological and functional outcome in Nipah virus infection. Ann Neurol 2007. https://doi.org/10.1002/ana.21178.

19. Rahman MA, Hossain MJ, Sultana S, et al. Date palm sap linked to Nipah virus outbreak in Bangladesh, 2008. Vector Borne Zoonotic Dis 2012;12(1):65–72.

20. Ching PKG, de los Reyes VC, Sucaldito MN, et al. Outbreak of henipavirus infection, Philippines, 2014. Emerg Infect Dis J 2015;21:328.

21. Ruan S. Likelihood of survival of coronavirus disease 2019. Lancet Infect Dis 2020;3099:2019–20.

22. Umapathi T, Kor AC, Venketasubramanian N, et al. Large artery ischaemic stroke in severe acute respiratory syndrome (SARS). J Neurol 2004;251: 1227–31.

23. Koh JS, De Silva DA, Quek AML, et al. Neurology of COVID-19 in Singapore. J Neurol Sci 2020;418(0): 117118. https://doi.org/10.1016/j.jns.2020.117118.

24. Fan BE, Umapathi T, Chua K, et al. Delayed catastrophic thrombotic events in young and asymptomatic post COVID-19 patients. J Thromb Thrombolysis 2021;51(4):971–7.

25. Poyiadji N, Shahin G, Noujaim D, et al. COVID-19–associated acute hemorrhagic necrotizing encephalopathy: imaging features. Radiology 2020;296: E119–20.

26. Lim PL, Kurup A, Gopalakrishna G. Laboratory-acquired severe acute respiratory syndrome. N Engl J Med 2004;350:1740–5. Available at: https://www.nejm.org/doi/full/10.1056/NEJMoa032565.

27. Normile D. Infectious diseases. SARS experts want labs to improve safety practices. Science 2003; 302(5642):31.

28. De Wit E, Van Doremalen N, Falzarano D, et al. SARS and MERS: recent insights into emerging coronaviruses. Nat Rev Microbiol 2016;14: 523–34.

29. Arabi YM, Harthi A, Hussein J, et al. Severe neurologic syndrome associated with Middle East respiratory syndrome corona virus (MERS-CoV). Infection 2015;43:495–501.

30. Puenpa J, Wanlapakorn N, Vongpunsawad S, et al. The history of enterovirus A71 outbreaks and molecular epidemiology in the Asia-Pacific region. J Biomed Sci 2019;26:75. Available at: https://jbiomedsci.biomedcentral.com/articles/10.1186/s12929-019-0573-2.

31. Huang C-C. Neurologic complications in children with enterovirus 71 infection. N Engl J Med 1999; 341:936–42.

32. Ormitti F, Ventura E, Summa A, et al. Acute necrotizing encephalopathy in a child during the 2009 influenza A(H1N1) pandemia: MR imaging in diagnosis and follow-up. AJNR Am J Neuroradiol 2010; 31:396–400.

33. Prerna A, Lim JYX, Tan NWH, et al. Neurology of the H1N1 pandemic in Singapore: a nationwide case series of children and adults. J Neurovirol 2015;21:491–9.

34. Howlett PJ, Walder AR, Lisk DR, et al. Case series of severe neurologic sequelae of Ebola virus disease during epidemic, Sierra Leone. Emerg Infect Dis 2018;24(8):1412–21.

35. Jacobs M, Rodger A, Bell DJ, et al. Late Ebola virus relapse causing meningoencephalitis: a case report. Lancet 2016;388:498–503.

36. Chertow DS, Nath A, Suffredini AF, et al. Severe meningoencephalitis in a case of Ebola virus disease: a case report. Ann Intern Med 2016;165(4): 301–4.

37. Campbell GL, Hills SL, Fischer M, et al. Estimated global incidence of Japanese encephalitis: a systematic review. Bull World Health Organ 2011; 89(10):766–774E.

38. Dengue vaccine: WHO position paper, September 2018—Recommendations, Vaccine, 37 (35), 2019, 4848-4849.

39. Vyas S, Ray N, Maralakunte M, et al. Pattern recognition approach to brain MRI findings in patients with dengue fever with neurological complications. Neurol India 2020;68:1038–47.

40. Vanjare HA, Mannam P, Mishra AK, et al. Brain imaging in cases with positive serology for dengue with neurologic symptoms: a clinicoradiologic correlation. AJNR Am J Neuroradiol 2018;39(4): 699–703.

41. Paliwal VK, Garg RK. Neurological complications of dengue: beware of striking similarities with severe COVID-19. Ann Indian Acad Neurol 2021;24:645–7.

42. Mehta R, Gerardin P, de Brito CAA, et al. The neurological complications of chikungunya virus: a systematic review. Rev Med Virol 2018;28(3):e1978.

43. Ganesan K, Diwan A, Shankar SK, et al. Chikungunya encephalomyeloradiculitis: report of 2 cases with neuroimaging and 1 case with autopsy findings. AJNR Am J Neuroradiol 2008;29(9):1636–7.

44. Duong V, Dussart P, Buchy P. Zika virus in Asia. Int J Infect Dis 2017;54:121–8. Available at: https://www.sciencedirect.com/science/article/pii/S120197121631640X.

45. Kauffman CA, Malani AN. Fungal infections associated with contaminated steroid injections. Microbiol Spectr 2016;4(2). https://doi.org/10.1128/microbiolspec.EI10-0005-2015.

46. Ryall FTE, Beeching C, Joekes NJ, et al. The benefits of an infectious disease/radiology multidisciplinary team meeting. J Infect 2012;65(Issue 4): 363–5.

47. Bitnun A, Yeh EA. Acute flaccid paralysis and enteroviral infections. Curr Infect Dis Rep 2018;20: 34.

48. Murphy OC, Messacar K, Benson L, et al. Acute flaccid myelitis: cause, diagnosis, and

management. Lancet 2021;397(10271):334–46. Available at: https://www.ncbi.nlm.nih.gov/pmc/articles/PMC7909727/#__ffn_sectitle doi: 10.1016/S0140-6736(20)32723-9.

49. Acute flaccid paralysis associated with circulating vaccine-derived poliovirus—Philippines, 2001. JAMA 2002;287(3):311.

50. Thakur KT, Boubour A, Saylor D, et al. Global HIV neurology: a comprehensive review. AIDS 2019; 33(2):163–84.

51. Novak RT, Kambou JL, Diomandé FV, et al. Serogroup A meningococcal conjugate vaccination in Burkina Faso: analysis of national surveillance data. Lancet Infect Dis 2012;12(Issue 10):757–64.

52. Mbaeyi SA, McNamara LA. Meningococcal disease. Chapter 4, travelers health, CDC. Available at: https://wwwnc.cdc.gov/travel/yellowbook/2020/travel-related-infectious-diseases/meningococcal-disease#4670. Accessed May 24, 2022.

53. Randis TM, Baker JA, Ratner AJ. Group B streptococcal infections. Pediatr Rev 2017;38(6):254–62.

54. Tan K, Wijaya L, Chiew H-J, et al. Diffusion-weighted MRI abnormalities in an outbreak of Streptococcus agalactiae Serotype III, multilocus sequence type 283 meningitis. J Magn Reson Imaging 2017;45: 507–14.

55. Kalimuddin S, Chen SL, Lim CTK, et al. 2015 epidemic of severe streptococcus agalactiae sequence type 283 infections in Singapore associated with the consumption of raw freshwater fish: a detailed analysis of clinical, epidemiological, and bacterial sequencing data. Clin Infect Dis 2017;64: S145–52.

56. Gray J, Chandry PS, Kaur M, et al. Colonisation dynamics of Listeria monocytogenes strains isolated from food production environments. Sci Rep 2021; 11:12195.

57. Erdem H, Inan A, Guven E, et al. The burden and epidemiology of community-acquired central nervous system infections: a multinational study. Eur J Clin Microbiol Infect Dis 2017;36(9): 1595–611.

58. Peng Tan B, Choon Lim K, Geng Goh Y, et al. Radiology preparedness in the ongoing battle against COVID-19: experiences from large to small public hospitals in Singapore. Radiol Cardiothorac Imaging 2020;2:2. Available at: https://pubs.rsna.org/doi/10.1148/ryct.2020200140.

59. Tim-Ee Cheng L, Chan LP, Tan BH, et al. Déjà vu or jamais vu? How the severe acute respiratory syndrome experience influenced a Singapore radiology department's response to the coronavirus disease (COVID-19) epidemic. AJR Am J Roentgenol 2020; 214(6):1206–10.

60. Pop R, Hasiu A, Bolognini F, et al. Stroke thrombectomy in patients with COVID-19: initial experience in 13 cases. AJNR Am J Neuroradiol 2020. https://doi.org/10.3174/ajnr.A6750.

61. Parmar HA, Lim TCC, Goh JS-K, et al. Providing optimal radiology service in the severe acute respiratory syndrome outbreak: use of mobile CT. AJR Am J Roentgenol 2004;182(1):57–60.

62. Sheth KN, Mazurek MH, Yuen MM, et al. Assessment of brain injury using portable, low-field magnetic resonance imaging at the bedside of critically ill patients. JAMA Neurol 2021;78(1):41–7.

63. Ker J, Wang L, Rao J, et al. Deep learning applications in medical image analysis. IEEE Access 2018; 6:9375–89.

64. Gangopadhyay A, Morris M, Saboury B, et al. ID-IOMS: infectious disease imaging outbreak monitoring system. Digital Government: Res Pract 2021; 2(1):1–5.

65. Do Amaral LLF, Ferreira RM, Da Rocha AJ, et al. Neurocysticercosis: evaluation with advanced magnetic resonance techniques and atypical forms. Top Magn Reson Imaging 2005;16(2):127–44.

66. Flanagan EP, Hinson SR, Lennon VA, et al. Glial fibrillary acidic protein immunoglobulin G as biomarker of autoimmune astrocytopathy: analysis of 102 patients. Ann Neurol 2017;81:298–309.

67. Pittock SJ, Debruyne J, Krecke KN, et al. Chronic lymphocytic inflammation with pontine perivascular enhancement responsive to steroids (CLIPPERS). Brain 2010;133(9):2626–34.

Neuroimaging Patterns of Intracranial Infections
Meningitis, Cerebritis, and Their Complications

Michael Tran Duong, PhD[a], Jeffrey D. Rudie, MD, PhD[b], Suyash Mohan, MD, PDCC[a],*

KEYWORDS

- Central nervous system • Infection • Meningitis • Cerebritis • Abscess • Ventriculitis
- Neuroimaging • Glymphatics

KEY POINTS

- Neuroimaging can confirm clinical suspicion for infection, rule out mimics, assist/replace/complement lumbar puncture and assess for complications including abscess, ventriculitis, extra-axial collections, hydrocephalus, herniation, cranial neuropathy, thrombosis, infarct and vasculitis.
- In acute bacterial meningitis, meningeal enhancement is often located along the cerebral convexity. Chronic and atypical forms of meningitis are usually prominent in the basal cisterns.
- Cerebritis can progress to abscess, which is commonly noted for ring enhancement and centrally restricted diffusion.
- Meningitis, cerebritis, and abscess are included in a wide variety of differential diagnoses related to altered mental status and headaches, so it is imperative to integrate radiographic and clinical information.
- Advanced neuroimaging techniques such as MRS, PET, and artificial intelligence may improve diagnosis of intracranial infections.

INTRODUCTION

Neuroimaging is essential for the diagnosis, management, and monitoring of central nervous system (CNS) infections.[1,2] Although some radiographic features are shared across infectious and noninfectious causes, CNS infections often exhibit specific or classic imaging patterns. During the last 3 decades, mortality from meningitis has decreased by 21% despite incidence rising by 13%, demonstrating the positive impact of accessibility to clinical care and decision-making guided by noninvasive and perioperative neuroimaging.[3]

Here, we provide an overview of classic imaging patterns of meningitis, cerebritis, intracranial abscess, and ventriculitis. We survey techniques such as computed tomography (CT), MR imaging, MR spectroscopy (MRS), diffusion-weighted imaging (DWI) with apparent diffusion coefficient (ADC) maps, PET, and recent advances in neuroimaging, including the potential role of artificial intelligence (AI) in diagnosing CNS infections. Then we survey specific infectious causes organized by location: extra-axial, intra-axial, and mixed. Finally, we present complications and mimics of CNS infections, including noninfectious meningitis, neoplastic, autoimmune, and inflammatory processes. We encourage the reader to reference other articles in this issue of *Neuroimaging Clinics* for further information about certain specific organisms, locations, or situations.

[a] Division of Neuroradiology, Department of Radiology, Perelman School of Medicine at the University of Pennsylvania, 3400 Spruce Street, Philadelphia, PA 19104, USA; [b] Department of Radiology, Scripps Clinic and University of California San Diego, 10666 Torrey Pines Road, La Jolla, CA 92037, USA
* Corresponding author.
E-mail address: suyash.mohan@pennmedicine.upenn.edu

Neuroimag Clin N Am 33 (2023) 11–41
https://doi.org/10.1016/j.nic.2022.07.001
1052-5149/23/© 2022 Elsevier Inc. All rights reserved.

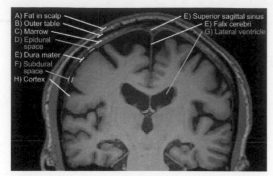

Fig. 1. Coronal T1-weighted MR imaging shows the meningeal layers and spaces in an older adult. Fat in scalp (A) and outer table (B). Bone marrow (C). Epidural space (D). Dura mater (E), including the superior sagittal sinus and falx cerebri. Subdural space (F). Arachnoid mater is not visualized on imaging. Subarachnoid space including the lateral ventricles (G). Cerebral cortex (H).

ANATOMY

The brain is covered by 3 connective tissue membranes, or "meninges." The outermost layer is the dura mater (or *pachymeninges*, meaning "tough membrane"), which includes the venous sinuses and the falx and tentorium. Underneath is the arachnoid and pia mater (which together comprise the *leptomeninges*, meaning "thin membrane"). The potential space between the inner table of the skull and dura is the epidural space. The potential space between the dura and arachnoid is the *subdural space*, which contains the delicate cortical bridging veins and arachnoid granulations. The space between the arachnoid mater and the pial vessels attached to the cortex is the *subarachnoid space*, which is bathed in cerebrospinal fluid (CSF; Fig. 1); all are prone to infected pus collections.

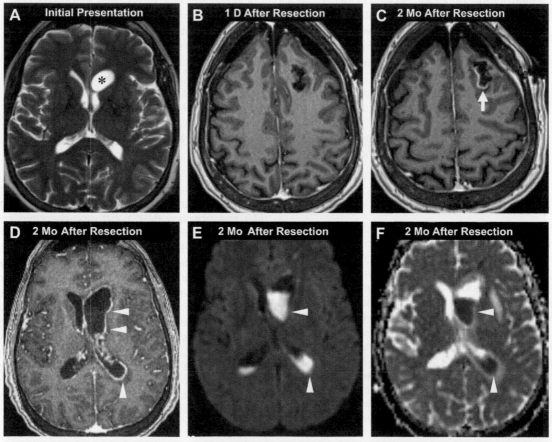

Fig. 2. Postsurgical CNS infection. T2-weighted MR imaging shows a low-grade cystic glioma abutting the left frontal horn (*asterisk*, *A*) before craniotomy/resection (*A*). Postoperative day one, axial T1 postcontrast image shows bilateral pneumocephalus with no enhancement around the resection cavity (*B*). Two months later, the patient presented with a seizure. T1 postcontrast MR imaging now depicts peripheral enhancement around the cavity (*arrow*, *C*) meningitis and ependymitis (*arrowheads*, *D*) and diffusion restricting, gravity-dependent pus-fluid meniscus levels (*arrowheads*, *E*, *F*) in the ventricles on DWI (*E*) and ADC (*F*), suggestive of meningitis, ventriculitis, and abscess.

PATHOPHYSIOLOGY OF CENTRAL NERVOUS SYSTEM INFECTION

There are 4 main routes of infectious spread to the brain and meninges.

(1) Hematogenous dissemination from a distal infectious source is the most common path.
(2) Direct inoculation (**Fig. 2**) occurs from trauma, iatrogenic lumbar puncture (LP), or neurosurgical interventions.
(3) Local extension of infection is seen with sinusitis, orbital cellulitis, mastoiditis (**Fig. 3**), otitis media, or dental infection.
(4) Spread along cranial nerves can occur by rabies, herpes simplex virus (HSV), and *Naegleria fowleri*.

Local extension is less common than hematogenous dissemination, although relatively straightforward to identify on imaging. Otomastoiditis is associated with adjacent abscesses of the temporal lobe and cerebellum (see **Fig. 3**), whereas frontal and ethmoid sinusitis and odontogenic infections are linked to frontal lobe abscess.[2]

There are additional, uncommon routes for infection as up to 40% of brain abscesses are cryptogenic.[4] The calvarial emissary veins are valveless and promote bacterial localization from superficial face and scalp infections to the CNS via retrograde thrombophlebitis causing subdural empyema and cavernous sinus thrombosis.[5] Iatrogenic spread includes neurosurgical incision, dural

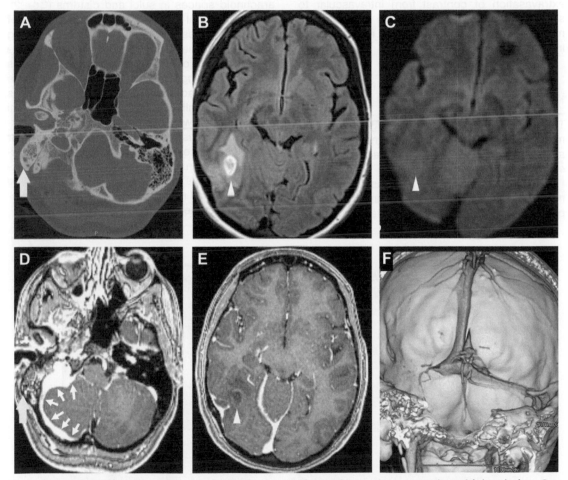

Fig. 3. Mastoiditis with intracranial complications of CNS infection in a patient presenting with headaches. Opacification of right mastoid air cells on CT (*yellow arrow, A*) is consistent with mastoiditis. Evidence of intracranial complications includes an FLAIR hyperintense lesion (*arrowhead, B*) that does not diffusion restrict on DWI (*arrowhead, C*). On T1 postcontrast (*D*), there is enhancement in the opacified mastoid air cells (*yellow arrow, D*) with adjacent pachymeningitis (*multiple white arrows, D*). Note the faintly ring-enhancing lesion in the posterior temporal lobe (*arrowhead, E*) on T1 postcontrast, indicative of cerebritis. Venous sinus thrombosis and thrombophlebitis of the right transverse sinus is seen on 3D shaded surface display volume rendering of CT venogram (*F*).

graft transplant, and LP with spread through meningeal spaces (see Fig. 2). The recently discovered brain meningeal lymphatic system in humans,[6] running alongside the dural venous sinuses, might provide a previously unrecognized route of infectious transmission. Such "glymphatics" are demonstrated by their enhancement with gadobutrol, a contrast agent with proclivity to extravasate into tissue but not with an intravascular contrast dye such as gadofosveset.[6] These venous and lymphatic routes may converge at the choroid plexus, wherein microbes can spread through subarachnoid and perivascular spaces via purulent or inflammatory exudates. Tissue invasion may trigger cytokine release by microglia and immune cells, which alters the integrity of the blood–brain barrier (BBB) and promotes extravasation of contrast from intravascular to subarachnoid spaces, leading to characteristic meningeal enhancement present in many CNS infections.[1,7,8]

MENINGEAL ENHANCEMENT AND MENINGITIS

There are several types of meningeal enhancement: from normal dural enhancement (Fig. 4) to abnormal enhancement (Fig 5). *Pachymeningeal enhancement* involves the dura (see Fig. 3; Figs. 6 and 7) and is more often associated with noninfectious processes such as intracranial hypotension, meningiomas, metastasis, and granulomatous disease (Box 1). Intracranial hypotension can result in pachymeningeal enhancement post-LP in about 1% of patients,[9] whereby a reduction in CSF pressure causes a compensatory hydrostatic shift of fluid volume into subarachnoid space veins. This phenomenon arises from the *Monro-Kellie doctrine*.[10] With contrast administration, this expanded subarachnoid volume seems as either local or diffuse pachymeningeal enhancement as well as distended dural venous sinuses. Certain CNS infections (neurosyphilis, tuberculous meningitis) may seem as more focal areas of pachymeningeal enhancement.[1,11]

Leptomeningeal enhancement (Fig. 8), when pathologic, is thicker, longer, asymmetric and extends into the depth of the sulci and fills the subarachnoid spaces in sulci and cisterns (Box 2). Leptomeningeal enhancement is seen in 50% of meningitis cases and has characteristic imaging features, sometimes extending to involve enhancement of the cranial nerve surfaces (Box 3). *Meningitis* is the inflammation of the meninges; bacterial and viral meningitis commonly exhibit thin, linear leptomeningeal enhancement, whereas fungal and atypical bacterial meningitis display thicker, irregular, or nodular enhancement.[1,11] Carcinomatous meningitis related to meningeal spread of primary/secondary tumors also seems as enhancing leptomeningeal nodules, often with pachymeningeal enhancement.[1,12]

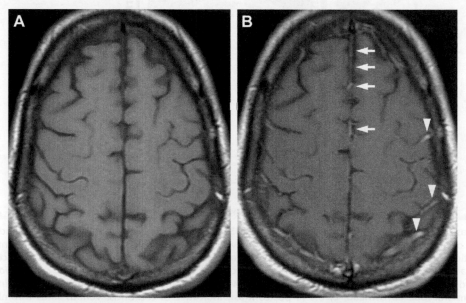

Fig. 4. Patterns of normal enhancement in precontrast (*A*) and postcontrast MR imaging (*B*) along the anterior falx (*arrows*) and normal meningeal vessels/cortical veins running in the cerebral sulci (*arrowheads*).

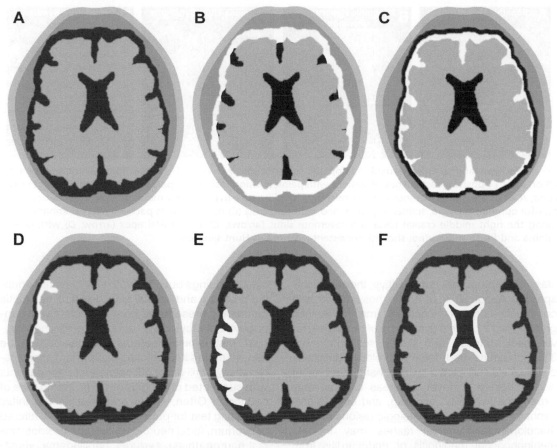

Fig. 5. Patterns of meningeal contrast enhancement (*white outlines*). Normal meninges (*A*). Diffuse pachymeningeal (*B*). Diffuse leptomeningeal (*C*) and localized leptomeningeal (*D*). Gyriform cortical (*E*). Ependymal (*F*).

Meningitis comprises about 15% of all annual CNS infections; bacterial causes account for about two-thirds of such cases.[13] Clinical features in adults include a classic triad of fever, nuchal rigidity, and altered mental status. Kernig's sign (pain elicited by passive knee extension) and Brudzinski's sign (hip/knee flexion elicited by passive neck flexion) may also be present. Although these

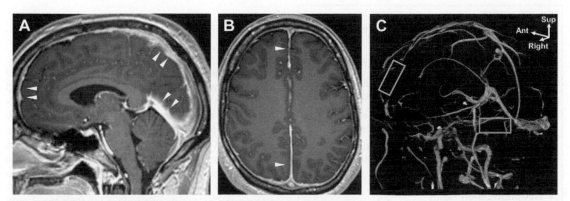

Fig. 6. Pachymeningeal enhancement in noninfectious granulomatosis with polyangiitis. (*arrowheads*, *A*, *B*). Diffuse pachymeningeal enhancement on MR imaging was complicated with chronic dural venous sinus thrombosis of the superior sagittal sinus (*empty green box*, *C*) and right transverse sinus (*empty blue box*, *C*) on an oblique view of CT venogram 3D reconstructions (*C*).

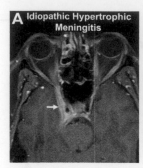 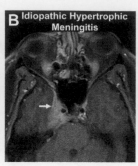 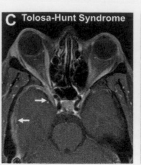 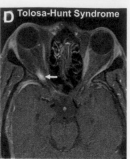

Fig. 7. Pachymeningeal enhancement in idiopathic hypertrophic meningitis (*A, B*) and Tolosa-Hunt syndrome (*C, D*) on axial T1 postcontrast images. A patient with painless vision loss shows pachymeningeal enhancement (*arrows, A, B*) of the right cavernous sinus, consistent with idiopathic hypertrophic meningitis. Another patient with painful ophthalmoplegia, sudden diplopia, and right proptosis (*C*) demonstrates pachymeningeal enhancement along the right middle cranial fossa and cavernous sinus (*arrows, C*) and orbital apex (*arrow, D*) with orbital edema and fat stranding (not shown), consistent with Tolosa-Hunt syndrome.

classic symptoms are not sensitive, they are highly specific. About 95% of adults hospitalized with community-acquired bacterial meningitis had greater than 2 of the 4 symptoms of headache, fever, neck stiffness, and altered sensorium, and 33% of adults had focal neurologic deficits.[14] Older adults may present with lethargy but without nuchal rigidity or fever, whereas children may experience irritability, vomiting, and even hydrocephalus (Box 4).[15] Dermatologic lesions such as maculopapular/petechial rashes may indicate meningococcal meningitis or endocarditis from staphylococci or pneumococci.[15,16]

In the clinical workup of suspected meningitis, CSF analysis by LP is a mainstay for diagnosing the pathogen and determining antimicrobial sensitivity. For bacterial meningitis, CSF analysis may reveal neutrophilic pleocytosis, elevated protein, and low glucose. Fungal meningitis has similar findings but often with very elevated opening pressure and normal glucose. Viral meningitis commonly presents as normal glucose with lymphocytic pleocytosis.[15] Although guidelines suggest that clinical features are deemed to be fairly accurate in predicting mass effect, many clinicians will still order CT before an LP for patients with suspected meningitis out of an abundance of caution.[16] Often, CT is preferred as the initial screening test for patients presenting with altered sensorium, focal neurologic deficits (besides cranial neuropathies), seizures, papilledema, vomiting, Cheyne-Stokes respirations or other signs of mass effect, and high intracranial pressure due to risk of herniation.[15,17] Additional factors favoring CT before LP include immunocompromised status and/or history of neurologic disorders. Imaging can also rule out meningitis mimics and elevated intracranial pressure before LP and assess for complications, such as edema and hydrocephalus.[1,15,18]

IMAGING OF MENINGITIS
Computed Tomography

Unenhanced CT can display mild dilatation of the ventricles with effaced subarachnoid spaces and suggestion of diffuse cerebral swelling. Obliteration of the normal basilar or convexity cisterns by exudates (of soft-tissue density) may also be seen (Fig. 9).[1] For older adults with large ventricles and effaced sulci/cisterns (as in ventriculo-sulcal discordance from normal pressure hydrocephalus), it may be necessary to consider acute conditions such as meningitis before labeling them with chronic diagnoses such as normal pressure hydrocephalus or age-related volume loss, in the appropriate clinical setting.

Box 1
Conditions with pachymeningeal versus leptomeningeal enhancement

Pachymeningeal	Leptomeningeal
• Intracranial hypotension	• Infectious meningitis
• Infection (syphilis, tuberculosis)	• Inflammatory (sarcoidosis)
• Inflammatory (sarcoidosis)	• Neoplastic meningitis
• Lymphoma/leukemia	
• Neoplastic meningitis	
• Granulomatosis with polyangiitis	

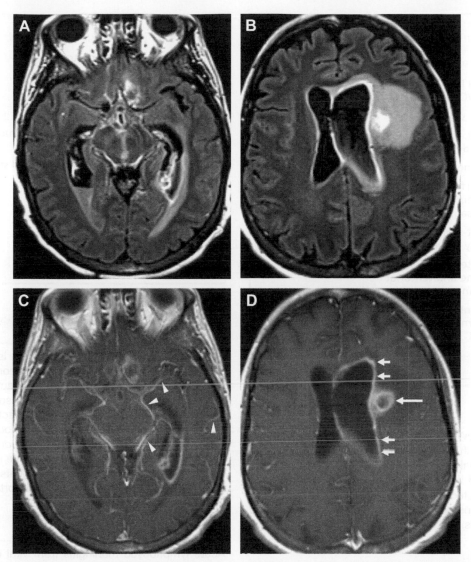

Fig. 8. Leptomeningeal and ependymal enhancement in bacterial meningitis. FLAIR (*A, B*) and T1 postcontrast MR imaging (*C, D*) in a patient status-post craniotomy shows leptomeningeal enhancement around the midbrain, adjacent sulci and cisterns (*arrowheads, C*) and ependymal surface of the left lateral ventricle (*arrows, D*). Note the ring-enhancing lesion (*long arrow, D*) consistent with abscess.

MR Imaging

Given its superior soft tissue contrast, MR imaging is much more sensitive at detecting meningitis and visualizing the soft tissue contrast in the basal cisterns, sylvian fissure, and sulcal regions. T1-weighted MR imaging may show obliteration of the basilar cisterns with enhancing inflammatory exudates (see **Fig. 9**H). Further, fluid attenuated inversion recovery (FLAIR) sulcal hyperintensities and leptomeningeal enhancement (see **Figs. 8** and **9**) may occur from elevated protein content in infectious exudates. FLAIR MR imaging is likely more sensitive than contrast enhancement in detecting leptomeningitis,[12] although the differential diagnosis is still broad (**Box 5**).[19]

Based on disease *chronicity*, meningeal enhancement of acute meningitis has a predilection for the cerebral convexity while chronic meningitis often involves the basilar cisterns. Enhancement in chronic meningitis is associated with dural thickening and sometimes popcorn-shaped dural calcifications.[1,20]

Diffusion-Weighted Imaging

Diffusion restriction is noted when there is increased DWI (b1000) signal and reduced ADC

Box 2
Differentiation between normal meningeal vessels versus abnormal leptomeningeal enhancement

Normal Meningeal Vessels/Cortical Veins	Abnormal Leptomeningeal Enhancement
• Thin, smooth	• Thick, nodular, irregular
• Short, discontinuous, well-demarcated	• Long, continuous, poorly demarcated
• Symmetric	• Asymmetric
• Superficial, most prominent parasagitally	•Extends deep to base of sulci
• Short-segment convexity enhancement	• Long-segment (>3cm) or diffuse convexity enhancement
• Isolated fine linear falcine and tentorial enhancement	
• No enhancement of cisterns, ventricular walls	• If meningeal enhancement present on 3 contiguous axial spin echo MR images

Box 4
Common clinical findings in meningitis

Infants	Adults
• Fever	• Fever
• Irritability	• Headache
• Constipation	• Nuchal rigidity
• Vomiting	• Brudzinski/Kernig sign
• Kernig sign	
• Seizures	• Altered mental status
• Altered sensorium	• Photophobia
• Bulging fontanelle	• Rash
	Older Adults
• Anorexia	• Fever
• Failure to thrive	• Lethargy

signal. DWI can demonstrate vascular complications such as infarcts from associated vasculitis,[1] meningeal and ependymal involvement in meningitis and ventriculitis,[21] and subtle, tiny amounts of restricted diffusion typically representing small collections of pus in the subarachnoid space and ventricles.[22]

Box 3
Imaging features of bacterial meningitis

- Most common finding is a normal scan
- Effaced CSF spaces
- Poorly visualized basilar cisterns
- Generalized cerebral edema
- Diffuse leptomeningeal enhancement
- Communicating hydrocephalus
- Subdural effusion (in children)/empyema
- Hyperintense sulcal signal abnormalities on FLAIR
- Subtle subarachnoid/ventricular high signal pus on DWI
- Sometimes associated with cranial nerve enhancement

CAUSES FOR INFECTIOUS MENINGITIS
Acute Pyogenic Meningitis

Acute pyogenic infections display diffuse leptomeningeal involvement and are more common in children. Purulent infections are often bacterial in origin, although enteroviruses can also cause acute meningitis. Frequent causes of bacterial infections are reviewed in Box 6. Immunocompromised patients may encounter *Pseudomonas*, *Klebsiella*, and fungal infections. Despite initiating empiric treatment, about 15% of patients experience neurologic complications and mortality remains around 20%.[1,15,20]

Acute Lymphocytic Meningitis

Acute lymphocytic meningitis from viral origin is generally benign and self-limited. History often includes travel, exposures, and new medications. Clinical signs are nonspecific, such as headache, fever, and meningismus.[15] Pathogens involved include enteroviruses, HSV, and mumps. Imaging findings are often normal but may demonstrate subtle, thin, linear, leptomeningeal enhancement (with parenchymal enhancement if there is associated encephalitis).[1,20]

Eosinophilic Meningitis

Eosinophilic meningitides are rare disorders defined by the presence of 10 or more eosinophils per cubic millimeter in CSF or CSF eosinophilia greater than 10%. It is generally caused by helminthic parasites endemic to the tropics and contracted by ingestion of contaminated food (Box 7). For example, angiostrongyliasis is associated with ingestion of raw seafood or

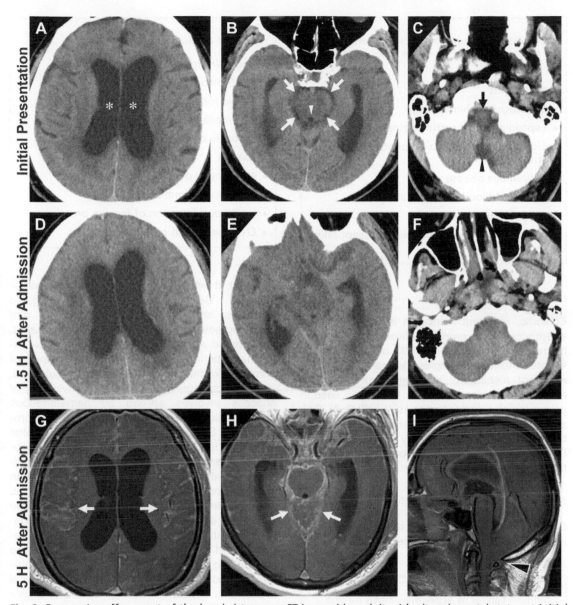

Fig. 9. Progressive effacement of the basal cisterns on CT in an older adult with altered mental status at initial presentation (*A, B, C*) with interval changes on follow-up CT (*D, E, F*) and MR imaging (*G, H, I*). On admission, there is prominence of bilateral lateral ventricles (*asterisks, A*) with narrower yet still visible CSF-density in perimesencephalic cisterns (*white arrows, B*), cerebral aqueduct (*white arrowhead, B*), perimedullary cistern (*black arrow, C*) and cisterna magna (*black arrowhead, C*). Within 1.5 hours of admission, patient deteriorated clinically and a follow-up head CT demonstrated similar appearance of lateral ventricles (*D*) but interval marked effacement of perimesencephalic and perimedullary cisterns (*E, F*). By 5 hours after admission, T1 postcontrast MR imaging noted diffuse enhancement of cerebral sulci (*arrows, G*), around the brainstem and posterior fossa (*arrows, H*). Notice significant worsening mass effect and cerebral swelling with tonsillar herniation on sagittal T1-weighted MR imaging (*black arrowhead, I*). Mental status decline corresponded to progressive cerebral swelling and herniations and the patient subsequently passed away.

contaminated vegetables. CSF studies indicate a raised eosinophil count with normal glucose levels. MR imaging depicts prominent perivascular spaces, periventricular T2 hyperintensities and enhancing subcortical lesions. Proton magnetic resonance spectroscopy (^{1}H-MRS) may show reduced choline within lesions, associated with neuronal damage.[1] Diagnosis is confirmed by presence of antibodies against *Angiostrongylus*, etc.[23]

Box 5
Differential diagnosis of sulcal hyperintensity on fluid attenuated inversion recovery MR imaging

- Meningitis
- Subarachnoid hemorrhage
- Leptomeningeal carcinomatosis
- Slow flow through pial collaterals in acute stroke
- Moyamoya disease
- Increased blood pool/CSF ratio
- Supplemental oxygen
- Artifact: Pulsation, magnetic susceptibility, motion

Box 7
Causes of eosinophilic meningitis

- *Angiostrongylus cantonensis*
- *Gnathostoma spinigerum*
- *Taenia solium*
- *Trichinella spiralis*
- *Toxocara canis*
- *Loa loa*
- *Mansonella perstans*
- *Coccidioides immitis*
- Intrathecal injection of foreign proteins
- CNS insertion of rubber tubing

Recurrent and Mollaret Meningitis

Episodic, recurrent meningitis is often linked to streptococci and gram-negative bacilli and can be responsible for up to 16% of all meningitis events.[1] Mollaret meningitis (also called idiopathic recurrent meningitis), is a rare syndrome with recurring episodes of aseptic meningitis seen in young females and linked to HSV (HSV2>1). Episodes are associated with reactivation and positive CSF markers for HSV2 by polymerase chain reaction analysis.[24,25] Specific imaging features have yet to be described.[26]

CEREBRITIS AND INTRACRANIAL ABSCESS

Cerebritis is a region of poorly defined acute brain inflammation with increased permeability of local

---

Box 6
Common causes of acute meningitis by age

Newborn <4 weeks	Adults
• Group B streptococci	• *S pneumoniae*
• *Escherichia coli*	• *N meningitidis*
• *Listeria monocytogenes*	• Enteroviruses
	• Herpes simplex
Children	**Older Adults**
• *H influenzae* type b	• *S pneumoniae*
• *N meningitidis*	• *N meningitidis*
• *S pneumoniae*	• *L monocytogenes*
• Enteroviruses	• Aerobic Gram-negative bacilli

---

vessels but without neovascularization or angiogenesis.[11] Cerebritis can arise from pyogenic infections and inflammatory conditions and may progress to form an abscess if left untreated. A pyogenic *abscess* is a focal area of parenchymal infection consisting of a central cavity of purulent exudate and surrounding vascularized, collagenous capsule.[2,27] The pathophysiology of abscess involves spread by hematogenous dissemination, direct invasion, or iatrogenic complications. Similar to metastasis, hematogenous dissemination typically results in multiple abscesses near the gray–white junction within middle cerebral artery territories bilaterally. Children with abscess may have underlying congenital heart disease. Other infectious sources include pulmonary abscess and arteriovenous malformation, bacterial endocarditis, intra-abdominal abscess, and dental infection. Abscesses can be adjacent to untreated otitis media and odontogenic infections. Abscess from neurosurgical procedures is also increasing, related to higher procedure frequency.[2]

Intracranial abscess constitutes about 4% of all CNS infections annually.[13] Brain abscess is more prevalent in men than in women and more commonly occurs in the first 4 decades of life. Predisposing factors include diabetes, alcoholism, intravenous drug use, pulmonary lesions, and immunosuppression.[4]

Symptoms vary by abscess location, extent of mass effect, and associated complications. Developing abscesses result in neurologic symptoms[15] (Box 8) that overlap with meningitis including headache (50%–90%), fever (60%), and altered sensorium (30%–70%). Abscesses with high intracranial pressure may present with papilledema. Laboratory tests are often unrevealing; indeed, the absence of leukocytosis or pathogens in the

Box 8
Clinical features suspicious of developing abscess

- Relentless headache
- Fever
- Worsening neurologic deficits
- Altered mental status
- Nausea and vomiting
- New seizures
- Developing papilledema

CSF does not preclude the diagnosis of abscess.[4] LP is often discouraged and even contraindicated in order to avoid herniation or ventricular rupture when neuroimaging demonstrates surrounding edema, mass effect, or increased intracranial pressure.[15] Blood cultures may reveal the underlying cause of abscess in the setting of hematogenous dissemination, although direct aspiration is often required for establishing accurate diagnosis and subsequent treatment.

IMAGING OF CEREBRITIS AND ABSCESS

The advent of CT and MR imaging has enabled rapid localization, accurate diagnosis, stereotactic aspiration, and serial postoperative evaluation of abscesses while improved newer generation antibiotics have enabled better empiric and selective therapy.[2,27] There should be a low threshold for performing neuroimaging when complications of meningitis are suspected and treatment planning can be further clarified. Intracranial abscesses greater than 1 cm are stereotactically aspirated while patients are on broad-spectrum antimicrobials and steroids.[28,29] Careful consideration is needed before biopsy of presumed cerebritis. Follow-up imaging is performed if there is clinical decline, a lack of improvement after 1 to 2 weeks and after recovery.[29]

Meningitis with Cerebritis and Abscess

Meningitis is accompanied by abscess in about 2% of patients with CNS infection. There are 3 common scenarios: (1) community-acquired bacterial meningitis can be complicated by cerebritis and abscess, (2) patients with infective endocarditis concurrently develop meningitis and focal abscess via mycotic emboli, and (3) abscess capsules rupture causing ependymal/meningeal spread and sudden decline.[2,30]

Computed Tomography

CT with contrast can evaluate the 4 stages of pyogenic infection: early cerebritis, late cerebritis, early capsule formation, and mature abscess.[30,31] In early cerebritis, bacteria enter the parenchyma, triggering an immune response resulting in perivascular swelling. On CT, this is seen as an ill-defined low attenuation with variable contrast enhancement. In late cerebritis, central necrosis is flanked by stromal matrix, leading to low attenuation with rim enhancement that is stable on delayed images. During full abscess formation stages, a collagenous surrounding capsule forms, appearing as ring enhancement that decays on delayed images (which corresponds to granulation tissue). Because the medial or ventricular wall of an abscess is thinner than the lateral wall, due to the blood supply gradient, an untreated abscess near the ventricles often ruptures, causing satellite abscesses and ventriculitis.[2,31]

MR Imaging

As with meningitis, abscess is better diagnosed with MR imaging compared with CT, especially due to sensitivity of MR imaging to water diffusion. Moreover, MR imaging is vital to the longitudinal evaluation of abscess. Cerebritis shows nonspecific, ill-defined T2/FLAIR hyperintensity and mild T1 hypointensity with poorly demarcated enhancement. In contrast, mature abscesses show central low intensity on T1 and central high intensity on T2 with surrounding vasogenic edema.[2,20] Most importantly, abscesses are a canonical *ring enhancing* lesion. On postcontrast T1-weighted MR imaging, the capsule seems as an enhancing, smooth, thin, circumferential rim that is T1 hyperintense and T2 hypointense relative to white matter (see Fig. 8; Fig. 10).[2] In fact, the T2 hypointense abscess capsule may seem as a "dual rim sign" of concentric circles (either complete or incomplete), which is a useful imaging clue to distinguish from necrotic gliomas (see Fig. 10).[32] The differential diagnosis for ring enhancement is described further in the "Mimics" section.

Diffusion-Weighted Imaging

Central diffusion restriction is a hallmark feature of most forms of untreated abscess, due to proteinaceous contents of inflammatory exudates/pus,[22] with high signal on DWI maps and low signal on ADC maps (see Fig. 10). Although cerebritis does not contain frank pus and often does not exhibit diffusion restriction (see Fig. 3), abscess does restrict water diffusion, reflecting the inflammatory

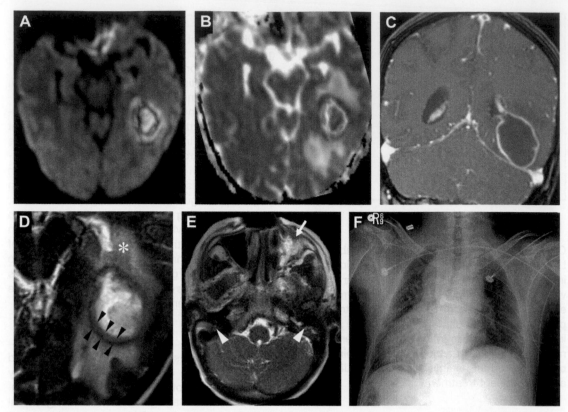

Fig. 10. Abscess in a patient with primary ciliary dyskinesia (Kartagener syndrome). The left temporal lesion shows restricted diffusion on DWI (*A*) and ADC (*B*) and peripheral-enhancement on T1 postcontrast (*C*). A close-up of the T2-weighted MR imaging portrays a capsule with 2 T2 hypointense layers suggestive of the "dual rim sign" (*black arrowheads, D*) and vasogenic edema (*asterisk, D*). On axial T2 image, notice the left maxillary sinus inflammatory disease (*white arrow, E*) and underdeveloped bilateral mastoid air cells (*white arrowheads, E*) from ciliary dysfunction. Chest X-ray (*F*) portrays situs inversus totalis, typical of primary ciliary dyskinesia.

milieu of necrotic debris, highly viscous proteinaceous exudates, and viable bacterial and immune cells in abscess cavities. Conversely, the central nonenhancing regions of a peripherally enhancing necrotic high-grade glioma contain fewer inflammatory cells and less viscous, clearer serous fluid that shows facilitated diffusion. Hence, DWI can accurately distinguish abscess from necrotic gliomas.[1,2,29] Although most bacterial abscesses seem centrally diffusion restricting,[33] other ring-enhancing entities such as toxoplasmosis may lack this critical finding.[34,35]

Quantification of ADC values can further assist in the differential diagnosis of enhancing mass lesions. Compared with cerebral white matter, which has a mean ADC value near 0.9×10^{-3} mm²/s,[36] pyogenic abscesses usually have mean ADC values 30% to 40% lower, at 0.5 to 0.6×10^{-3} mm²/s.[37,38] Compared with the low mean ADC values of spontaneous brain

abscesses,[37,38] other mass lesions often have mean ADC values higher than 1.3×10^{-3} mm²/s, including gliomas,[37–39] toxoplasmosis,[39] and iatrogenic postoperative brain abscesses.[40] Nevertheless, diffusion restriction in abscess often become less prominent on treatment initiation and may help distinguish between therapeutic success and the reaccumulation of infectious material/pus.[38]

MR Spectroscopy

Mature brain abscesses have certain spectroscopic profiles that distinguish them from neoplasms on ¹H-MRS (Box 9). Although abscess and tumors share features such as decreased normal neuronal metabolites, choline (3.2 ppm) is elevated in brain tumors and can be used to distinguish from pyogenic abscess (Fig. 11). In addition, pyogenic abscesses demonstrate signal from cytosolic, branched chain amino acids (valine,

<table>
<tr><td colspan="2">Box 9
MR spectroscopy findings of pyogenic abscess</td></tr>
<tr><td>Decreased or not
Elevated neuron
metabolites</td><td>Increased
inflammation</td></tr>
</table>

Decreased or not Elevated neuron metabolites	Increased inflammation
• N-acetyl-aspartate (2.0 ppm)	• Lactate (1.33 ppm)
	• Lipids (0.9-1.3 ppm)
• Creatine (3.0 ppm)	**Elevated and specific to infection**
• Choline (3.2 ppm)	• Valine, leucine, isoleucine (0.9 ppm)
	• Succinate (2.4 ppm)
	• Acetate (1.9 ppm)

leucine, isoleucine, 0.9 ppm) and succinate (2.4 ppm), which diminish on successful therapy.[2] Because acetate is a product and substrate in anaerobic bacterial metabolism,[41] elevated acetate peaks (1.9 ppm) are also often present in anaerobic abscesses (Fig. 12).[2,42,43] Although these are general MRS findings typically associated with abscess, exceptions exist.[44] Overall, ^{1}H-MRS is more supportive than determinative and has 72% to 100% sensitivity and 30% to 100% specificity.[45,46]

In immunocompromised patients, ^{1}H-MRS can assist in distinguishing toxoplasmosis from primary CNS lymphoma. The increase in lipid and lactate peaks (1.3 ppm) is usually much more substantial in toxoplasmosis than lymphoma while the increase of choline (3.2 PM) is higher in lymphoma and often decreased in toxoplasmosis.[46]

Nuclear Medicine

Focal intracranial infections can also be evaluated using metabolic PET tracers, although this is not widely used in clinical practice. Although ^{18}F-fluorodeoxyglucose (^{18}F-FDG) uptake can detect hypermetabolism associated with infections such as rhinocerebral mucormycosis,[47] infections generally have less metabolic activity than tumors.

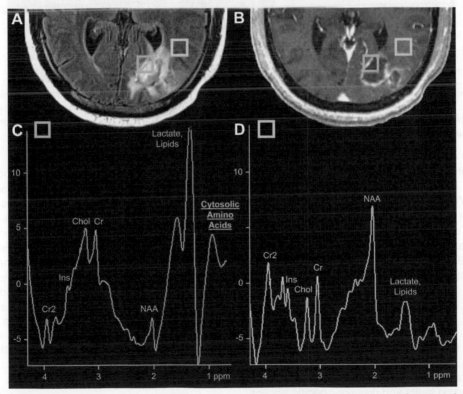

Fig. 11. Fungal abscess on MR imaging and MRS. An FLAIR hyperintense (A), peripherally enhancing abscess (B) in the left occipital lobe. The orange square denotes placement of voxel including the abscess cavity while the green square depicts an unaffected region adjacent to the edematous abscess. Comparison of MRS peaks from the abscess cavity (C) and perilesional edematous region (D) reveals elevated cytosolic amino acids (0.9 ppm) and lactate/lipids (1.3 ppm) with decreased N-acetyl-aspartate (NAA, 2.0 ppm), choline (Cho, 3.0 ppm) and creatine (Cr, 3.2 ppm), consistent with an abscess.

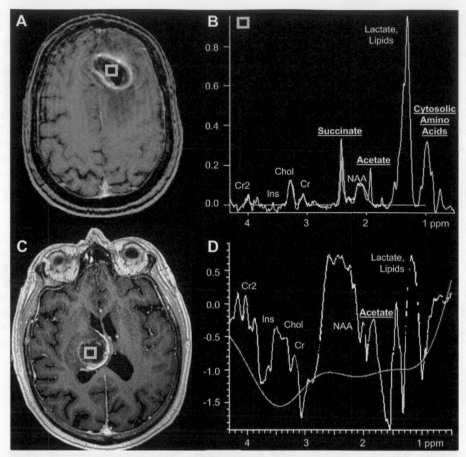

Fig. 12. Two patients with bacterial abscesses displaying acetate peaks on MRS. T1 postcontrast shows a left fron-tal abscess with (voxel, *A*). MRS (*B*) depicts elevated succinate (2.4 ppm), acetate (1.9 ppm), amino acids (0.9 ppm), and lactate/lipid (1.3 ppm) peaks and low NAA (2.0 ppm). In a second patient, T1 postcontrast MR imaging depicts a right thalamic abscess (voxel, *C*) with acetate peak and low NAA on MRS (*D*).

When differentiating lymphoma from toxoplas-mosis in patients with human immunodeficiency virus (HIV), note that lymphoma exhibits significant uptake of radiotracers in ^{18}F-FDG PET and [201]Th and ^{99m}Tc-sestamibi single-photon emission CT. These tracers also have ~100% sensitivity and 60% to 90% specificity in identifying lymphoma over toxoplasmosis.[48,49]

Artificial Intelligence for Central Nervous System Infections

With the increasing adoption of deep learning in medicine, AI models have demonstrated remark-able accuracy and efficiency on an assortment of neuroimaging tasks and disease-specific applica-tions.[50–54] For instance, neural networks could distinguish between bacterial and viral meningi-tis.[55] Recent convolutional neural networks (such as U-Net) can perform at the level of radiologists on FLAIR lesion detection.[56] Moreover, the

integration of these deep learning models with Bayesian inference enables accurate and inter-pretable probabilistic differential diagnoses for an array of CNS infections (including abscess, toxo-plasmosis, cryptococcosis) and their mimics[57] as well as HIV encephalopathy and progressive multi-focal leukoencephalopathy.[58] Because neural net-works can identify and predict signature imaging findings in cerebral infections, including ring enhancement and FLAIR hyperintensities,[59] clin-ical validation and integration studies are the next phase in translating this research into aug-menting the radiologist's workflow in the future (Fig. 13).

CAUSES FOR CEREBRITIS, ABSCESS, AND CEREBRAL INVOLVEMENT
Bacterial Abscess

Most intracranial abscesses are polymicrobial in composition, including aerobic and/or anaerobic

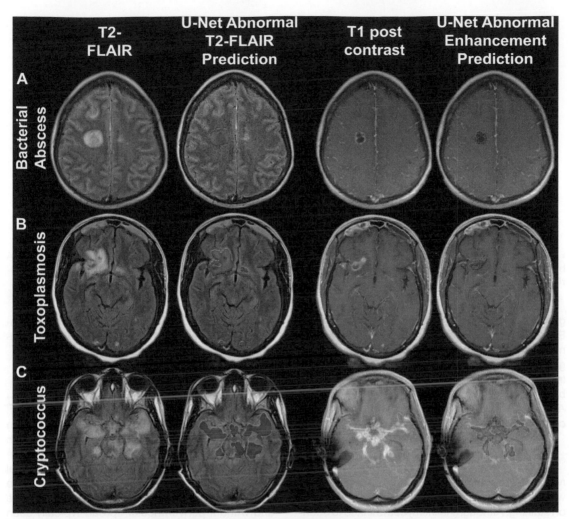

Fig. 13. Predictions of T2 FLAIR (*left*) and T1 postcontrast (*right*) MR imaging lesions of CNS infections with a deep learning U-net model. Abscess (*A*), toxoplasmosis (*B*), cryptococcosis (*C*).

bacteria (**Box 10**). Immunocompetent patients may develop bacterial abscesses due to infective endocarditis, pulmonary shunts, trauma, and dental/sinus infections,[28] whereas immunocompromised patients typically present with fungal and *Nocardia* abscesses.[15] Note that abscess in immunocompromised patients may not display the typical ring enhancement, restricted diffusion, and/or vasogenic edema, and the lack of inflammatory response is usually associated with worse outcomes.[2]

Aspergillosis

Cerebral aspergillosis is a common cause of abscess in immunocompromised cohorts with a mortality of about 90%.[60] Along with candidiasis, aspergillosis is one of the most common sources of intracranial fungal abscess (aspergilloma) and arises in the settings of neutropenia, transplantation, and HIV infection.[20,29] Aspergillomas are usually ring enhancing and T1 hypointense with central diffusion restriction on DWI.[33,61] Angioinvasive aspergillosis tends to infiltrate and occlude smaller perforating vessels supplying the basal

Box 10 Common causes of brain abscess	
Immunocompetent	Immunocompromised
• S aureus	• Aspergillus
• E coli	• Cryptococcus
• Enterobacter	• Toxoplasma
• Actinomyces	• Nocardia
• Bacteroides	• Candida
• Prevotella	• Mucor, Rhizopus

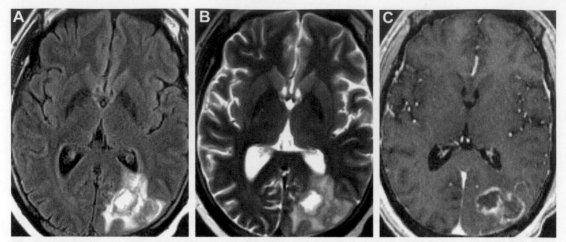

Fig. 14. Aspergillosis in a patient with graft-versus-host disease presenting with right inferior quadrantanopia. A bilobed abscess in the left occipital region seems FLAIR hyperintense (A) with T2 hypointense capsule (B) and peripheral enhancement (C) and perilesional edema (A, B).

ganglia, thalami, corpus callosum, and brainstem. Because hemorrhage occurs in 25% of aspergillomas and even more commonly in invasive aspergillosis, ferromagnetic blood products in such lesions might seem T1 hyperintense and susceptible on gradient echo (GRE) sequence (Fig. 14).[61] Aspergillus meningitis rarely occurs in immunocompetent individuals.[60]

Nocardiosis

Nocardia is a branching, filamentous bacteria that is weakly acid fast, distinguishing it from Actinomyces on staining. Although Actinomyces is linked to odontogenic abscess, nocardiosis is related to HIV infection and immunosuppression.[29] Importantly, pulmonary nocardiosis in immunocompromised

patients should undergo screening intracranial imaging.[15] Compared with other causes, nocardial abscess is usually multiloculated (Fig. 15).[62]

Toxoplasmosis

Toxoplasmosis is caused by Toxoplasma gondii. It is the most frequent opportunistic infection linked to HIV and occurs in 33% of patients with HIV,[34] toxoplasmosis lesions often seem as multifocal nodules in the basal ganglia or frontoparietal regions (Fig. 16A–C), with disproportionate extent of vasogenic edema and/or hemorrhage and without periventricular spread typically seen in lymphoma.[1,47] Differences may be noted on MRS[46] and ^{18}F-FDG PET.[48] Although the "eccentric target sign" for cerebral toxoplasmosis only

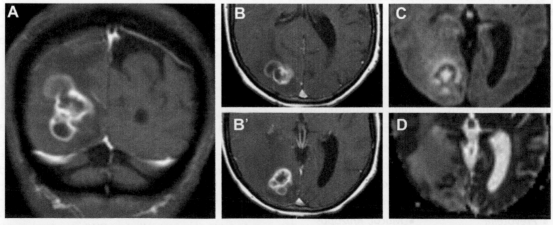

Fig. 15. Nocardiosis in a patient with leukemia complicated by graft-versus-host disease. T1 postcontrast MR imaging in coronal (A) and axial (B, B') planes visualize a multiloculated ring enhancing nocardial abscess in the right parietooccipital region with restricted diffusion on DWI (C) and ADC (D).

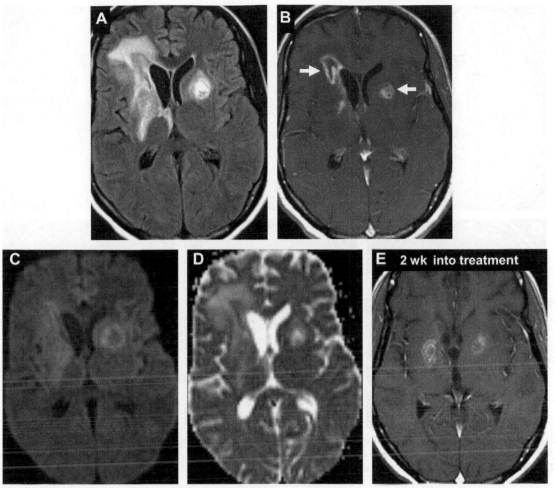

Fig. 16. Toxoplasmosis in an HIV-positive patient. Ill-defined heterogenous lesions on FLAIR with surrounding vasogenic edema (*A*) and peripheral enhancement (*B*) are evident in the bilateral basal ganglia (*arrows, B*). Unlike typical abscess, there is facilitated diffusion on DWI (*C*) and ADC (*D*). Two weeks after initiating antitoxoplasma treatment (*E*), there is interval reduction in enhancement of the lesions, with decreased vasogenic edema (not shown). Note, "eccentric target sign" (*arrow, B*).

has 25% sensitivity and is seen in only 30% of cases, it is greater than 95% specific.[63] The eccentric target sign is seen on postcontrast images as irregular ring enhancement with eccentric nodularity, likely from invagination of the abscess wall with inflamed vessels in its groove, surrounded by perilesional edema, inflammation, and demyelination.[64] Although abscess and toxoplasmosis both have peripheral enhancement, the central diffusion restriction seen in abscess is generally absent in toxoplasmosis (Fig. 16D, E).[34] Compared with parenchymal infection, toxoplasma meningitis is rare in HIV infection or transplant recipients,[65] and cryptococcal/tuberculous meningitis and lymphoma should be considered in the differential diagnosis of abnormal meningeal enhancement.[66]

CAUSES WITH MIXED MENINGEAL AND CEREBRAL INVOLVEMENT
Chronic Meningitis and Abscess: Tuberculosis and Cryptococcosis

Exudates from chronic meningitides (tubercular or fungal) seem as thick, nodular leptomeningeal enhancement and often coalesce into localized forms of infection such as tuberculoma, cryptococcoma, and so forth.[20]

Tuberculous meningitis occurs through hematogenous dissemination. CSF findings are often nonspecific and only show the pathogen in about 30% of cases.[15,67] On imaging, tuberculous meningitis displays basal and posterior fossa leptomeningeal enhancement associated with hydrocephalus. Vasculitis, thrombosis, and infarction may also be seen (Fig. 17).[68,69] Tuberculomas

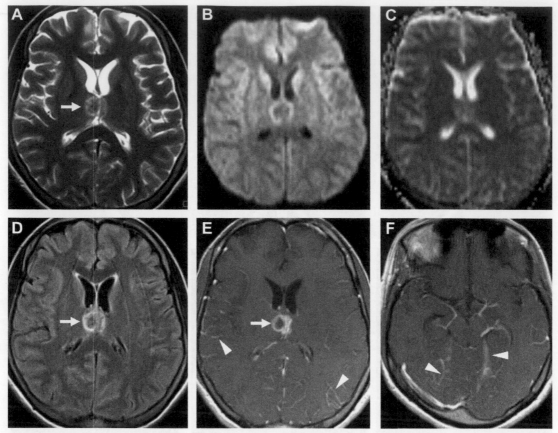

Fig. 17. Tuberculoma with meningitis. A thalamic lesion with central T2 hypointensity (*arrow, A*), characteristic for tuberculoma, with no restricted diffusion on DWI (*B*) and ADC (*C*) but with FLAIR hyperintensity (*arrow, D*). On T1 postcontrast, there is ring enhancement (*arrow, E*) and associated meningitis (*arrowheads, E, F*).

are ring-enhancing lesions that are heterogeneously T2 hypointense.[70] Unlike typical abscesses, tuberculomas usually do not exhibit central diffusion restriction due to caseous necrosis, although the periphery may.[35] On ^{1}H-MRS, tuberculomas exhibit elevated lipid peaks (1.3 ppm), derived from mycolic acid, yet lack cytosolic amino acids (0.9 ppm).[2,20]

Cryptococcosis has a predilection for the neuraxis in immunocompromised patients.[1,20] On contrast-enhanced MR imaging, cryptococcosis results in enhancement of the leptomeninges and perivascular spaces (Fig. 18). Parenchymal lesions frequently occur around the basal ganglia and include ring-enhancing cryptococcomas and diffusion-restricting gelatinous pseudocysts that are associated with edema and infarcts. The gelatinous pseudocysts represent spread of the fungi via perivascular spaces, leading to dilation and enhancement of these pial-lined, fluid-filled structures.[71] Serial LP, ventriculoperitoneal shunts and steroids mitigate elevated intracranial pressures, hydrocephalus and edema.[72]

Immunocompromised patients have worse outcomes and may not present with edema and enhancement.[73]

Neurocysticercosis

Neurocysticercosis is the most prevalent CNS infection worldwide, accounting for 83% of all CNS infections annually. It is endemic in Asia, Africa and Latin America, where it is the commonest cause of seizures and CSF eosinophilia.[13] There are 3 types of disease: meningobasilar (most common), ventricular and parenchymal.[74] About 60% of patients also demonstrate parenchymal cysts.[75,76] There are 4 classic stages of disease. In the early vesicular stage of parenchymal cysticercosis, cysts often manifest as a "dot in a hole" attributed to a visible scolex or hooked mouth of the parasite inside the lesion (Fig. 19). The scolex inner "dot" seems T2 hypointense, FLAIR hyperintense, and enhancing[76] and may be well visualized on 3D constructive interference in steady state MR sequence (see Fig. 19B).[77] This stage is followed by the vesicular-colloidal, granular nodular, and calcified nodular stages. As

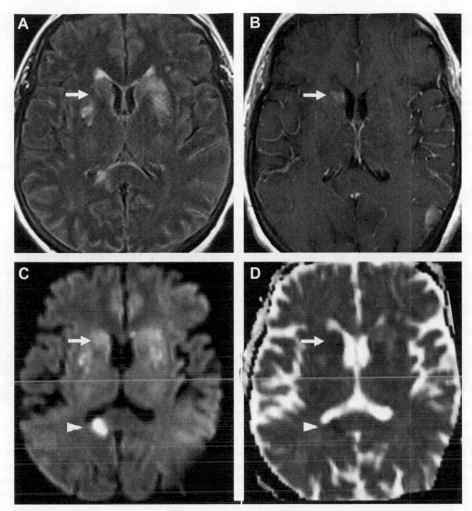

Fig. 18. Cryptococcosis with meningitis and acute infarction. Multifocal FLAIR hyperintense cryptococcomas are seen in the basal ganglia (*arrows, A*) and corpus callosum with enhancement in the right caudate nucleus (*arrow, B*) and bilateral cerebral sulci (*B*). Diffusion restriction in a right splenium of corpus callosum suggesting acute infarct (*arrowhead, C, D*) and faint diffusion abnormality in the basal ganglia (*arrow, C, D*) on DWI (*C*) and ADC (*D*).

the parasite dies, the cyst ruptures, recruiting inflammatory cells with edema, altering signal intensity and ultimately causing calcification.[1,20]

OTHER COMPLICATIONS OF MENINGITIS, CEREBRITIS, AND ABSCESS
Ventriculitis

Ventriculitis (or ependymitis) is the involvement of the ependyma, choroid plexus, and/or ventricles and is a very severe complication that occurs in 30% of patients with CNS infections. Organisms such as *Staphylococcus aureus* and *Enterobacter* can breach the ventricular system via (1) direct extension from trauma or neurosurgical intervention, (2) meningeal spread into the ventricles, (3)

hematogenous dissemination through the subependyma and choroid plexus, (4) CSF backflow from extraventicular to intraventricular spaces, and (5) abscess rupture. Clinical progression is insidious, so it is paramount to treat the underlying source assiduously.[1,15]

Chronic viral infections can produce periventricular calcifications.[7] Cranial ultrasound in children is often superior to CT and may reveal irregular, echogenic ependyma, intraventricular debris, and stranding associated with ventricular dilatation.[1] MR imaging is most revealing; the ependyma enhances while the ventricles are dilated and filled with T2/FLAIR hyperintense, diffusion restricting purulent exudate (see Fig. 2; Fig. 20). Notably, higher ADC values

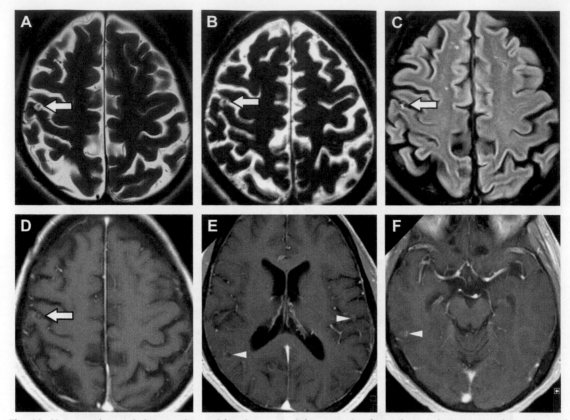

Fig. 19. Neurocysticercosis in a patient with seizures. A right posterior frontal cystic lesion seen along the pial surface seems with a T2 hypointense inner "dot in a hole" sign (arrows, A, B) on T2-weighted (A) and T2-weighted thin-section 3D constructive interference in steady state (B) images, pathognomonic for the scolex in neurocysticercosis. This cyst is FLAIR hyperintense (arrow, C) with central and ring enhancement (arrow, D). T1 postcontrast MR imaging reveals leptomeningeal enhancement (D, E, F) and additional ring enhancing cysts in the right parietal lobe (arrowhead, E), left frontal operculum (arrowhead, E) and right lateral temporal lobe (arrowhead, F).

might be observed from mixing of CSF and pus.[7,21]

Hydrocephalus and Herniation

Hydrocephalus in CNS infections varies from mild/transient (81% of cases) to severe (5%),[78,79] which can lead to brain herniation and sudden death (see Fig. 9). Hydrocephalus arises when (1) debris impedes CSF resorption, (2) infections infiltrate the ventricular system, or (3) mass lesions compress drainage structures.[79] Moreover, ruptured cysticercal scolex lesions and mycobacterial antigens are immunogenic in 30%[80] and 65% of cases, respectively.[69] Hydrocephalus also occurs in up to 60% of patients with cryptococcosis and is associated with very-high LP opening pressures (>350 mm H_2O in 50% of cases; Fig. 21). Large abscesses create inflammatory exudate, vasogenic edema and mass effect, midline shift, and

herniation. In cryptococcosis, CSF shunting or sequential LP can prevent herniation.[72]

Extra-Axial Collections

Extra-axial fluid collections associated with infections can be sterile (effusion) or purulent (empyema). Microbes can induce inflammation of the dura and subdural veins, creating subdural effusions. Most sterile effusions seem along the frontal and temporal convexities and tend to resolve spontaneously within months. If such findings produce mass effect, drainage may be warranted.[7] Typically, imaging of subdural effusions reveals crescentic collections of similar density/intensity as CSF. Some effusions may resemble empyema after accruing fibrin deposits and proteinaceous collections, possibly demonstrating enhancement on postcontrast MR imaging and failure of FLAIR suppression.[81,82] Presence of

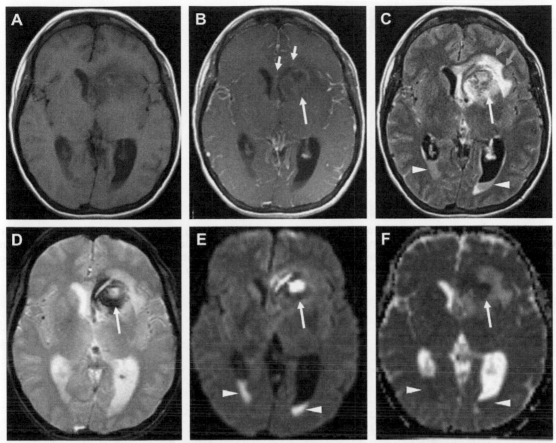

Fig. 20. Ventriculitis associated with ruptured abscess (*long arrow, B–D*). Axial T1-weighted precontrast (*A*) and postcontrast MR images (*B*) demonstrate a peripherally enhancing left caudate abscess (*long arrow, B*) with subtle linear enhancement of the ependyma of the left frontal horn and midline septum (*short arrows, B*) and diffuse leptomeningeal enhancement. The left caudate abscess is surrounded by vasogenic edema (*short blue arrows, C*), and has ruptured in the ventricles, susceptibility from blood products on GRE (*long arrow, D*) and restricted diffusion (*long arrows, E, F*) on DWI (*E*) and ADC (*F*). Notice a lack of susceptibility of the dependent debris in the occipital horns on GRE, with corresponding FLAIR hyperintensity (*arrowheads, C*) and restricted diffusion (*arrowheads, E, F*), consistent with layering pus.

diffusion restriction, however, favors empyema over effusion.[83]

Empyemas are life-threatening and should be drained. Streptococci are the most common pathogens, followed by *S aureus* and anaerobes. The clinical presentation is more severe and persistent than effusion.[15] Subdural empyema is located between the dura and arachnoid mater over the convexities or between hemispheres (Fig. 22). It is often due to thrombophlebitis from emissary veins. CT depicts a hypodense/isodense crescentic or lenticular collection while MR imaging shows a diffusion restricting crescentic collection with surrounding enhancement.[7] Perilesional T2/FLAIR hyperintensities of the cortex and concomitant venous thrombosis and infarct are specific to empyema compared with

effusions. Epidural empyema seems between the dura and calvaria and is more insidious and benign. Similar to subdural empyema, epidural empyema has FLAIR hyperintensities but is biconvex in shape (Fig. 23) and may occasionally have low/mixed DWI signal as the pus is less viscous and inflammatory.[81]

Cranial Nerve Involvement

Cranial nerve enhancement is almost always pathologic. Differential diagnosis includes infection, inflammation, demyelination, toxic-metabolic, genetic, neoplastic, and idiopathic (ie, Tolosa-Hunt syndrome, Fig. 7).[84] Basal meningeal exudates can cause compression, strain, and ischemia of cranial nerves, leading to

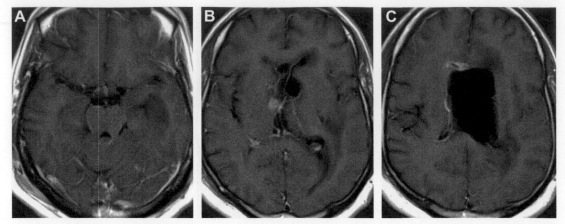

Fig. 21. Cryptococcosis and hydrocephalus. T1 postcontrast MR imaging visualizes subtle perimesencephalic and bilateral posterior leptomeningeal enhancement (*A*). Enhancement along an obstructed foramen of Monro (*B*). Ependymal enhancement with enlarged left lateral ventricle (*C*). The right lateral ventricle is reduced in volume due to left ventricle compression and drainage by a ventriculostomy catheter.

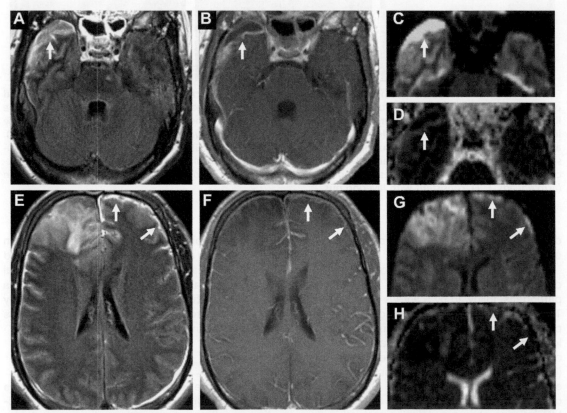

Fig. 22. Subdural empyema in a patient with bacterial meningitis and cerebritis. A crescentic subdural collection in the right middle cranial fossa (*arrows*) is FLAIR hyperintense (*A*) with enhancement (*B*) and restricted diffusion on DWI (*C*) and ADC (*D*). In the left anterior convexity (*arrows*), a thin FLAIR hyperintense collection (*E*) with leptomeningeal enhancement (*F*) shows diffusion restriction on DWI (*G*) and ADC (*H*). Note also diffuse leptomeningitis (*F*) and frontal cerebritis, right worse than left (*E–H*).

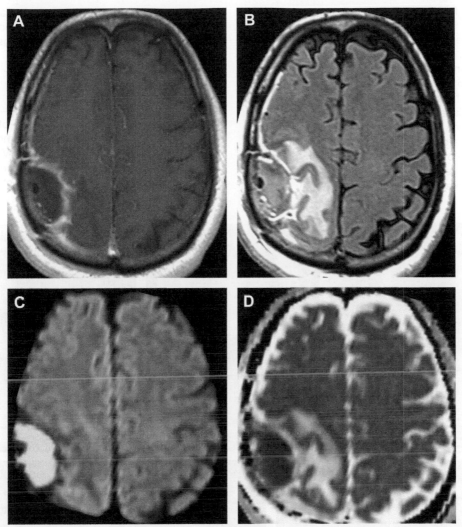

Fig. 23. Epidural empyema in bacterial meningitis. This seems as a biconvex collection with thick peripheral enhancement (*A*) subjacent the craniotomy site with FLAIR hyperintensity (*B*) and diffusion restriction on DWI (*C*) and ADC (*D*) maps.

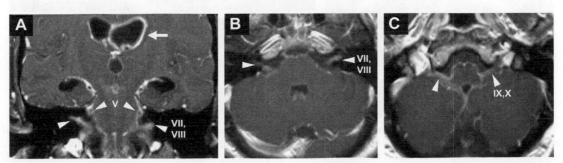

Fig. 24. Cranial neuropathy in a patient with bacterial leptomeningitis presenting with dilated, fixed pupils lacking several cranial nerve (CN) reflexes. T1 postcontrast images demonstrate enhancement of bilateral trigeminal nerves (CN V, *arrowheads*, *A*), facial/vestibulocochlear nerves (CN VII, VIII, *arrowheads*, *A*, *B*) and glossopharyngeal/vagus nerves (CN IX, X, *arrowheads*, *C*). Thick ependymal enhancement is noted (*arrow*, *A*).

diplopia, facial palsy, hearing loss, and so forth (Fig. 24). Meningitis associated with otitis media from *Streptococcus pneumoniae*, *Haemophilus influenza*, and *Neisseria meningitidis* can result in transient and permanent sensorineural hearing loss in 15% to 30% of cases.[85,86] Local involvement such as labyrinthitis with inner ear sclerosis may be visualized on CT and T2-weighted MR imaging. Note that meningitis-induced hearing loss should be differentiated from hearing loss secondary to ototoxic antibiotics.[7] Additional cranial neuropathies impair the optic, oculomotor, and facial nerves. Cranial neuropathy may seem as

cranial nerve and perineural enhancement and classically presents in neuroborreliosis, tuberculous meningitis, cryptococcosis, and schistosomiasis.[84]

Venous Sinus Thrombosis, Vasculitis, and Infarction

Venous sinus thrombosis occurs in 1% of patients with meningitis.[87] Cerebral venous thrombosis can evolve into infarct in 30% of patients.[7] Venous sinus thrombosis can also develop secondary to bacterial meningitis, pyogenic infection (see Fig. 3; Fig. 25) and mastoiditis.

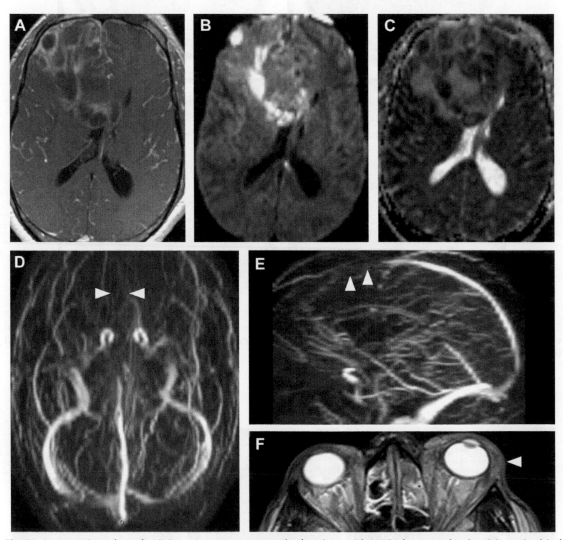

Fig. 25. Venous sinus thrombosis in an immunocompromised patient with MRSA bacteremia, sinusitis, and orbital cellulitis. Axial T1 postcontrast MR imaging (*A*) shows leptomeningeal and irregular peripheral enhancement, suggestive of meningitis. Diffusion restriction DWI (*B*) and ADC (*C*) maps indicate multiple abscesses. Time-of-flight venogram MIP images (*D*, *E*) demonstrate loss of flow-related enhancement of the anterior superior sagittal sinus, consistent with venous sinus thrombosis (*arrowheads*, *D*, *E*). Notice extensive preseptal and postseptal inflammation in the left orbit (*arrowhead*, *F*) and opacified ethmoid air cells (*F*). MIP, maximum intensity projection.

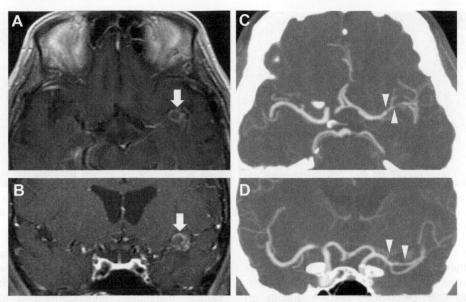

Fig. 26. Vasculitis in tuberculous meningitis. In a patient with HIV and left-sided retroorbital headaches, T1 post-contrast axial (A) and coronal MR images (B) reveal a peripherally enhancing lesion in the left perisylvian region (arrows, A, B) and faint basilar enhancement, consistent with tuberculous meningitis with tuberculoma. CT angiography (CTA) via axial (C) and coronal thin MIP images (D) show focal narrowing and irregularity of the distal M1, M2, and proximal M3 segments of the left middle cerebral artery (arrowheads, C, D), suggestive of vasculitis secondary to tuberculous meningitis.

Infectious vasculitis can complicate syphilis, tuberculous meningitis (Fig. 26), angioinvasive aspergillosis and other infections. Ischemic strokes associated with vasculitis occur in 14% of patients with neurosyphilis.[88]

Infarction occurs in up to 30% of adults with bacterial meningitis,[89] especially chronic meningitis: 13% to 32% of patients with cryptococcal meningitis[90,91] (see Fig. 18) and about 25% to 40% of patients with tuberculous meningitis.[92,93] Tuberculosis-associated infarcts predominantly localize to the basal ganglia and thalamus, which are supplied by small Circle of Willis branches including the medial lenticulostriate and thalamo-perforating arteries, as well as lateral lenticulostriate, anterior choroidal, and thalamogeniculate arteries,[94] although the exact frequencies are debated.[92] Hence, the risk of infarct in tuberculous meningitis is more correlated with the presence of basal meningeal enhancement and vasospasm and less with the encapsulation of mycobacteria in a tuberculoma.[68,95]

MIMICS OF CENTRAL NERVOUS SYSTEM INFECTION

Radiographic features associated with CNS infections, such as meningeal or ring enhancement, are shared with many noninfectious disorders (see Box 1).

Meningeal Enhancement in Chemical/Drug-Induced Meningitis

In particular, subacute noninfectious meningeal inflammation can share symptoms with infectious meningitis. Chemical meningitis occurs in response to nonmicrobial irritants in the subarachnoid space (blood, dermoid cyst rupture, intrathecal drug instillation), often in the setting of neurosurgery or neurointervention. CSF reveals leukocytosis, elevated protein, and low glucose but negative cultures.[96] Drug-induced meningitis is rarely associated with certain nonsteroidal anti-inflammatory drugs (NSAIDs), intravenous immunoglobulin (IV-IG), and other therapies (Box 11). MR imaging findings are nonspecific,

---

Box 11
Causes of drug-induced meningitis

- NSAIDs: ibuprofen, celecoxib, naproxen
- Antibiotics: trimethoprim/sulfamethoxazole, amoxicillin, metronidazole, ciprofloxacin
- Immunomodulatory agents: sulfasalazine, azathioprine, capecitabine, methotrexate
- Immunotherapies: IV-IG, cetuximab, adalimumab, infliximab, nivolumab, pembrolizumab, ipilimumab, muromonab
- Antiepileptics: lamotrigine, carbamazepine

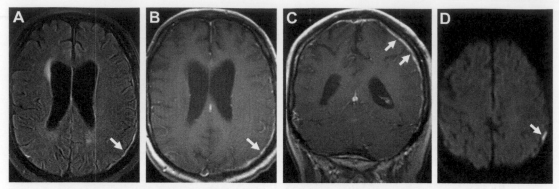

Fig. 27. Carcinomatous meningitis with dural enhancement in a patient with acute myeloid leukemia. Notice FLAIR hyperintensity (*arrow, A*), and thick dural-based enhancement on T1 postcontrast (*arrows, B, C*) with restricted diffusion (*arrow, D*).

including pial and dural enhancement. Immunotherapy-induced meningitis may resemble infectious or carcinomatous meningitis.[97] Symptoms and CSF pleocytosis resolve quickly on drug withdrawal.[98]

Meningeal Enhancement in Neoplasia

Leptomeningeal enhancement or *carcinomatous meningitis* is the spread of neoplasm across the subarachnoid space (Fig. 27). Timely imaging and diagnosis are critical because carcinomatous meningitis is a marker of advanced disease and the median survival time without treatment is about 4 to 6 weeks. Metastases, lymphoma, and primary CNS tumors impair the BBB and promote contrast leakage, typically appearing as nodular leptomeningeal enhancement.[97] Some tumors are also associated with focal pachymeningeal enhancement. Meningioma tumor cells recruit blood vessels, promoting vasocongestion and

interstitial edema resulting in thickened dura, pachymeningeal enhancement and the classic "dural tail sign."[99] Schwannomas can show perineural meningeal enhancement.[11] Meningeal involvement in paraneoplastic limbic encephalitis is reported but uncommon (<10%).[100]

Meningeal Enhancement in Neurosarcoidosis

Neurosarcoidosis is an archetypal neuroinflammatory granulomatous disease with a predilection for meningeal enhancement. It occurs in about 10% of patients with sarcoidosis. Granulomatous basal leptomeningitis, ependymitis, and inflammation of the perivascular spaces can result in edema, causing headache, nuchal rigidity, cranial neuropathy, visual symptoms, and motor weakness. Given the variable presentation of neurosarcoidosis, diagnosis requires a high degree of clinical suspicion.[15] Hallmark basal meningeal enhancement can be focal or diffuse with nodular

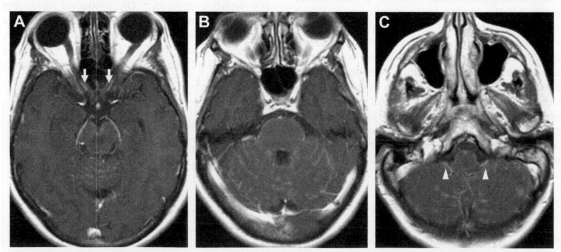

Fig. 28. Neurosarcoidosis. T1 postcontrast MR imaging demonstrates enhancement of both prechiasmatic optic nerves (*arrows, A*) with patchy linear and nodular enhancement around the brainstem and cerebellum (*B*) and bilateral enhancement of the glossopharyngeal/vagus nerves (*arrowheads, C*).

> **Box 12**
> **Differential diagnosis of ring and peripheral enhancement**
>
> - Metastasis
> - Abscess
> - Glioma, Lymphoma
> - Infarct
> - Contusion
> - Demyelination
> - Resolving hematoma
> - Radiation necrosis

leptomeningeal or pachymeningeal enhancement.[100,101] Enhancement of the pituitary stalk, cranial nerves, and perivascular spaces with white matter changes and hydrocephalus can occur (Fig. 28). Enhancement coincides with lesion activity and generally improves with steroid therapy.[102] Systemic involvement with ^{18}F-FDG avid nodules of the lungs, heart, lymph nodes, and skin are highly supportive of neurosarcoidosis.[103] Additional causes of neuroinflammatory conditions include posterior reversible encephalopathy syndrome and chronic lymphocytic inflammation with pontine perivascular enhancement responsive to steroids.[104,105]

Ring-Enhancing Lesions

Ring-like contrast enhancement is a sensitive though nonspecific radiologic feature for intracranial abscess (Box 12, Fig. 29). In a series of 221 ring-enhancing lesions, the most frequent diseases were glioma (40%), followed by metastasis (30%), abscess (8%), and multiple sclerosis (6%).[106] Tumors tend to be solitary, necrotic

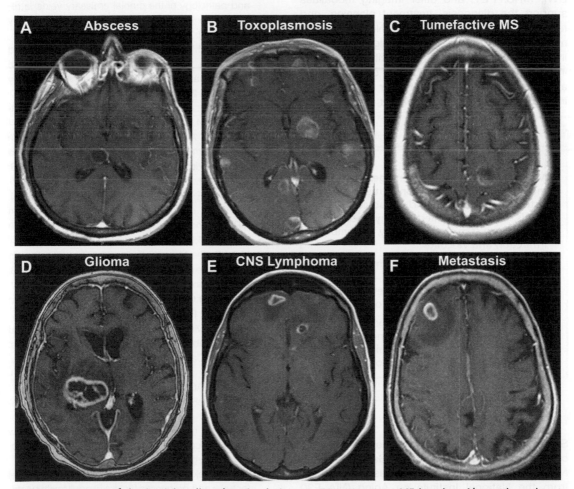

Fig. 29. Assortment of ring/peripherally enhancing lesions on T1 postcontrast MR imaging. Abscess in an immunocompromised patient (*A*). Multicentric toxoplasmosis (*B*). New demyelinating lesion in tumefactive multiple sclerosis (*C*). Necrotic high-grade glioma (*D*). Multifocal primary CNS lymphoma in an immunocompromised patient with congenital lymphangiectasia (*E*). Junctional metastasis with surrounding edema (*F*).

lesions, whereas abscess and demyelinating lesions were more often multifocal. In immunocompromised patients, diseases that traditionally seem as single masses, such as primary CNS lymphoma, may manifest as multifocal ring-enhancing lesions (**Fig. 29**).[107] Demyelinating lesions generally exhibit incomplete ring enhancement. Abscesses generally elicit a greater foreign immune response and edema, with smooth, circumferential capsules with central diffusion restriction.[2,11,108]

SUMMARY

Numerous infectious and noninfectious conditions share enhancement and diffusion restriction patterns in the meninges and brain parenchyma. Therefore, a solid foundation of anatomy, pathophysiology, and clinical medicine guides appropriate neuroimaging interpretation of meningitis, abscess, and their mimics. CT, MR imaging, DWI, MRS, PET, and other imaging modalities support the diagnosis, treatment planning, and monitoring for CNS infections. Newer imaging methods and deep learning algorithms may improve diagnostic imaging capacity. Overall, the integration of neuroimaging with clinical history and laboratory results is vital for suitable CNS infection workup and management.

CLINICS CARE POINTS

- Meningitis appears as meningeal enhancement along the cerebral convexities and basal cisterns. Complications include abscess, ventriculitis, extra-axial collections, hydrocephalus, herniation, cranial neuropathy, thrombosis, infarction and vasculitis.

- Cerebritis leads to abscess, which is supported by ring enhancement, central diffusion restriction on DWI and often elevated amino acids, succinate and/or acetate on MRS.

- The differential diagnosis for meningeal enhancement and ring enhancement patterns is broad and should be guided by additional imaging and clinical factors.

DISCLOSURE

S. Mohan has grant funding from the National Cancer Institute (NCI R01 CA262584), Galileo CDS and Novocure, USA. M. T. Duong has research funding from the National Institute on Aging (NIA F30 AG074524). J. D. Rudie has research support from the National Institute of Biomedical Imaging and Bioengineering (NIBIB T32 EB004311) and Radiological Society of North America (RSNA RR1778) research grant. There are no additional disclosures to report.

REFERENCES

1. Mohan S, Jain KK, Arabi M, et al. Imaging of Meningitis and Ventriculitis. Neuroimaging Clin N Am 2012;22(4):557–83.
2. Rath TJ, Hughes M, Arabi M, et al. Imaging of Cerebritis, Encephalitis, and Brain Abscess. Neuroimaging Clin N Am 2012;22(4):585–607.
3. Global Burden of Disease 2016 Meningitis Collaborators. Global, regional, and national burden of meningitis, 1990–2016: a systematic analysis for the Global Burden of Disease Study 2016. Lancet Neurol 2018;17(12):1061–82.
4. Patel K, Clifford DB. Bacterial Brain Abscess. Neurohospitalist 2014;4(4):196–204.
5. Mortazavi MM, Tubbs RS, Riech S, et al. Anatomy and pathology of the cranial emissary veins: a review with surgical implications. Neurosurgery 2012;70(5):1312–8.
6. Absinta M, Ha S-K, Nair G, et al. Human and nonhuman primate meninges harbor lymphatic vessels that can be visualized noninvasively by MRI. eLife 2017;6:e29738.
7. Castillo M. Imaging of meningitis. Semin Roentgenol 2004;39(4):458–64.
8. Montagne A, Toga AW, Zlokovic BV. Blood-brain Barrier Permeability and Gadolinium: Benefits and Potential Pitfalls in Research. JAMA Neurol 2016;73(1):13–4.
9. Wesley SF, Garcia-Santibanez R, Liang J, et al. Incidence of meningeal enhancement on brain MRI secondary to lumbar puncture. Neurol Clin Pract 2016;6(4):315–20.
10. Mokri B. The Monro-Kellie hypothesis: applications in CSF volume depletion. Neurology 2001;56(12):1746–8.
11. Smirniotopoulos JG, Murphy FM, Rushing EJ, et al. Patterns of Contrast Enhancement in the Brain and Meninges. RadioGraphics 2007;27:551–626.
12. Koksel Y, McKinney AM. Potentially Reversible and Recognizable Acute Encephalopathic Syndromes: Disease Categorization and MRI Appearances. AJNR Am J Neuroradiol 2020. https://doi.org/10.3174/ajnr.A6634.
13. Robertson FC, Lepard JR, Mekary RA, et al. Epidemiology of central nervous system infectious diseases: a meta-analysis and systematic review with implications for neurosurgeons worldwide. J Neurosurg 2018;130(4):1039–408.
14. van de Beek D, de Gans J, Spanjaard L, et al. Clinical features and prognostic factors in adults with bacterial meningitis. N Engl J Med 2004;351(18):1849–59.
15. Srinivasan J, Chaves CJ, Scott BJ, et al. Netter's Neurology. 3rd ed. Philadelphia: Elsevier; 2020.

16. van de Beek D, Cabellos C, Dzupova O, et al. ESC-MID guideline: diagnosis and treatment of acute bacterial meningitis. Clin Microbiol Infect 2016;22: S37–62.

17. Hasbun R, Abrahams J, Jekel J, et al. Computed tomography of the head before lumbar puncture in adults with suspected meningitis. N Engl J Med 2001;345(24):L1727–33.

18. Salazar L, Hasbun R. Cranial Imaging Before Lumbar Puncture in Adults With Community-Acquired Meningitis: Clinical Utility and Adherence to the Infectious Diseases Society of America Guidelines. Clin Infect Dis 2017;64(12):1657–62.

19. Shang WJ, Shu CLM, Liao HW, et al. The Association between FLAIR Vascular Hyperintensity and Stroke Outcome Varies with Time from Onset. AJNR Am J Neuroradiol 2019;40:1317–22.

20. Shih RY, Koeller KK. Bacterial, Fungal, and Parasitic Infections of the Central Nervous System: Radiologic-Pathologic Correlation and Historical Perspectives. Radiographics 2015;35(5):1141–69.

21. Pezzullo JA, Tung GA, Mudigonda S, et al. Diffusion-Weighted MR Imaging of Pyogenic Ventriculitis. AJR Am J Roentgenol 2003;180:71–5.

22. Tung GA, Rogg JM. Diffusion-weighted imaging of cerebritis. AJNR Am J Neuroradiol 2003;24(6):1110–3.

23. Senthong V, Chindaprasirt J, Sawanyawisuth K. Differential Diagnosis of CNS Angiostrongyliasis: A Short Review. Hawaii J Med Public Health 2013;72:52–4.

24. Shalabi M, Whitley RJ. Recurrent Benign Lymphocytic Meningitis. Clin Infect Dis 2006;43(9):1194–7.

25. Min Z, Baddley JW. Mollaret's meningitis. Lancet Infect Dis 2014;14:1022. https://doi.org/10.1016/S1473-3099(14)70874-6.

26. Prandota J. Mollaret meningitis may be caused by reactivation of latent cerebral toxoplasmosis. Int J Neurosci 2009;119(10):1655–92.

27. Villanueva-Meyer JE, Cha S. From Shades of Gray to Microbiologic Imaging: A Historical Review of Brain Abscess Imaging. RadioGraphics 2015;35:1555–62.

28. Sonneville R, Ruimy R, Benzonana N, et al. An update on bacterial brain abscess in immunocompetent patients. Clin Microbiol Infect 2017;23(9):614–20.

29. Brouwer MC, Tunkel AR, McKhann GM, et al. Brain Abscess. N Engl J Med 2014;371:447–56.

30. Jim KK, Brouwer MC, van der Ende A, et al. Cerebral abscesses in patients with bacterial meningitis. J Infect 2012;64:236–8.

31. Britt RH, Enzmann DR, Yeager AS. Neuropathological and computerized tomographic findings in experimental brain abscess. J Neurosurg 1981; 55(4):590–603.

32. Toh CH, Wei K-C, Chang C-N, et al. Differentiation of pyogenic brain abscesses from necrotic glioblastomas with use of susceptibility-weighted imaging. AJNR Am J Neuroradiol 2012;33(8):1534–8.

33. Gaviani P, Schwartz RB, Hedley-Whyte E, et al. Diffusion-Weighted Imaging of Fungal Cerebral Infection. AJNR Am J Neuroradiol 2005;26(5):1115–21.

34. Lee GT, Antelo F, Mlikotic AA. Cerebral Toxoplasmosis. RadioGraphics 2009;29(4):1200–5.

35. Shetty B, Balla, S, Reddy S. Radiological Society of North America 2005 Scientific Assembly and Annual Meeting, November 27 - December 2, 2005 ,Chicago IL. http://archive.rsna.org/2005/4418443.html.

36. Sener RN. Diffusion MRI: apparent diffusion coefficient (ADC) values in the normal brain and a classification of brain disorders based on ADC values. Comput Med Imaging Graph 2001;25(4):299–326.

37. Guzman R, Barth A, Lövblad K-O, et al. Use of diffusion-weighted magnetic resonance imaging in differentiating purulent brain processes from cystic brain tumors. J Neurosurg 2002;97(5). https://doi.org/10.3171/jns.2002.97.5.1101.

38. Cartes-Zumelzu FW, Stavrou I, Castillo M, et al. Diffusion-Weighted Imaging in the Assessment of Brain Abscesses Therapy. Am J Neuroradiol AJNR 2004;25(8):1310–7.

39. Chang SC, Lai PH, Chen WL, et al. Diffusion-weighted MRI features of brain abscess and cystic or necrotic brain tumors: comparison with conventional MRI. Clin Imaging 2002;26:227–36.

40. Lotan E, Hoffmann C, Fardman A, et al. Postoperative versus Spontaneous Intracranial Abscess: Diagnostic Value of the Apparent Diffusion Coefficient for Accurate Assessment. Radiology 2016; 281(1):168–74.

41. Diekert G. CO2 reduction to acetate in anaerobic bacteria. FEMS Microbiol Rev 1990;7(3–4): 391–5. https://doi.org/10.1111/j.1574-6968.1990.tb04942.x.

42. Pal D, Bhattacharyya A, Husain M, et al. In Vivo Proton MR Spectroscopy Evaluation of Pyogenic Brain Abscesses: A Report of 194 Cases. AJNR Am J Neuroradiol 2010;31(2):360–6.

43. Öz G, Alger JR, Barker PB, et al. Clinical Proton MR Spectroscopy in Central Nervous System Disorders. Radiology 2014;270(3):658–79.

44. Verma A, Kumar I, Verma N, et al. Magnetic resonance spectroscopy — Revisiting the biochemical and molecular milieu of brain tumors. BBA Clin 2016;5:170–8.

45. Hsu S-H, Chou M-C, Ko C-W, et al. Proton MR spectroscopy in patients with pyogenic brain abscess: MR spectroscopic imaging versus single-voxel spectroscopy. Eur J Radiol 2013;82(8):1299–307.

46. Chang L, Cornford ME, Chiang FL, et al. Radiologic-Pathologic Correlation: Cerebral Toxoplasmosis and Lymphoma in AIDS. AJNR Am J Neuroradiol 1995;16:1653–63.

47. Sharma P, Mukherjee A, Karunithi S, et al. Potential Role of ^{18}F-FDG PET/CT in Patients With

Fungal Infections. AJR Am J Roentgenol 2014; 203:180–9.

48. Marcus C, Feizi P, Hogg J, et al. Imaging in Differentiating Cerebral Toxoplasmosis and Primary CNS Lymphoma With Special Focus on FDG PET/CT. AJR Am J Roentgenol 2021;216(1):157–64.

49. El Omri H, Hascsi Z, Taha R, et al. Tubercular Meningitis and Lymphadenitis Mimicking a Relapse of Burkitt's Lymphoma on 18F-FDG-PET/CT: A Case Report. Case Rep Oncol 2015;8:226–32.

50. Zaharchuk G, Gong E, Wintermark M, et al. Deep Learning in Neuroradiology. AJNR Am J Neuroradiol 2018;39(10):1776–84.

51. Rudie JD, Rauschecker AM, Bryan RN, et al. Emerging Applications of Artificial Intelligence in Neuro-Oncology. Radiology 2019;290:607–18.

52. Rudie JD, Duda J, Duong MT, et al. Brain MRI Deep Learning and Bayesian Inference System Augments Radiology Resident Performance. J Digit Imaging 2021;34:1049–58.

53. Duong MT, Rauschecker AM, Mohan S. Diverse Applications of Artificial Intelligence in Neuroradiology. Neuroimaging Clin N Am 2020;30(4):505–16.

54. Duong MT, Rauschecker AM, Rudie JD, et al. Artificial intelligence for precision education in radiology. Br J Radiol 2019;92(1103):20190389.

55. Ene M, Gorunescu M, Gorunescu F, et al. A Machine Learning Approach to Differentiating Bacterial From Viral Meningitis. IEEE John Vincent Atanasoff Int Symp Mod Comput 2006;155–62.

56. Duong MT, Rudie JD, Wang J, et al. Convolutional neural network for automated FLAIR lesion segmentation on clinical brain MR imaging. AJNR Am J Neuroradiol 2019;40(8):1282–90.

57. Rudie JD, Rauschecker AM, Xie L, et al. Subspecialty-level deep gray matter differential diagnoses with deep learning and Bayesian networks on clinical brain MRI: a pilot study. Radiol Artif Intelligence 2020;2(5):e190146. https://doi.org/10.1148/ryai.2020190146.

58. Rauschecker AM, Rudie JD, Xie L, et al. Artificial Intelligence System Approaching Neuroradiologist-level Differential Diagnosis Accuracy at Brain MRI. Radiology 2020;295(3):626–37.

59. Rudie JD, Colby JB, Laguna B, et al. Automated Detection and Segmentation of Abnormal Enhancement Across 15 Neurological Diseases using a 3D U-Net Convolutional Neural Network. Society for Imaging Informatics in Medicine Virtual Meeting 2020.

60. Antinori S, Corbellino M, Meroni L, et al. Aspergillus meningitis: A rare clinical manifestation of central nervous system aspergillosis. Case report and review of 92 cases. J Infect 2013;66(3):218–38.

61. Almutairi BM, Nguyen TB, Jansen GH, et al. Invasive Aspergillosis of the Brain: Radiologic-Pathologic Correlation. RadioGraphics 2009;29:375–9.

62. Mamelak AN, Obana WG, Flaherty JF, et al. Nocardial Brain Abscess: Treatment Strategies and Factors Influencing Outcome. Neurosurgery 1994; 35(4):622–31.

63. Ramsey RG, Geremia GK. CNS complications of AIDS: CT and MR findings. AJR Am J Roengenol 1988;151(3):449–54.

64. Kumar GGS, Mahadevan A, Guruprasad AS, et al. Eccentric Target Sign in Cerebral Toxoplasmosis – neuropathological correlate to the imaging feature. J Magn Reson Imaging 2010;31(6):1469–72.

65. Fernàndez-Sabé N, Cervera C, Fariñas MC, et al. Risk factors, clinical features, and outcomes of toxoplasmosis in solid-organ transplant recipients: a matched case-control study. Clin Infect Dis 2012;54(3):355–61.

66. Ganiem AR, Dian S, Indriati A, et al. Cerebral Toxoplasmosis Mimicking Subacute Meningitis in HIV-Infected Patients; a Cohort Study from Indonesia. PLOS Negl Trop Dis 2013;7(1):e1994.

67. Rock RB, Olin M, Baker CA, et al. Central Nervous System Tuberculosis: Pathogenesis and Clinical Aspects. Clin Microbiol Rev 2008;21(2):243–61.

68. Chan KH, Cheung RT, Lee R, et al. Cerebral infarcts complicating tuberculous meningitis. Cerebrovasc Dis 2005;19(6):361–5.

69. Raut T, Garg RK, Jain A, et al. Hydrocephalus in tuberculous meningitis: Incidence, its predictive factors and impact on the prognosis. J Infect 2013;66(4):330–7.

70. Kim TK, Chang KH, Kim CJ, et al. Intracranial Tuberculoma: Comparison of MR with Pathologic Findings. AJNR Am J Neuroradiol 1995;16:1903–8.

71. Rudie JD, Rauschecker AM, Nabavizadeh SA, et al. Neuroimaging of Dilated Perivascular Spaces: From Benign to Pathologic Causes to Mimics. J Neuroimaging 2017;28(2):139–49.

72. Liliang P-C, Liang C-L, Chang W-N, et al. Shunt Surgery for Hydrocephalus Complicating Cryptococcal Meningitis in Human Immunodeficiency Virus-Negative Patients. Clin Infect Dis 2003; 37(5):673–8.

73. Saag MS, Graybill RJ, Larsen RA, et al. Practice Guidelines for the Management of Cryptococcal Disease. Clin Infect Dis 2000;30(4):710–8.

74. La Mantia L, Costa A, Eoli M, et al. Racemose neurocysticercosis after chronic meningitis: effect of medical treatment. Clin Neurol Neurosurg 1995; 97(1):50–4.

75. Zhao J-L, Lerner A, Shu Z, et al. Imaging spectrum of neurocysticercosis. Radiol Infect Dis 2015;1(2):94–102.

76. Kimura-Hayama ET, Higuera JA, Corona-Cedillo R, et al. Neurocysticercosis: Radiologic-Pathologic Correlation. RadioGraphics 2010;30(6):1705–19.

77. Verma A, Madhavi, Patwari S, et al. Use of 3D CISS as part of a routine protocol for the evaluation of

intracranial granulomas. Indian J Radiol Imaging 2011;21(4):311.

78. Cabral DA, Flodmark O, Farrell K, et al. Prospective study of computed tomography in acute bacterial meningitis. J Pediatr 1987;111(2):201–5.

79. Kasanmoentalib ES, Brower MC, van der Ende A, et al. Hydrocephalus in adults with community-acquired bacterial meningitis. Neurology 2010; 75(10):918–23.

80. Sotelo J, Guerrero V, Rubio F. Neurocysticercosis: a new classification based on active and inactive forms: a study of 753 cases. Arch Intern Med 1985;145(3):442–5.

81. Ferreira NP, Otta GM, do Amaral LL, et al. Imaging aspects of pyogenic infections of the central nervous system. Top Magn Reson Imaging 2005; 16(2):145–54.

82. van de Beek D, Campeau NG, Eelco W. The clinical challenge of recognizing infratentorial empyema. Neurology 2007;69(5):477–81.

83. Wong AM, Zimmerman RA, Simon EM, et al. Diffusion-weighted MR imaging of subdural empyemas in children. AJNR Am J Neuroradiol 2004;25:1016–21.

84. Saremi F, Helmy M, Farzin S, et al. MRI of Cranial Nerve Enhancement. AJR Am J Roentgenol 2005; 185(6):1487–97.

85. Richardson MP, Reid A, Tarlow MJ, et al. Hearing loss during bacterial meningitis. Arch Dis Child 1997;76(2):134–8.

86. Reijen J, Casselman J, Joosten F, et al. Magnetic resonance imaging in patients with meningitis induced hearing loss. Eur Arch Otorhinolaryngol 2009;266(8):1229–36.

87. Deliran SS, Brouwer MC, Coutinho JM, et al. Bacterial meningitis complicated by cerebral venous thrombosis. Eur Stroke J 2020;5(4):394–401.

88. Liu L-L, Zheng W-H, Tong M-L, et al. Ischemic stroke as a primary symptom of neurosyphilis among HIV-negative emergency patients. J Neurol Sci 2012;317(1–2):35–9.

89. Kastenbauer S, Pfister HW. Pneumococcal meningitis in adults: spectrum of complications and prognostic factors in a series of 87 cases. Brain 2003;126:1015–25.

90. Mishra AK, Arvind VH, Muliyil D, et al. Cerebrovascular injury in cryptococcal meningitis. Int J Stroke 2018;13(1):57–65.

91. Lan SH, Chang WN, Lu CH, et al. Cerebral infarction in chronic meningitis: a comparison of tuberculous meningitis and cryptococcal meningitis. QJM 2001;94(5):247–53.

92. Tai M-LS, Viswanathan S, Rahmat K, et al. Cerebral infarction pattern in tuberculous meningitis. Sci Rep 2016;6:38802.

93. Wasay M, Khan M, Farooq S, et al. Frequency and Impact of Cerebral Infarctions in Patients With Tuberculous Meningitis. Stroke 2018;49:2288–93.

94. Hsieh FY, Chia LG, Shen WC. Locations of cerebral infarctions in tuberculous meningitis. Neuroradiology 1992;34(3):197–9.

95. Zhang L, Zhang X, Li H, et al. Acute ischemic stroke in young adults with tuberculous meningitis. BMC Infect Dis 2019;19:362.

96. Forgacs P, Geyer CA, Freidberg SR. Characterization of Chemical Meningitis after Neurological Surgery. Clin Infect Dis 2001;32(2):179–85.

97. Bier G, Klumpp B, Roder C, et al. Meningeal enhancement depicted by magnetic resonance imaging in tumor patients: neoplastic meningitis or therapy-related enhancement? Neuroradiology 2019;61(7):775–82.

98. Morís G, Garcia-Monco JC. The challenge of drug-induced aseptic meningitis revisited. JAMA Intern Med 2014;174(9):1511–2.

99. Wilms G, Lammens M, Marchal G, et al. Thickening of dura surrounding meningiomas: MR features. J Comput Assist Tomogr 1989;13(5):763–8.

100. Delgado-García G, Ramirez-Bermudez J, Flores-Rivera J, et al. Pachymeningeal Enhancement in Anti-NMDA Receptor Encephalitis. Neurology 2020;94(15):2567.

101. Degnan AJ, Levy LM. Neuroimaging of Rapidly Progressive Dementias, Part 2: Prion, Inflammatory, Neoplastic, and Other Etiologies. AJNR Am J Neuroradiol 2014;35(3):424–31.

102. Dumas JL, Valeyre D, Chapelon-Abric C, et al. Central nervous system sarcoidosis: follow-up at MR imaging during steroid therapy. Radiology 2000;214(2):411–20.

103. Ganeshan D, Menias CO, Lubner MG, et al. Sarcoidosis from Head to Toe: What the Radiologist Needs to Know. RadioGraphics 2018;38(4): 1180–200.

104. Pittock SJ, Debruyne J, Krecke KN, et al. Chronic lymphocytic inflammation with pontine perivascular enhancement responsive to steroids (CLIPPERS). Brain 2010;133(9):2626–34.

105. Tobin WO, Guo Y, Krecke KN, et al. Diagnostic criteria for chronic lymphocytic inflammation with pontine perivascular enhancement responsive to steroids (CLIPPERS). Brain 2017;140(9): 2145–425.

106. Schwartz KM, Erickson BJ, Lucchinetti C. Pattern of T2 hypointensity associated with ring enhancing brain lesions can help to differentiate pathology. Neuroradiology 2006;48:143–9.

107. Haldorsen IS, Espeland A, Larsson JL. Central Nervous System Lymphoma: Characteristic Findings on Traditional and Advanced Imaging. Am J Neuroradiol 2011;32(6):984–92.

108. Hartmann M, Jansen O, Heiland S, et al. Restricted Diffusion within Ring Enhancement Is Not Pathognomonic for Brain Abscess. Am J Neuroradiol AJNR 2001;22(9):1738–42.

Structured Imaging Approach for Viral Encephalitis

Norlisah Mohd Ramli, MBBS, FRCR[a],*, Yun Jung Bae, MD, PhD[b]

KEYWORDS

- Magnetic resonance imaging (MRI) • Neuroimaging • Viral encephalitis
- Acute encephalitis syndromes (AES) • Infectious encephalitis

KEY POINTS

- Understanding the typical MR imaging (MRI) patterns caused by archetype viral pathogens is important, despite considerable overlap, diagnostic uncertainty, and unknown etiologies among patients with acute encephalitis syndrome.
- Acute encephalitis caused by herpes simplex virus type 1 typically affects the temporal lobe.
- In patients with bi-thalamic involvement, Japanese encephalitis and influenza-associated encephalitis should be considered.
- Enterovirus and rabies virus infections can involve the brainstem.
- Varicella-zoster virus infection can cause vasculopathy. Dengue virus can be present with various MRI patterns.

INTRODUCTION

Acute encephalitis syndrome (AES) is defined as acute inflammatory processes affecting the brain, resulting in neurologic manifestations, such as fever, seizures, psychiatric/behavioral/speech disorders, disturbances of consciousness/memory, focal neurologic deficit, involuntary movement, and ataxia; the cause can be both infective and noninfective (such as immune-mediated encephalitis).[1] In many population studies, up to 50% of AES cases have an unknown etiology. There are ongoing global efforts to identify new and emerging infectious agents and new forms of immune-mediated encephalitis.[2] The estimated incidence of presumed cases of infectious encephalitis is approximately 1.5 to 7 cases per 100,000 people per year, with a higher incidence among the elderly, pediatric, and immunocompromised patients.[3] Table 1 shows the wide variety of viruses known to cause human disease, including herpes simplex virus (HSV, 11%–22% of cases in some studies), varicella-zoster virus (VZV, 4%–14%), enteroviruses (1%–4%), arboviruses (arthropod-borne pathogens spread by mosquitos, ticks, and other vectors, usually with geographic and seasonal variability in incidence) such as Japanese encephalitis virus (JEV), dengue virus (DENV), and Zika viruses. Outbreak viruses, such as Hendra, Nipah, Middle East respiratory syndrome, severe acute respiratory syndrome coronavirus 1, and severe acute respiratory syndrome coronavirus 2 are uncommon but cause disproportionate public health damage, while cytomegalovirus is an essential consideration for immunocompromised patients.[4] Readers are encouraged to refer to articles 4 and 5 for neuroimaging features of Coronavirus disease.

[a] Department of Biomedical Imaging, Faculty of Medicine, University of Malaya, Jln Profesor Diraja Ungku Aziz, 50603 Kuala Lumpur, Malaysia; [b] Department of Radiology, Seoul National University Bundang Hospital, Seoul National University College of Medicine, 82, Gumi-ro 173 Beon-gil, Bundang-gu, Seongnam-si, Gyeonggi-do 13620, Republic of Korea
* Corresponding author. Department of Biomedical Imaging, University of Malaya Medical Centre, 12B South Tower, Kuala Lumpur 50603, Malaysia.
E-mail address: norlisahramli@gmail.com

Neuroimag Clin N Am 33 (2023) 43–56
https://doi.org/10.1016/j.nic.2022.07.002
1052-5149/23/© 2022 Elsevier Inc. All rights reserved.

Abbreviations	
ADEM	acute disseminated encephalomyelitis
AES	acute encephalitis syndrome
CE	chronic viral encephalitis
CNS	central nervous system
CSF	cerebrospinal fluid
DENV	dengue virus
DWI	diffusion-weighted imaging
FLAIR	fluid-attenuated inversion recovery
GRE	gradient-echo recalled
HHS	human herpesvirus
HSE	HSV encephalitis
HSV	herpes simplex virus
JE	Japanese encephalitis virus
JEV	Japanese encephalitis virus
PCR	polymerase chain reaction
PML	progressive multifocal leukoencephalopathy
VZV	varicella-zoster virus

However, chronic viral encephalitis (CE) is rare. Chronicity can be defined as a period of 4 weeks, but no consensus has been reached on the definition. Clinically, CE can present similarly to AES, but the course can be protracted, and neurologic syndromes can be unspecific[5]; viruses responsible for CE include John Cunningham virus and measles viruses.

There are three broad mechanisms by which viruses cause central nervous system (CNS) disease: infection limited to the meninges (also called "aseptic meningitis"; this mild, self-limiting disease has a good prognosis); brain invasion resulting in encephalitis; and immune-mediated processes [such as acute disseminated encephalomyelitis (ADEM)].[4] Correct and timely diagnosis of infectious encephalitis (Box 1) and identifying the causative pathogen are necessary for patient management, especially since patients with AES often undergo prolonged hospitalization and can have poor outcomes resulting in disability or death.[6] However, the clinical diagnosis can be challenging for the following reasons: (a) cerebrospinal fluid (CSF) examination can show normal glucose and normal protein and may not conform to the typical pattern of increased protein with predominantly lymphocytic pleocytosis,[7] (b) confirmatory polymerase chain reaction (PCR) is time-consuming, expensive, and scarce[8,9]; and (c) a negative test result does not rule out the diagnosis. Furthermore, it is difficult to differentiate viral from immune-mediated encephalitis on imaging alone. The antibodies responsible for autoimmune encephalitis are broadly categorized into neuronal surface antibodies, such as NMDAR,

Table 1
Viruses that can cause encephalitis

DNA viruses	
ssDNA viruses	Anelloviridae Parvoviridae Parvovirus • Parvovirus B19
Partially ssDNA viruses	Hepadnaviridae
dsDNA viruses	Adenoviridae Adenovirus • Adenovirus serotypes 7, 12, 32 Herpesviridae Human herpes virus • Herpes simplex virus (HSV)* • Varicella-zoster virus (VZV)* • Epstein-Barr virus (EBV)* • Cytomegalovirus (CMV)* • Human herpesvirus 6 (HHV-6)* • Human herpesvirus 7 (HHV-7)* Papillomaviridae Polyomaviridae Polyomavirus • JC virus (JCV)* Poxviridae
RNA viruses	
+ssRNA viruses	Astroviridae Coronavirida Flaviviridae Flavivirus • West Nile virus • Japanese encephalitis virus* • Tick-borne encephalitis virus • Dengue virus types 1-4* Hepacivirus • Hepatitis C virus* Hepeviridae Picornaviridae Enterovirus* • Poliovirus types 1-3 • Coxsackievirus A and B • Enterovirus 70, 71* Retroviridae Lentivirus • Human immunodeficiency virus 1-2* Deltaretrovirus

(*continued on next page*)

Table 1 (continued)		
	DNA viruses	
	• Human T-lymphotropic virus 1-2*	
	Togaviridae	
	Alphavirus	
	Rubellavirus	
-ssRNA viruses	Arenaviridae	
	Arenavirus	
	Bornaviridae	
	Orthomyxoviridae*	
	Influenzavirus A	
	• Influenza A virus	
	Influenzavirus B	
	• Influenza B virus	
	Paramyxoviridae	
	Henipavirus	
	Hendra virus	
	• Morbillivirus	
	• Measle virus*	
	Rubulavirus	
	• Mumps virus*	
	Respirovirus	
	• Human parainfluenza virus	
	Pneumoviridae	
	Rhabdoviridae	
dsRNA viruses	Picobirnaviridae	
	Reoviridae	
	Collivirus	
	Seadornavirus	
	Rotavirus	
	• Rotavirus*	

Abbreviations: +ssRNA, positive-sense single-stranded RNA; dsDNA, double-stranded DNA; dsRNA, double-stranded RNA; ssDNA, single-stranded DNA; -ssRNA, negative-sense single-stranded RNA;
  Common viruses are highlighted with *

Box 1
Diagnostic criteria for presumed infectious or autoimmune encephalitis

Major criterion *(required)*:

  Altered mental status (ie, decreased or altered level of consciousness, lethargy, or personality change) lasting $\geq$ 24 hours with no identifiable alternative cause

Minor criteria *(two required for possible encephalitis, more than three required for probable or confirmed[a] encephalitis)*:

  Fever $\geq$ 38°C within 72 hours before or after presentation

  New onset of focal neurologic findings

  CSF WBC count $\geq$ 5 mm^3

  [b]Abnormality of brain parenchyma on neuroimaging suggestive of encephalitis that is either new from prior studies or appears acute in onset.

  Abnormality on electroencephalography consistent with encephalitis and not attributable to another cause

Abbreviations: CSF, cerebrospinal fluid; WBC, white blood cell. [a]Confirmed encephalitis requires pathologic examinations or laboratory tests that can strongly suggest autoimmune encephalitis. [b]MR imaging is the modality of choice for the evaluation of the encephalitis.
Adapted from Venkatesan A, Tunkel AR, Bloch KC, Lauring AS, Sejvar J, Bitnun A, Stahl JP, Mailles A, Drebot M, Rupprecht CE, Yoder J, Cope JR, Wilson MR, Whitley RJ, Sullivan J, Granerod J, Jones C, Eastwood K, Ward KN, Durrheim DN, Solbrig MV, Guo-Dong L, Glaser CA; International Encephalitis Consortium. Case definitions, diagnostic algorithms, and priorities in encephalitis: consensus statement of the international encephalitis consortium. Clin Infect Dis. 2013 Oct;57(8):1114-28.

CASPR2, LGI-1, and GABA, versus intracellular antibodies, such as Hu (ANNA 1), Ri (ANNA2), CRMP5, Amphiphysin, MA2, and GAD 65. Some patients with autoimmune or paraneoplastic limbic encephalitis may show unilateral or bilateral increased T2/fluid-attenuated inversion recovery (FLAIR) signal in the medial temporal lobes, mimicking HSV-1 encephalitis.[10]

STRUCTURED APPROACH TO IMAGE ANALYSIS

MR imaging has demonstrated its value in assessing viral encephalitis.[11] This article proposes a structured diagnostic approach using MR imaging-based neuroanatomical localization and pattern recognition (Fig. 1). First, the course of the disease should be determined: if it is acute (ie, AES) or chronic (ie, CE). The next step involves the assessment of MR imaging abnormalities based on the anatomic location. It forms a framework to understand viruses that preferentially show MR imaging changes in the temporal lobes, thalami, brainstem, splenium of the corpus callosum, and other viruses that may be more variable in appearance, such as VZV and DENV. Although different pathogens may share similar imaging features (eg, HSV-1 and HHV-6), and a single virus can cause a variety of MR imaging abnormalities (for instance, DENV), we believe this approach may have value if we accept its inherent limitations in overlap and over-simplification, and bear in mind that neuroimaging alone cannot definitively identify the pathogen but needs corroborative clinical and laboratory evidence.

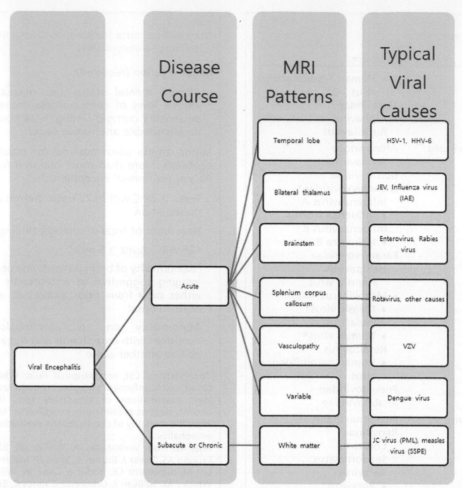

Fig. 1. Diagnostic algorithm using the structured approach to the viral encephalitis. HHV, human herpesvirus; HSV, herpes simplex virus; JEV, Japanese encephalitis virus; PML, progressive multifocal leukoencephalopathy; SSPE, subacute sclerosing panencephalitisl VZV, Varicella-Zoster virus.

ACUTE ENCEPHALITIS SYNDROME
Temporal Lobe Location

Herpes simplex virus type-1

The annual incidence of HSV encephalitis (HSE) has been estimated to be ~2 to 4 individuals/million population worldwide.[12] More than 90% of HSE results from HSV type-1 (HSV-1) infection in adults, while HSV-2 infection usually occurs in neonates or immunocompromised patients.[13] In addition, about 30% of HSE cases occur from a primary HSV-1 infection, whereas the remaining cases are attributed to viral reactivation or reinfection.[14] The incidence of HSE from HSV-1 infection has a bimodal age peak, with the first in the pediatric population and the second in adults over 50 years of age.[15,16] CSF examination with PCR should be performed for confirmation.[17]

MR imaging is sensitive and specific for HSE diagnosis even in the early stages of the disease,[18] showing brain abnormalities in 80% to 100% of cases.[19] T2-and (FLAIR)-high signal intensities with swelling preferentially affecting unilateral or bilateral asymmetric cortical and subcortical areas of the anterior and medial temporal lobes and insular cortex are typical (Fig. 2). HSV infection can also involve other parts of the limbic system, subfrontal area, and cingulate gyrus; isolated brainstem involvement is rare.[19] The lesions can be either unilateral or bilateral and are mostly asymmetric. It can be combined with hemorrhage, which can be well depicted as hypointensity on T2*-gradient-echo recalled (GRE) imaging or susceptibility-weighted imaging. There may be contrast enhancement in the parenchyma or meninges. In the early stage, diffusion-weighted imaging (DWI) can detect diffusion restriction before the onset of T2-/FLAIR-signal changes,[20] and T2-/FLAIR-signal abnormalities seem more prominent later in the course. In addition, one

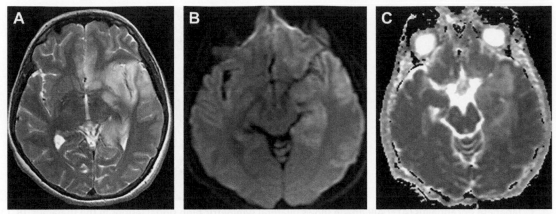

Fig. 2. Herpes simplex virus encephalitis (*A*) T2-weighted image shows multiple hyperintense lesions in cortical and subcortical areas of the left temporal lobe and left insular cortex. (*B*, *C*) Diffusion-weighted imaging (DWI) shows high signal intensity of the involving lesions with mixed apparent diffusion coefficient (ADC) values.

study showed that the presence of restricted diffusion was associated with poor outcomes at discharge, but T2-/FLAIR-abnormalities did not influence functional outcomes.[21] In addition, bilateral temporal lobe involvement or more extensive brain involvement at admission can be associated with a poor prognosis.[22] In immunocompromised patients, the lesions can be widespread and affect regions other than the temporal lobes.

Human herpesvirus type 6

Encephalitis caused by HHV-6 is rare but often has devastating sequelae.[23] HHV-6A and HHV-6B are globally dispersed DNA viruses.[24] Although HHV-6 infection is generally asymptomatic, its acute infection or reactivation in immunocompromised individuals can be associated with encephalitis and other diseases, such as Alzheimer's disease or cognitive dysfunction,[25] several types of cancer, multiple sclerosis, progressive multifocal leukoencephalopathy (PML), seizure, heart/lung/liver diseases, and epilepsy.[26] HHV-6 encephalitis can also be diagnosed using CSF tests.[17]

HHV-6 encephalitis typically affects the mesial temporal lobe, thus resembling HSE.[26–28] MRI may also show T2-/FLAIR-high signal intensities in the thalamus, hypothalamus, brainstem, cerebellum, or basal ganglia.[29] In 2010, Noguchi and colleagues[26] compared HHV-6 encephalitis and HSE; they found that mesial temporal lobes were exclusively affected in HHV-6 encephalitis but, in HSE, extratemporal regions could be additionally involved. They also found that sequential MRI showed that, in the late period, abnormal signal intensities resolved in HHV-6 encephalitis but persisted in HSE. Although these subtle differences may distinguish HHV-6 infection from HSV infection, there is significant overlap; additionally,

HHV-6 encephalitis, like HSE in the early and middle stages, can present diffusion restriction in the affected area.[30]

Bilateral Thalamic Location

Japanese Encephalitis virus

Japanese Encephalitis (JE) is caused by infection by the JEV, which is endemic in East and Southeast Asia.[31] JEV mainly affects children but can also involve adults and is transmitted through a zoonotic cycle between mosquitoes, pigs, and water birds. Humans are accidently infected and are dead-end hosts because of low levels of transient viremia.[32] Although transmission occurs year-round, seasonal epidemics during the rainy season occur when the mosquito density is at its maximum.[33] Approximately 35,000 to 50,000 people develop JE each year, with an annual mortality rate of 10,000 to 15,000. Its incidence and morbidity have substantially decreased due to the wide application of the JE vaccine. However, outbreaks still occur, with adult infections also increasing.[34]

It is common to have bilateral thalamic involvement[35] (**Fig. 3**). Thus, when patients with AES residing in endemic regions present with bilateral thalamic lesions, PCR testing should focus on JEV.[17] Lesions can also be observed in the substantia nigra, brainstem, cerebellum, cerebral cortex, basal ganglia, and white matter.[36] MR imaging is sensitive for evaluating the lesions and demonstrates higher diagnostic value. Typically, lesions are hypointense on T1-weighted imaging and hyperintense on T2-weighted imaging and FLAIR images. Thalamic lesions may show mixed intensity on T1- and T2-weighted imaging in the subacute phase, suggestive of hemorrhagic

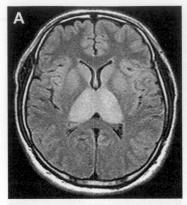
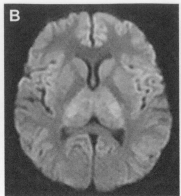
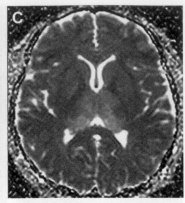

Fig. 3. Japanese encephalitis (*A*) FLAIR image shows bilateral symmetric high signal lesions in the thalamus. (*B, C*) Most of the lesions show high signal on DWI and mixed ADC values.

changes.[37] The involvement of the temporal lobe has also been observed in some studies, but all reported patients also demonstrated abnormalities of the thalamus and substantia nigra. This may help differentiate JE from the HSE.[35] On DWI, the lesions may show diffusion restriction in the acute phase[38] but most often show high apparent diffusion coefficient values.[35] In addition, JE in association with cerebral venous sinus thrombosis has been reported with the help of MRI and MR venography.[39]

Influenza-associated encephalopathy

Influenza-associated encephalopathy (IAE) is most common in children (those under 5 years of age), the elderly, and people who are immunocompromised or have chronic renal, cardiac, or respiratory diseases. The incidence of IAE from 1999 to 2000 was reported as 6 to 11 cases per 1,000,000 population aged less than 15 years (12–29 per 1,000,000 aged <4 years) in Japan. A/H2N3 was the most frequently identified influenza subtype among these cases, although A/h1N1 and influenza B have also been reported.[40,41] IAE should be considered in the differential diagnosis in patients with influenza-like symptoms and altered mental status. For the diagnosis, CSF analysis and laboratory-confirmed respiratory tract infection may be necessary.[42]

The neuroradiologic findings in patients with IAE were divided into five categories:

1. Category 1—diffuse brain edema
2. Category 2—symmetric involvement of the thalamus, brainstem, and cerebellum; the so-called acute necrotizing encephalopathy (**Fig. 4**)
3. Category 3—normal findings in the acute phase followed by the appearance of diffuse brain edema and mild brain atrophy

4. Category 4—post-infectious focal encephalitis
5. Category 5—no abnormal lesions

Hence, category 2 IAE may mimic JE on MR imaging, causing bilateral thalamic abnormalities. In addition, reversible diffusion-restricted splenial lesions have also been reported in the corpus callosum (see later).[43,44]

Brainstem Location

Enterovirus

Enteroviruses are classified into four groups (polioviruses, Coxsackie A viruses, Coxsackie B viruses, and echoviruses) and multiple serotypes.[45] As vaccination efforts have almost eradicated poliovirus, Enterovirus-A71 has become the most frequent one that causes severe CNS infections among the non-polioviruses.[46,47] Enteroviruses are responsible for large-scale, periodic epidemics in pediatric cohorts, particularly in East and Southeast Asia.[8] In China alone, between 2008 and 2012, 6.5 million children were diagnosed with hand, foot, and mouth disease (HFMD) caused by the enterovirus family, and more than 2200 died. Chinese and Malay children in Singapore are more susceptible to developing HFMD than Indian children.[48] With prodromal respiratory disease preceding the onset of CNS symptoms, CSF PCR tests may help confirm the diagnosis of enteroviruses.[35]

MR imaging typically shows abnormalities located in the dorsal pons and pontine tegmentum, especially in the nuclei of the abducens and facial nerve (**Fig 5**). The cortico-spinal tracts, located ventrally, are often not affected, while the caudate nucleus may be involved.[35] DWI is more sensitive in detecting abnormalities (89.7%) than T2-weighted image (48.7%), FLAIR (41.0%), and T1-weighted image (35.9%), and its

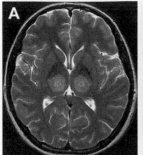
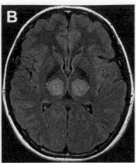
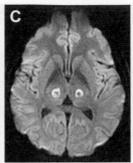
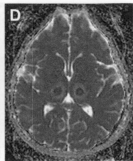

Fig. 4. Influenza-associated encephalopathy (IAE) manifested as ANEC (acute necrotizing encephalopathy of childhood) (*A, B*) T2-weighted and FLAIR images show bilateral symmetric high signal in the thalamus. (*C, D*) Focal diffusion-restricted portion is noted in the center of the lesions.

positive ratio was significantly higher than other sequences.[43] In patients with aseptic meningitis, findings are nonspecific; however, subdural effusion, meningeal enhancement, and hydrocephalus can be indirect signs.[49]

Acute flaccid paralysis associated with Enterovirus-D68 can demonstrate diffuse spinal cord edema, affecting the entire gray matter, evolving over several days with T2-hyperintensity restricted to the anterior horn.[44] In addition, contrast enhancement of the caudal roots and sometimes of the cranial nerves can be seen.

Rabies
Among the bullet-shaped Rhabdoviridae family, at least six serotypes in the genus *Lyssavirus* cause diseases clinically related to rabies, including rabies virus and multiple bat viruses.[50] The viruses can be transmitted through the bite of infected bats or other infected mammals, resulting in fever, agitation, excessive salivation, and hydrophobia. Rabies has a dismal prognosis and limited treatment options once symptoms set in, with only 12 reported survivors globally.[51] Diagnosis can be made by skin biopsy with PCR testing.[52]

The MR imaging changes in rabies may be due to viral infection per se, host response, or complications such as hypoxia, bleeding, shock, and metabolic abnormalities. Rabies encephalitis may show T2-hyperintense signal changes in the brainstem, hippocampus, limbic cortex, thalamus, or hypothalamus regions (Fig. 6). It can also involve the spinal cord, and the degree of abnormality may vary widely depending on the stage of progression. In the late stages, the lesion may increase due to the alteration in the blood–brain barrier.[36,38] Rabies encephalitis typically shows almost exclusive gray matter involvement in ADEM, which predominantly involves white matter.

For the rare survivors, mainly those promptly treated with immunoglobulin and rabies vaccine, MR imaging showed progressive brain atrophy, leukoencephalopathy, persistent T2 hyperintensities in the basal ganglia, and gliosis. In addition, some have reported blooming artifacts in bilateral basal ganglia suggestive of mineralization.[39]

Splenial Location

Rotavirus
Rotavirus is a leading cause of acute gastroenteritis worldwide, with a high hospitalization rate and

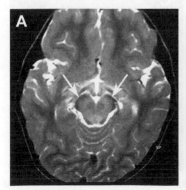
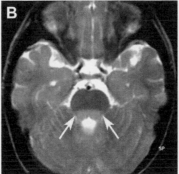
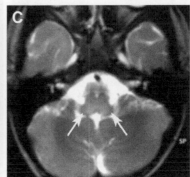

Fig. 5. Enterovirus encephalitis (*A–C*) T2-weighted images shows typical bilateral hyperintensity in dorsal pons tegmentum area, midbrain, and medulla (*arrows*).

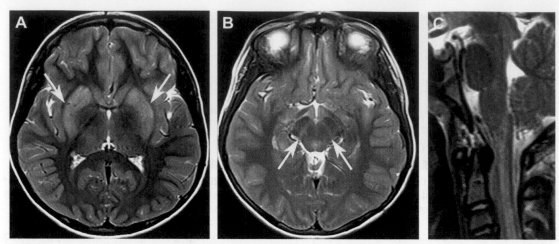

Fig. 6. Rabies encephalitis (*A*, *B*) T2-weighted images show typical involvement of bilateral basal ganglia and midbrain (*arrows*). (*C*) On sagittal T2-weighted image, T2-high signal lesions involving medulla and upper cervical spinal cord are seen. Courtesy of Jitender Saini, MD, NIMHANS, Bengaluru, Karnataka

mortality for children under 5 years of age.[53] Simultaneous CNS involvement has been reported in patients with rotavirus gastroenteritis. The clinical findings include encephalopathy, febrile and afebrile convulsions, hemorrhagic shock, Guillain–Barré syndrome, and Reye syndrome after primary intestinal infection.[54,55]

Brain MR imaging can show hyperintensities in the splenium of the corpus callosum and/or bilateral dentate nuclei on T2-weighted imaging or DWI with diffusion restriction (Fig. 7). These lesions are reported to disappear rapidly, the shortest being 12 days and the longest being 51 days.[56,57] Therefore, especially in pediatric AES cases with gastroenteritis, rotavirus encephalitis should be a differential diagnosis when MR imaging demonstrates reversible splenial and/or dentate lesions. However, reversible splenial

abnormalities are not specific. They can be caused by other infectious agents, including Epstein–Barr virus, *Staphylococcus*, *Escherichia coli*, and noninfectious causes such as drug therapy, malignancy, metabolic disorders, and trauma.[58]

Vasculopathy and Ischemic Infarction in Children

Varicella-zoster virus
VZV causes chickenpox (varicella) and shingles (zoster) and was once responsible for over 4 million infections in the United States annually. After the resolution of the acute varicella episode, the virus can remain latent in the dorsal ganglia of the spine and reactivate with declining immunity, causing herpes zoster, often complicated by post-herpetic neuralgia (chronic pain), VZV vasculopathy, meningoencephalitis, meningoradiculitis,

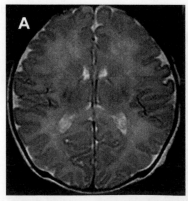
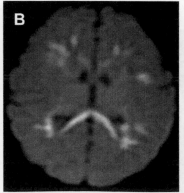
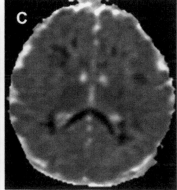

Fig. 7. Rotavirus encephalitis T2-weighted image (*A*), DWI (*B*), and ADC map (*C*) of a neonate show multifocal white matter involvement with diffusion restriction including corpus callosum splenium and genu. (*Courtesy of S Kumar MD, Bangalore South, India.*)

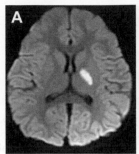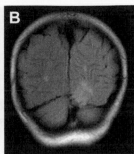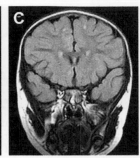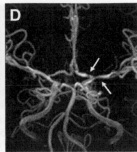

Fig. 8. Varicella-zoster virus (VZV) related vasculopathy (*A–C*) Axial DWI and coronal FLAIR image demonstrate multifocal acute infarctions with restricted diffusion in left globus pallidus, left occipital cortex and frontal white matter. (*D*) MR angiography (MRA) shows several short stenosis at left M1 and A1 segments (*arrows*).

cerebellitis, myelopathy, and ocular disease.[59,60] In addition to CSF analysis, other pathogen tests, including virology tests, antibody detection, and molecular biology tests, may help confirm VZV encephalitis.[61]

In children, VZV vasculopathy accounts for 31% of all arterial ischemic strokes; moreover, stroke was preceded by chickenpox in 44% of children with transient cerebral arteriopathy.[61] Ischemic lesions involving gray–white matter junctions and deep gray matter of the thalamus could also be seen[60] (Fig. 8). Angiography revealed abnormalities in 70% of subjects, with large and small arteries involved in 50%, with small arteries only in 37% and large arteries only in 13%.[60] Other complications of VZV vasculopathy include cerebral aneurysm, subarachnoid and intracerebral hemorrhage, ectasia, and dissection.[61] The DWI image can detect ischemic lesions associated with VZV vasculopathy, and the GRE image can detect hemorrhagic lesions.[62] Also, DWI can be better than conventional MR imaging for spinal cord involvement to detect spinal cord ischemia and infarction.[63] Therefore, MR imaging can play a significant role in diagnosing neurologic manifestations of VZV, and DWI and GRE sequences should be included.

VZV meningitis may also present as normal brain images, or very rarely, it can cause rhombencephalomyelitis involving the pons and spinal cord, with T2-/FLAIR-high signal and variable contrast enhancement.[64] The involved cranial nerves (trigeminal, facial, and/or vestibulocochlear) can be enhanced.[65]

Variable Imaging Pattern

Dengue virus

The *Aedes* mosquito transmits multiple serotypes of DENV, which is prevalent in 128 countries, with 2.5 billion individuals at risk each year.[66] Three neuropathogenic mechanisms are associated with DENV infection: (1) invasion of the CNS and peripheral nervous system leading to meningitis, encephalitis, myelitis, and paresis; (2) metabolic and vascular disorders leading to encephalopathy, vasculitis, and bleeding in the CNS; and (3) immune-mediated dengue syndromes, including ADEM, neuromyelitis optica, neuritis, myelitis, encephalopathy, and Guillain–Barré syndrome.[67] The diagnostic criteria for dengue encephalitis include fever, AES symptoms, and the detection of anti-dengue IgM antibodies or genomic materials in the serum or CSF.[68]

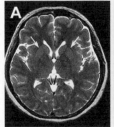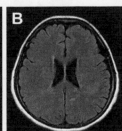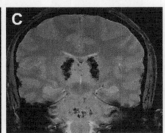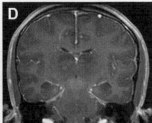

Fig. 9. Dengue encephalitis (*A, B*) T2-weighted and FLAIR images show multifocal lesions in bilateral basal ganglia (*arrows*) and cerebral white matter. Hypointense hemorrhage on coronal T2*-gradient recalled echo image (*C*) and diffuse leptomeningeal enhancement on coronal contrast-enhanced T1-weighted image are noted (*D*).

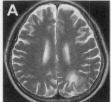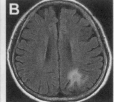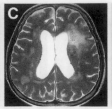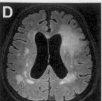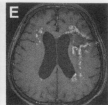

Fig. 10. Classic progressive multifocal leukoencephalopathy (PML) and PML-IRIS (*A, B*) Classic PML shows focal T2- and FLAIR-hyperintense lesion without mass effect or contrast enhancement located in the subcortical white matter. Unlike classic PML, (*C–E*) PML-IRIS shows multifocal T2-and FLAIR-hyperintense lesions in bilateral cerebral subcortical white matter with contrast enhancement.

Neuroimaging in dengue encephalitis shows variable features, with normal findings in most cases. Multifocal confluent and ill-defined increased T2-weighted signal abnormalities are reported in the cerebral white matter, hippocampus, basal ganglia, and thalamus, with or without cortical involvement.[66,69] There can be hemorrhage, edema, patchy focal diffusion restriction, and meningeal enhancement (**Fig. 9**).[70]

Most post-dengue ADEM cases are similar to ADEM from other etiologies, with white- and gray matter abnormalities on T2-weighted and FLAIR images. These demyelinating lesions may be disseminated to multiple sites, including the periventricular area, corona radiata, internal capsule, and cerebral peduncles, possibly showing hemorrhagic foci.[69,71]

SUBACUTE OR CHRONIC COURSE

Viruses can rarely present with a subacute or chronic course, particularly human immunodeficiency virus (HIV) and associated complications.

Readers are encouraged to refer to article 9 for neuroimaging features of HIV.

Progressive Multifocal Leukoencephalopathy Caused by John Cunningham Virus

MR imaging is the modality of choice for the diagnosis of PML. Typical PML lesions frequently involve subcortical hemispheric white matter (**Fig 10**), but they can also affect cerebellar white matter or gray matter structures, such as basal ganglia or thalamus. The lesions can be multifocal, showing T1-low, T2-and FLAIR-high signal intensities. Classic PML does not usually show any mass effect or contrast enhancement. However, inflammatory PML or progressive multifocal leukoencephalopathy immune reconstitution inflammatory syndrome (PML-IRIS) lesions (see **Fig 10**) can show substantial contrast enhancement due to inflammation and blood–brain barrier disruption. It can also accompany edema, swelling, or mass effects.[72]

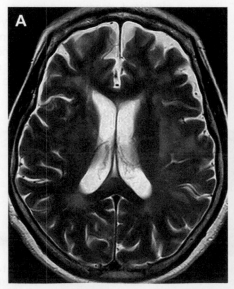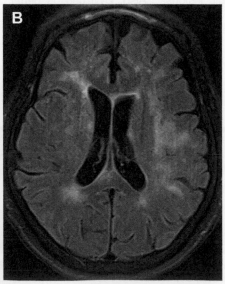

Fig. 11. Subacute sclerosing panencephalitis (SSPE) (*A, B*) Multifocal T2-and FLAIR-high signal lesions are demonstrated in bilateral periventricular and subcortical white matter.

Table 2
Summary of MR imaging patterns in typical acute viral encephalitis

Preferential Anatomic Involvement	Viral Pathogens	Radiological Features	Clinical Features
Temporal lobe	Herpes simplex virus type-1	Typically insula and limbic system, frontal lobe. More widespread in HSV-2	HSV-1 infection in adults, HSV-2 in children
	Human herpes virus type-6	Typically exclusive mesial temporal lobe	Immunocompromised patients
Bilateral thalami	Japanese encephalitis virus	May show hemorrhage	Especially children in endemic area
	Influenza virus	Acute necrotizing encephalopathy	Antecedent respiratory infection especially in children
Brainstem	Enterovirus	Medulla, pons, midbrain, callosal splenium, and ventral spinal cord	Associated with hand–foot–mouth disease or outbreaks in children
	Rabies virus	Brainstem, hippocampus, limbic system, hypothalamic and spinal cord (predominant in gray matter)	History of rabid animal bite
Splenium of corpus callosum	Rotavirus	Typically reversible on DWI	Associated with acute gastroenteritis in children

Subacute Sclerosing Panencephalitis Caused by the Measles Virus

Subacute sclerosing panencephalitis (SSPE) is a rare, progressive, chronic inflammatory encephalitis secondary to a measles virus infection that causes widespread demyelination in children and adolescents.[73] In the developed world, the prevalence of SSPE has steadily declined since the introduction of the measles virus vaccine in the 1960s. The incidence of SSPE is inversely related to the rate of measles vaccination.[74] Overall, 4 to 11 cases of SSPE are expected for every 100,000 cases of measles, with a higher incidence among children aged less than 5 years (18/100,000, compared with 1.1/100,000 after 5 years of age).[75] The highest incidence of SSPE relative to measles is reported in the Middle East, where the rate is 360/100,000 in individuals infected before 1 year of age. The incidence varies dramatically depending on the measles infection's age and vaccination status.[76]

MR imaging findings mainly depend on the disease duration.[77] MR imaging findings can be normal in the early stages. As the disease progresses, periventricular and subcortical T2-high signal lesions are seen[78] (Fig. 11). The cerebral cortex, corpus callosum, and deep structures can be involved in the more advanced stages. These lesions may show contrast enhancement and high signal intensities on DWI.[79] In the chronic phase, the lesions may disappear, new lesions can occur, and progressive brain atrophy can develop.

SUMMARY

Clinical diagnosis of the cause of viral encephalitis can be difficult. Nonetheless, an accurate and timely diagnosis is essential to guide management and appropriate treatment. In this article, a diagnostic algorithm based on MR imaging features is proposed to systematically aid the differential diagnosis of viral encephalitis. The typical MR imaging patterns should not be overlooked (Table 2).

The proposed MR imaging findings must be interpreted in the correct clinical context, and thus, making a diagnosis solely based on the MR imaging findings has limitations. Nonetheless, using this simple systemic approach based on the visual assessment of structural imaging can help both radiologists and clinicians evaluate MR imaging to support the correct diagnosis. We believe that future validation of the diagnostic algorithm is necessitated. Future studies using advanced techniques, such as automated classifier algorithms may play a complementary role in clinical practice.

CLINICS CARE POINTS

- Viruses can cause central nervous system disease via three broad mechanisms: aseptic meningitis, encephalitis, and immune-mediated processes; adopting a structured but simplified diagnostic approach based on typical MR imaging patterns can assist in suggesting a viral pathogen, even though there is considerable overlap.

- By aggregating imaging, clinical and laboratory evidence, radiologists can contribute to multidisciplinary teams caring for patients, leading to the appropriate treatment and better outcomes.

DISCLOSURE

The authors have nothing to disclose.

REFERENCES

1. Kar A, Dhanaraj M, Dedeepiya D, et al. Acute encephalitis syndrome following scrub typhus infection. Indian J Crit Care Med 2014;18(7): 453–5.
2. Granerod J, Tam CC, Crowcroft NS, et al. Challenge of the unknown. A systematic review of acute encephalitis in non-outbreak situations. Neurology 2010;75(10):924–32.
3. Boucher A, Herrmann JL, Morand P, et al. Epidemiology of infectious encephalitis causes in 2016. Med Mal Infect 2017;47(3):221–35.
4. Bookstaver PB, Mohorn PL, Shah A, et al. Management of Viral Central Nervous System Infections: A Primer for Clinicians. J Cent Nerv Syst Dis 2017;9. 1179573517703342.
5. Bechter K. Encephalitis, Mild Encephalitis, Neuroprogression, or Encephalopathy-Not Merely a Question of Terminology. Front Psychiatry 2019;9:782.
6. Goel S, Chakravarti A, Mantan M, et al. Diagnostic Approach to Viral Acute Encephalitis Syndrome (AES) in Paediatric Age Group: A Study from New Delhi. J Clin Diagn Res 2017;11(9):Dc25–dc29.
7. Chaudhuri A, Kennedy PG. Diagnosis and treatment of viral encephalitis. Postgrad Med J 2002;78(924): 575–83.
8. Gonzalez G, Carr MJ, Kobayashi M, et al. Enterovirus-Associated Hand-Foot and Mouth Disease and Neurological Complications in Japan and the Rest of the World. Int J Mol Sci 2019;20(20):5201.
9. Kumar R. Understanding and managing acute encephalitis. F1000Res 2020;9.
10. Dalmau J, Graus F, Villarejo A, et al. Clinical analysis of anti-Ma2-associated encephalitis. Brain 2004; 127(Pt 8):1831–44.
11. Jayaraman K, Rangasami R, Chandrasekharan A. Magnetic Resonance Imaging Findings in Viral Encephalitis: A Pictorial Essay. J Neurosci Rural Pract 2018;9(4):556–60.
12. Granerod J, Ambrose HE, Davies NW, et al. Causes of encephalitis and differences in their clinical presentations in England: a multicentre, population-based prospective study. Lancet Infect Dis 2010; 10(12):835–44.
13. Aurelius E, Johansson B, Sköldenberg B, et al. Encephalitis in immunocompetent patients due to herpes simplex virus type 1 or 2 as determined by type-specific polymerase chain reaction and antibody assays of cerebrospinal fluid. J Med Virol 1993;39(3):179–86.
14. Piret J, Boivin G. Immunomodulatory Strategies in Herpes Simplex Virus Encephalitis. Clin Microbiol Rev 2020;33(2).
15. Kolski H, Ford-Jones EL, Richardson S, et al. Etiology of acute childhood encephalitis at The Hospital for Sick Children, Toronto, 1994-1995. Clin Infect Dis 1998;26(2):398–409.
16. Glaser CA, Honarmand S, Anderson LJ, et al. Beyond viruses: clinical profiles and etiologies associated with encephalitis. Clin Infect Dis 2006;43(12): 1565–77.
17. Venkatesan A, Tunkel AR, Bloch KC, et al. Case definitions, diagnostic algorithms, and priorities in encephalitis: consensus statement of the international encephalitis consortium. Clin Infect Dis 2013;57(8): 1114–28.
18. Domingues RB, Fink MC, Tsanaclis AM, et al. Diagnosis of herpes simplex encephalitis by magnetic resonance imaging and polymerase chain reaction assay of cerebrospinal fluid. J Neurol Sci 1998; 157(2):148–53.
19. Stahl JP, Mailles A. Herpes simplex virus encephalitis update. Curr Opin Infect Dis 2019;32(3): 239–43.
20. Renard D, Nerrant E, Lechiche C. DWI and FLAIR imaging in herpes simplex encephalitis: a comparative and topographical analysis. J Neurol 2015; 262(9):2101–5.
21. Singh TD, Fugate JE, Hocker S, et al. Predictors of outcome in HSV encephalitis. J Neurol 2016; 263(2):277–89.
22. Sili U, Kaya A, Mert A. Herpes simplex virus encephalitis: clinical manifestations, diagnosis and outcome in 106 adult patients. J Clin Virol 2014; 60(2):112–8.

23. Fida M, Hamdi AM, Bryson A, et al. Long-term Outcomes of Patients With Human Herpesvirus 6 Encephalitis. Open Forum Infect Dis 2019;6(7):ofz269.

24. Santpere G, Telford M, Andrés-Benito P, et al. The Presence of Human Herpesvirus 6 in the Brain in Health and Disease. Biomolecules 2020;10(11): 1520.

25. Eimer WA, Vijaya Kumar DK, Navalpur Shanmugam NK, et al. Alzheimer's Disease-Associated β-Amyloid Is Rapidly Seeded by Herpesviridae to Protect against Brain Infection. Neuron 2018; 99(1):56–63.e3.

26. Noguchi T, Yoshiura T, Hiwatashi A, et al. CT and MRI findings of human herpesvirus 6-associated encephalopathy: comparison with findings of herpes simplex virus encephalitis. AJR Am J Roentgenol 2010;194(3):754–60.

27. Handley G, Hasbun R, Okhuysen P. Human herpesvirus 6 and central nervous system disease in oncology patients: A retrospective case series and literature review. J Clin Virol 2021;136:104740.

28. Noguchi T, Mihara F, Yoshiura T, et al. MR imaging of human herpesvirus-6 encephalopathy after hematopoietic stem cell transplantation in adults. AJNR Am J Neuroradiol 2006;27(10):2191–5.

29. Yassin A, Al-Mistarehi AH, El-Salem K, et al. Clinical, radiological, and electroencephalographic features of HHV-6 encephalitis following hematopoietic stem cell transplantation. Ann Med Surg (Lond) 2020;60: 81–6.

30. Liu D, Wang X, Wang Y, et al. Detection of EBV and HHV6 in the Brain Tissue of Patients with Rasmussen's Encephalitis. Virol Sin 2018;33(5):402–9.

31. Meng Q, Zou Y-L, Bu H, et al. Imaging and cytological analysis of 92 patients with Japanese encephalitis. Neuroimmunology and Neuroinflammation 2014;1(-1):29–34.

32. Misra UK, Kalita J. Overview: Japanese encephalitis. Prog Neurobiol 2010;91(2):108–20.

33. Umenai T, Krzysko R, Bektimirov TA, et al. Japanese encephalitis: current worldwide status. Bull World Health Organ 1985;63(4):625–31.

34. Zheng Y, Li M, Wang H, et al. Japanese encephalitis and Japanese encephalitis virus in mainland China. Rev Med Virol 2012;22(5):301–22.

35. Helfferich J, Knoester M, Van Leer-Buter CC, et al. Acute flaccid myelitis and enterovirus D68: lessons from the past and present. Eur J Pediatr 2019; 178(9):1305–15.

36. Pleasure SJ, Fischbein NJ. Correlation of clinical and neuroimaging findings in a case of rabies encephalitis. Arch Neurol 2000;57(12):1765–9.

37. Chuang YY, Huang YC. Enteroviral infection in neonates. J Microbiol Immunol Infect 2019;52(6):851–7.

38. Kalita J, Bhoi SK, Bastia JK, et al. Paralytic rabies: MRI findings and review of literature. Neurol India 2014;62(6):662–4.

39. Rao A, Pimpalwar Y, Mukherjee A, et al. Serial brain MRI findings in a rare survivor of rabies encephalitis. Indian J Radiol Imaging 2017;27(3):286–9.

40. Sugaya N. Influenza-associated encephalopathy in Japan. Semin Pediatr Infect Dis 2002;13(2):79–84.

41. Fujimoto S, Kobayashi M, Uemura O, et al. PCR on cerebrospinal fluid to show influenza-associated acute encephalopathy or encephalitis. Lancet 1998;352(9131):873–5.

42. Chen YC, Lo CP, Chang TP. Novel influenza A (H1N1)-associated encephalopathy/encephalitis with severe neurological sequelae and unique image features–a case report. J Neurol Sci 2010; 298(1–2):110–3.

43. Lian ZY, Huang B, He SR, et al. Diffusion-weighted imaging in the diagnosis of enterovirus 71 encephalitis. Acta Radiol 2012;53(2):208–13.

44. Maloney JA, Mirsky DM, Messacar K, et al. MRI findings in children with acute flaccid paralysis and cranial nerve dysfunction occurring during the 2014 enterovirus D68 outbreak. AJNR Am J Neuroradiol 2015;36(2):245–50.

45. Hixon AM, Frost J, Rudy MJ, et al. Understanding Enterovirus D68-Induced Neurologic Disease: A Basic Science Review. Viruses 2019;11(9):821.

46. World Health Organization. Regional Office for the Western, P., A guide to clinical management and public health response for hand, foot and mouth disease (HFMD). Manila: WHO Regional Office for the Western Pacific; 2011.

47. Casas-Alba D, de Sevilla MF, Valero-Rello A, et al. Outbreak of brainstem encephalitis associated with enterovirus-A71 in Catalonia, Spain (2016): a clinical observational study in a children's reference centre in Catalonia. Clin Microbiol Infect 2017;23(11): 874–81.

48. Jones E, Pillay TD, Liu F, et al. Outcomes following severe hand foot and mouth disease: A systematic review and meta-analysis. Eur J paediatric Neurol 2018;22(5):763–73.

49. Li J, Chen F, Liu T, et al. MRI findings of neurological complications in hand-foot-mouth disease by enterovirus 71 infection. Int J Neurosci 2012; 122(7):338–44.

50. Hankins DG, Rosekrans JA. Overview, prevention, and treatment of rabies. Mayo Clin Proc 2004; 79(5):671–6.

51. Netravathi M, Udani V, Mani Rs, et al. Unique clinical and imaging findings in a first ever documented PCR positive rabies survival patient: A case report. J Clin Virol 2015;70:83–8.

52. Mahadevan A, Suja MS, Mani RS, et al. Perspectives in Diagnosis and Treatment of Rabies Viral Encephalitis: Insights from Pathogenesis. Neurotherapeutics 2016;13(3):477–92.

53. Naghavi M, W.H., Lozano R, et al. Global, regional, and national age-sex specific all-cause and cause-

specific mortality for 240 causes of death, 1990-2013: a systematic analysis for the Global Burden of Disease Study 2013. Lancet 2015;385(9963): 117–71.

54. Lynch M, Lee B, Azimi P, et al. Rotavirus and central nervous system symptoms: cause or contaminant? Case reports and review. Clin Infect Dis 2001; 33(7):932–8.

55. Abe T, Kobayashi M, Araki K, et al. Infantile convulsions with mild gastroenteritis. Brain Dev 2000;22(5): 301–6.

56. Li C-Y, Li C-HJNA. Probable etiology of mild encephalopathy with reversible isolated lesions in the corpus callosum in children: A review of 20 cases from northern China 2018;23(2):153–8.

57. Paketçi C, Edem P, Okur D, et al. Rotavirus encephalopathy with concomitant acute cerebellitis: report of a case and review of the literature. Turk J Pediatr 2020;62(1):119–24.

58. Starkey J, Kobayashi N, Numaguchi Y, et al. Cytotoxic Lesions of the Corpus Callosum That Show Restricted Diffusion: Mechanisms, Causes, and Manifestations. Radiographics 2017;37(2): 562–76.

59. Shaw J, Gershon AA. Varicella Virus Vaccination in the United States. Viral Immunol 2018;31(2):96–103.

60. Nagel MA, Gilden D. Neurological complications of varicella zoster virus reactivation. Curr Opin Neurol 2014;27(3):356–60.

61. Gilden D, Cohrs RJ, Mahalingam R, et al. Varicella zoster virus vasculopathies: diverse clinical manifestations, laboratory features, pathogenesis, and treatment. Lancet Neurol 2009;8(8):731–40.

62. Prelack MS, Patterson KR, Berger JR. Varicella zoster virus rhombencephalomyelitis following radiation therapy for oropharyngeal carcinoma. J Clin Neurosci 2016;25:164–6.

63. Orme HT, Smith AG, Nagel MA, et al. VZV spinal cord infarction identified by diffusion-weighted MRI (DWI). Neurology 2007;69(4):398–400.

64. Becerra JC, Sieber R, Martinetti G, et al. Infection of the central nervous system caused by varicella zoster virus reactivation: a retrospective case series study. Int J Infect Dis 2013;17(7):e529–34.

65. Inagaki A, Toyoda T, Mutou M, et al. Ramsay Hunt syndrome associated with solitary nucleus, spinal trigeminal nucleus and tract, and vestibular nucleus involvement on sequential magnetic resonance imaging. J Neurovirol 2018;24(6):776–9.

66. Li GH, Ning ZJ, Liu YM, et al. Neurological Manifestations of Dengue Infection. Front Cell Infect Microbiol 2017;7:449.

67. Almeida Bentes A, Kroon EG, Romanelli RMC. Neurological manifestations of pediatric arboviral infections in the Americas. J Clin Virol 2019;116: 49–57.

68. Soares C, Puccioni-Sohler M. Dengue encephalitis: Suggestion for case definition. J Neurol Sci 2011; 306(1):165.

69. Wan Sulaiman WA, Inche Mat LN, Hashim HZ, et al. Acute disseminated encephalomyelitis in dengue viral infection. J Clin Neurosci 2017;43:25–31.

70. Jugpal TS, Dixit R, Garg A, et al. Spectrum of findings on magnetic resonance imaging of the brain in patients with neurological manifestations of dengue fever. Radiol Bras 2017;50(5):285–90.

71. Sundaram C, Uppin SG, Dakshinamurthy KV, et al. Acute disseminated encephalomyelitis following dengue hemorrhagic fever. Neurol India 2010; 58(4):599–601.

72. Cortese I, Reich DS, Nath A. Progressive multifocal leukoencephalopathy and the spectrum of JC virus-related disease. Nat Rev Neurol 2021;17(1): 37–51.

73. Cece H, Tokay L, Yildiz S, et al. Epidemiological findings and clinical and magnetic resonance presentations in subacute sclerosing panencephalitis. J Int Med Res 2011;39(2):594–602.

74. Anlar B, Köse G, Gürer Y, et al. Changing epidemiological features of subacute sclerosing panencephalitis. Infection 2001;29(4):192–5.

75. Campbell H, Andrews N, Brown KE, et al. Review of the effect of measles vaccination on the epidemiology of SSPE. Int J Epidemiol 2007;36(6):1334–48.

76. Zilber N, Kahana E. Environmental risk factors for subacute sclerosing panencephalitis (SSPE). Acta Neurol Scand 1998;98(1):49–54.

77. Gutierrez J, Issacson RS, Koppel BS. Subacute sclerosing panencephalitis: an update. Dev Med Child Neurol 2010;52(10):901–7.

78. Tuncay R, Akman-Demir G, Gökyigit A, et al. MRI in subacute sclerosing panencephalitis. Neuroradiology 1996;38(7):636–40.

79. Oguz KK, Celebi A, Anlar B. MR imaging, diffusion-weighted imaging and MR spectroscopy findings in acute rapidly progressive subacute sclerosing panencephalitis. Brain Dev 2007;29(5):306–11.

Acute Neurological Complications of Coronavirus Disease

Sanders Chang, MD[a], Michael Schecht, MD[a], Rajan Jain, MD[b,c], Puneet Belani, MD[a,d],*

KEYWORDS

- Coronavirus disease • Stroke • Large vessel occlusion • Venous sinus thrombosis
- Acute disseminated encephalomyelitis • Leukoencephalopathy
- Posterior reversible encephalopathy syndrome • Multisystem inflammatory syndrome

KEY POINTS

- Acute/subacute stroke is the most common neuroimaging finding seen in patients with coronavirus disease (COVID-19). Other vascular findings include dural venous sinus thrombosis, arterial dissection, and vasculitis.
- Intracerebral hemorrhage may manifest as a large hemorrhage or microhemorrhages, the latter being more predominant in the hemispheres or corpus callosum.
- Leukoencephalopathies may manifest as posterior reversible encephalopathy syndrome.
- Neuropathies may be multiple or single, ranging from anosmia, facial nerve palsy, to Guillain-Barré syndrome.
- Multisystem inflammatory syndrome can be seen in the pediatric population.

INTRODUCTION

The coronavirus disease (COVID-19) pandemic, caused by the severe acute respiratory syndrome coronavirus 2 (SARS-CoV-2) virus, has affected hundreds of millions people globally and led to several million deaths.[1] In addition to respiratory sequelae (eg, interstitial pneumonia and acute respiratory distress syndrome), neurologic manifestations have been observed with COVID-19, including encephalopathy, acute cerebrovascular disease, and sensory abnormalities.[2,3] The frequency of neurologic symptoms has been observed in up to 36.4% of COVID-19 patients and is more common in patients with severe stages of infection.[4]

Recognizing the neuroradiological features associated with COVID-19 is crucial, as they have implications on diagnosis and management. This article reviews the various acute neuroradiological patterns that have been observed with SARS-CoV-2 infections (Table 1).

STROKE

Stroke has been observed in 1% to 3% of all hospitalized patients with COVID-19.[5,6] From a meta-analysis of published articles detailing MRI neuroimaging findings during the peak of the pandemic, acute and subacute strokes were the most common neuro-radiological abnormality.[7] Development of strokes bears important

[a] Department of Diagnostic, Molecular and Interventional Radiology, Icahn School of Medicine at Mount Sinai, 1176 5th Avenue MC Level, New York, NY 10029, USA; [b] Department of Radiology, NYU Grossman School of Medicine, 660 1st Avenue, 1st Floor, New York, NY 10016, USA; [c] Department of Neurosurgery, NYU Grossman School of Medicine, 660 1st Avenue, 1st Floor, New York, NY 10016, USA; [d] Department of Neurosurgery, Icahn School of Medicine at Mount Sinai, 1176 5th Avenue MC Level, New York, NY 10029, USA
* Corresponding author. 1176 5th Avenue MC Level, New York, NY 10029.
E-mail address: puneet.belani@mountsinai.org

Neuroimag Clin N Am 33 (2023) 57–68
https://doi.org/10.1016/j.nic.2022.07.003
1052-5149/23/© 2022 Elsevier Inc. All rights reserved.

Table 1
Neuroimaging findings in acute coronavirus disease infection

Clinical Syndrome	Imaging Findings (Computed Tomography or MRI)	Proposed Pathogenesis
Stroke	• Anterior circulation most common • Multiterritorial involvement • Large vessel occlusions, especially in uncommonly affected vessels: subclavian artery and pericallosal gyrus • Higher prevalence among younger patients and those without traditional risk factors for stroke	• Endothelial cell dysfunction via immune-mediated cytokine storm or direct viral interactions • Indirect propagation of thrombosis and plaque rupture from immune response to the virus
Dural vein thrombosis	• Multifocal involvement: superior sagittal , transverse, and sigmoid sinuses, internal jugular vein • Associated parenchymal hemorrhage, cerebral edema, venous infarcts	• Indirect propagation of thrombosis and plaque rupture from immune response to the virus
Arterial dissection	• Extracranial carotid and vertebral arteries, commonly bilateral • Absence of typical risk factors such as connective tissue disorders or trauma	• Endothelial cell dysfunction via immune-mediated cytokine storm or direct viral interactions
Vasculitis	• Long segment vessel wall enhancement of multiple arteries • *Focal cerebral arteriopathy*: pediatric patient with focal stenosis, irregular narrowing, concentric contrast enhancement of a large vessel	• Endothelial cell dysfunction via immune-mediated cytokine storm or direct viral interactions
Intraparenchymal hemorrhage	• Unifocal or multifocal involvement with extension into subarachnoid and intraventricular spaces • Associated diffuse edema and mass effect • Microhemorrhages: cortical, juxtacortical, deep white matter (WM), perivenular, and corpus callosal involvement	• Dysregulation of blood pressure control through virus-related downregulation of ACE-2 receptors • Endothelial cell dysfunction via immune-mediated cytokine storm or direct viral interactions • Iatrogenic: anticoagulation, ECMO, mechanical ventilation • Hypoxic-induced injury to the blood-brain barrier
PRES	• CT hypoattenuation, T2/FLAIR signal abnormality, and diffusion restriction in the subcortical WM of posterior temporal and occipital lobes • Associated parenchymal hemorrhages and microhemorrhages	• Endothelial cell dysfunction via immune-mediated cytokine storm or direct viral interaction • Dysregulation of blood pressure control through virus-related downregulation of ACE-2 receptors
Leukoencephalopathy	• Multifocal WM lesions with diffusion restriction and T2/FLAIR hyperintensity, predominantly in the posterior WM • Central restricted diffusion greater for COVID-19 lesions	• Endothelial cell dysfunction via immune-mediated cytokine storm or direct viral interactions

(continued on next page)

Table 1
(continued)

Clinical Syndrome	Imaging Findings (Computed Tomography or MRI)	Proposed Pathogenesis
	• Associated enhancement and microhemorrhages • Severe: central expansile T2/FLAIR hyperintensity in the basal ganglia and thalami	
Cranial neuropathy • Anosmia/dysgeusia • Facial and abducens nerve palsy	• Anosmia/dysgeusia: T2/FLAIR signal abnormality in the gyrus rectus and olfactory bulbs • Facial and abducens nerve palsy: affected cranial nerves demonstrating STIR hyperintensity, gadolinium enhancement, and diffusion restriction	• Autoimmune-mediated

implications in the clinical course of the COVID-19 patient. Their detection signifies poor prognosis with reported rates of mortality up to 50%.[8] Severe disability has been seen in COVID-19 survivors with ischemic strokes upon discharge, significantly greater than those with non-COVID-19-related ischemic strokes.[9] Moreover, studies have shown that COVID-19 represents a significant independent risk factor in stroke development among hospitalized patients, even greater than traditional comorbidities such as cardiovascular disease and obesity.[10,11]

Certain neuroradiological characteristics are linked to COVID-19-related strokes. These features include multiterritorial involvement, involvement of atypical vessels, and large vessel occlusions.

Stroke Distribution

Strokes in COVID-19 patients more commonly involve the anterior circulation compared with the posterior circulation.[12–14] Multivascular distribution is a common feature, observed in up to 40% of cases.[12] This rate is higher than that observed in the prepandemic era (10.7%).[15] The high prevalence of multiterritorial strokes is consistent with the induced prothrombotic environment and increased embolic risk associated with the SARS-COV-2 virus, and had been reported in the previous 2003 outbreak of SARS-COV-1 virus infection.[16] Infection severity is also likely correlated with risk for multiterritorial strokes. In 1 study, multiterritorial strokes were significantly more frequent among hospitalized patients with severe infection compared to outpatients with less severe infections (56.4% vs 33.3%).[17]

Large Vessel Occlusions

Large vessel occlusions (LVOs) have been observed in up to around 60% of COVID-19 patients with ischemic infarctions.[18,19] In comparison, arterial occlusions were historically observed in up to 46% of ischemic strokes in the prepandemic era.[20] In 1 study, proximal large vessel occlusions were significantly more common among COVID-19 patients compared with historic controls.[6] The relatively high prevalence of LVOs among COVID-19-related acute ischemic strokes suggests the prothrombotic nature of the SARS-COV-2 virus.

LVOs in COVID-19 patients most commonly involve the anterior circulation, particularly the middle cerebral artery (MCA) and internal carotid artery (Fig. 1).[12,13] Other locations include the posterior cerebral artery (PCA), basilar artery, vertebral artery, and common carotid arteries.[12,21,22] Significant thrombotic burden and occlusions of otherwise uncommonly affected vessels have also been observed in the subclavian artery[12] and the pericallosal artery.[23] Occlusions can appear in tandem, which was seen in up to 40% of patients in 1 case series.[12]

Strokes in Younger Patients

Younger age onset of strokes has been observed in COVID-19 patients. In 1 study, 73.3% of patients with large vessel occlusions were younger than 50 years old.[12] Median age of stroke-onset in COVID-19 patients was found to be significantly lower than that of patients without COVID-19 (median age of 63 vs 70).[6] In addition, the mean age of COVID-19 patients with emergency large vessel

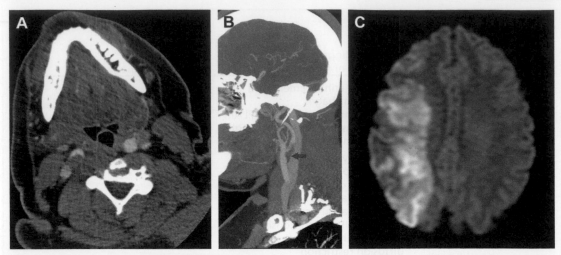

Fig. 1. 33-year-old woman with ongoing COVID-19 infection experienced sudden onset left hemiparesis and sensory loss. Axial CT angiography (CTA) image of the neck (*A*) and sagittal maximum intensity projection (MIP) (*B*) demonstrated a large noncalcified thrombus (*arrows*) in the proximal right internal carotid artery (ICA) causing moderate stenosis. Subsequent MRI diffusion weighted imaging (DWI) (*C*) demonstrated a large acute infarct involving the right MCA territory (*star*).

occlusions was also significantly less than that of patients without COVID-19 (mean age of 59 vs 74 years).[24]

Certain clinical factors are shared among younger patients with COVID-19 and stroke, such as the absence of traditional risk factors for stroke (eg, diabetes, hypertension, hyperlipidemia, and coronary artery disease),[12] and minimal to absent respiratory symptoms during the initial stage of the disease course.[25] In 1 study, a significantly higher number of patients younger than 50 years old experienced an ischemic stroke in the absence of any prior respiratory symptoms (50.0%, $P=.014$).[26]

Pathophysiology of Stroke

The mechanism behind the development of strokes in COVID-19 patients is presumed to be multifactorial. Interaction between the SARS-COV-2 virus with endothelial angiotensin converting enzyme 2 (ACE-2) receptors is thought to result in direct endothelial damage, predisposing to occlusive events.[27] Indirectly, a proinflammatory state induced by a misdirected immune response to the SARS-COV-2 virus can result in propagation of thrombosis and plaque rupture. Inflammatory infiltrates have been found within the intima of surgically removed thrombosis on pathology, consistent with endotheliitis.[28]

It is unclear whether arterial thrombosis is a de novo phenomenon or related to worsening of pre-existing atheromatous plaque. Many COVID-19-related strokes have been observed in patients with prior atherosclerotic disease.[22,27,28] However,

patients without any significant medical history, especially those younger than the observed population, have presented with strokes and large vessel occlusions. Direct endothelial damage may be the primary mechanism behind occlusive events in these patients. In addition, acute extracranial events, such as pulmonary embolism or cardiac arrests, may be triggers for strokes. In 1 meta-analysis, younger COVID-19 patients (<50 years) had a higher frequency of elevated cardiac troponin, suggesting that acute myocardial injury is a possible risk factor for the development of strokes.[26]

DURAL VEIN THROMBOSIS

Dural vein thrombosis is a relatively rare presentation among COVID-19 patients; in 1 large study, the prevalence was only 0.02% (Fig. 2).[29] When present, sinus vein thrombosis tends to involve multiple sites, most commonly the superior sagittal, transverse, and sigmoid sinuses.[30–32] Other sites include the cortical veins, vein of Galen, and internal cerebral veins.[33] Complications from the venous thrombosis may also be seen, such as surrounding parenchymal hemorrhage, cerebral edema, and hemorrhagic venous infarcts.[31,34]

Given the low number of cases, the relationship between the development of dural vein thrombosis and SARS-COV-2 virus has yet to be elucidated. In many case series, dural venous thrombosis and its associated complications were seen in patients with predisposing risk factors, such as hypertension, diabetes, obesity, oral contraceptive pill

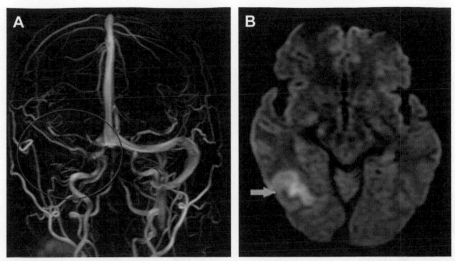

Fig. 2. 40-year-old man presented with severe headache in the setting of a recent COVID-19 diagnosis. MR venogram coronal MIP image (*A*) showed thrombosis of the left transverse and sigmoid sinuses (*circle*). MRI DWI (*B*) showed hyperintense acute venous infarct in the right temporal lobe (*arrow*) corresponding to the region of the venous thrombosis.

(OCP) use, and hormonal therapy for cancer. However, sinus thrombosis can present in patients without prior risk factors or inciting events.[35] Its pathogenesis is likely tied to the prothrombogenic state associated with COVID-19.

ARTERIAL DISSECTION

Arterial dissections are rarely observed among COVID-19 patients, typically occurring in the extracranial carotid and vertebral arteries, and often bilaterally.[18,36–38] One report noted extension of the dissection from the distal cervical part to the petrous segment of the internal carotid arteries.[37] Patients were also noted to lack typical risk factors for dissection, such as connective tissue disorders, or inciting events, such as trauma (Fig. 3).

Although the mechanism remains unclear, endothelial damage propagated by the cytokine storm and direct infection by the SARS-COV-2 virus likely play a role. Dissections at other sites, such as the aorta and coronary arteries, have been observed in the context of COVID-19 and likely follow a similar pathogenesis.[39,40]

VASCULITIS AND FOCAL CEREBRAL ARTERIOPATHY

Acute vasculitis is a rare neuroradiologic manifestation observed in COVID-19 patients. Typical imaging features include long segment vessel wall enhancement of multiple arteries. In 1 case of a 64-year-old patient, vasculitis was observed in

MCAs, anterior cerebral arteries (ACAs), vertebral arteries, and the basilar artery, and was associated with multiterritorial infarcts.[41]

In pediatric COVID-19 patients, several cases of focal cerebral arteriopathy of childhood-inflammatory type have been reported.[42,43] Imaging findings include focal stenosis and irregular narrowing of a large vessel, such as the M1 segment, with associated wall thickening and concentric contrast enhancement. In lieu of typical cardiovascular factors and pre-existing disease, focal cerebral arteriopathy may represent a possible mechanism for which strokes can develop in children. One case of stroke has been observed in a COVID-19 patient as young as 5 years old.[44]

INTRACEREBRAL HEMORRHAGE

Intracranial hemorrhage is a neurologic complication seen in approximately 0.2% of COVID-19 patients.[29] It has been observed in up to 42% of patients with abnormal neuroradiological findings.[14] Typical imaging features of intracranial hemorrhage include massive intraparenchymal hemorrhage, usually with extension into the subarachnoid and intraventricular spaces, multifocal intraparenchymal hemorrhages, and microhemorrhages.[8,23,31,32,45] Diffuse edema is often associated with foci of hemorrhage,[23,31] and may contribute to significant mass effect with increased risk of brain herniation.[46] Rarely, acute parenchymal hematomas can involve the bilateral basal ganglia.[47] The mechanism behind

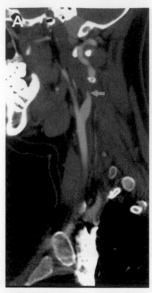
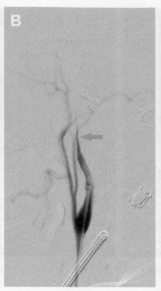
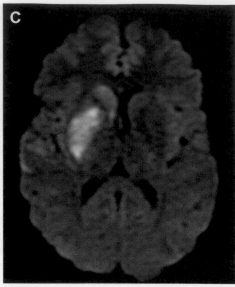

Fig. 3. 34-year-old woman with no significant past medical history and no recent trauma presented with acute onset of left facial droop, dysarthria, right gaze deviation, and left hemiparesis/hemisensory loss. Sagittal view from a CTA of the head and neck (*A*) and lateral view from a catheter angiogram arterial phase injection of the right ICA (*B*) demonstrated an acute dissection in the right ICA shortly after its origin (*arrows*). Axial DWI (*C*) showed an acute right ganglionic infarct. COVID-19 polymerase chain reaction (PCR) test was positive.

this distribution of hemorrhage is hypothesized to be disrupted drainage of the basal ganglia secondary to occlusion of the great cerebral vein.

Intracranial hemorrhage may result spontaneously, which typically occurs in critically ill patients with severe infections and multiorgan failure.[23,31] Hemorrhage can also result secondarily from other pathologic processes, such as hemorrhagic transformation of ischemic strokes,[8,17,18,46] rupture of dissecting aneurysms[48] and pseudoaneurysms,[49] hemorrhagic infarction associated with venous sinus thrombosis,[33,34] reversible cerebral vasoconstriction syndrome,[50] posterior reversible encephalopathy syndrome (PRES),[51,52] and iatrogenic causes.

Pathophysiology of Hemorrhage

The pathophysiology for the development of intracranial hemorrhage is multifactorial. COVID-19 is associated with coagulopathies, such as thrombocytopenia and disseminated intravascular coagulation, which increase the risk for hemorrhage.[53] More directly, SARS-COV-2 virus is known to bind to the angiotensin-converting enzyme 2 (ACE-2) receptor in order to enter host cells. ACE-2 receptors are expressed on various organs, including cerebrovascular endothelial cells, and are integral components of the renin-angiotensin pathway. SARS-COV-2-induced downregulation of ACE-2 receptors can result in dysregulation of blood pressure control and lead to blood pressure

spikes, potentially causing arterial wall rupture and hemorrhage in the brain.[45] Alternatively, the mechanism of diffuse thrombotic microangiopathy has been proposed.[54] Diffuse thrombosis and vascular endothelial damage can lead to breakdown of the blood-brain barrier, facilitating the development of microhemorrhages that eventually coalesce into large intraparenchymal hematomas.

Iatrogenic causes most likely play a role in the pathogenesis of intracranial hemorrhage. Anticoagulation therapy has been determined to be the cause of a substantial number of cases of intracranial hemorrhage in COVID-19 patients.[18,55] In 1 study, most parenchymal hemorrhages were attributed to anticoagulation (60%), whereas a few cases were related to indeterminate mechanisms (30%).[55] Other case series indicated that all patients with observed hemorrhagic transformation of ischemic strokes were on anticoagulation therapy.[18,46] Characteristic imaging features can help distinguish coagulopathic intracranial hemorrhages from other etiologies. The presence of a fluid-blood level, represented by a meniscus separating dependent hyperattenuating blood products from lighter hypoattenuating serous fluid, is a highly specific finding for anticoagulation or antiplatelet therapy in COVID-19 patients.[54,56]

High prevalence of intracranial hemorrhage has been reported in COVID-19 patients on extracorporeal membrane oxygenation (ECMO) therapy. In 1 case series, up to 41.7% of COVID-19 patients on veno-venous ECMO therapy had subarachnoid, intraparenchymal, or intraventricular hemorrhage.[57] ECMO therapy is associated with derangements of hematologic and coagulation pathways, resulting from continuous contact between the patient's blood and extracorporeal circuit.[58] These factors, possibly compounded by the coagulopathic environment associated with the SARS-COV-2 virus, promote the development of hemorrhagic complications.

Microhemorrhages

Microhemorrhages make up approximately 11.1% of abnormal neuroimaging findings in COVID-19 patients.[7] Distribution patterns are various and include cortical, juxtacortical, subcortical, deep white matter, perivenular, and corpus callosal involvement.[7,22,32] Microhemorrhages attributable to COVID-19 can be made by deduction through the exclusion of other etiologies, such as hypertensive coagulopathy, diffuse axonal injury, or cerebral amyloid angiopathy, based on atypical distribution patterns and absence of clinical factors, such as hypertension or trauma.[14]

Corpus callosum involvement, particularly the splenium, is a commonly reported finding in multiple case series of COVID-19 patients.[51,55,59] Microhemorrhages in the corpus callosum have been previously described in other patient populations, such as in delayed posthypoxic leukoencephalopathy from acute respiratory distress syndrome,[60,61] high-altitude cerebral edema,[62] and in critical illness-associated microbleeds,[63] in which there is additional involvement of the juxtacortical white matter with sparing of the deep and periventricular white matter. The underlying mechanism is multifactorial, related to hypoxic-induced injury to the blood-brain barrier and impaired cerebral venous return from increased intracranial pressures. COVID-19-related microhemorrhages likely follow similar mechanisms; however, the pervasive use of mechanical ventilation among COVID-19 patients represents a confounding factor. Increased intrathoracic pressures related to ventilator use can reduce cerebral venous return in critically ill patients, which may better explain the development of microhemorrhages than direct effects from the SARS-COV-2 virus.[55]

CORONAVIRUS DISEASE-RELATED LEUKOENCEPHALOPATHIES

Leukoencephalopathies have been observed in up to 27% of abnormal neuroimaging findings among COVID-19 patients.[14] These include white matter abnormalities that are similar imaging patterns described in the literature associated with other infectious diseases, PRES, acute disseminated encephalomyelitis (ADEM), and acute hemorrhagic leukoencephalitis (AHLE). There are several pathologic findings described in COVID-19-related leukoencephalopathy that may relate to the different imaging patterns. However, the definite mechanisms are as yet incompletely understood.[64]

Posterior Reversible Encephalopathy Syndrome

PRES manifestations are typically seen as reversible confluent white matter changes in the posterior cerebrum. These appear as striking areas of hypoattenuation on noncontrast computed tomography (CT), correlating with findings of T2/fluid attenuated inversion recovery (FLAIR) signal abnormality on MRI. The distribution is typically in the areas associated with PRES, predominantly the subcortical white matter of the posterior temporal and occipital lobes.[51,65,66] Corresponding high diffusivity is seen in these regions. Areas of hemorrhage are also described, including small parenchymal hemorrhages visible on CT and microhemorrhages best visualized on gradient echo (GRE)/susceptibility weighted imaging (SWI) (**Fig. 4**).[52,67,68] The pathologic mechanism is thought to be related to direct binding of the virus to surface ACE-2 receptors on neurovascular endothelial cells, leading to breakdown of the blood brain barrier.[55] Blood pressure dysregulation caused by ACE-2 dysfunction is also a possibility.[52] Interestingly, the PRES-like findings of COVID-19 may be associated with lower blood pressure elevations than seen in other PRES etiologies.[67,68]

Acute Leukoencephalopathy

Several ADEM-type lesions have been described secondary to COVID-19.[64,69,70] Findings generally include multifocal areas of white matter restricted diffusion (**Fig. 5**) with associated T2/FLAIR hyperintensity. These predominate in the posterior white matter, in a similar distribution to PRES-like findings. However, the less confluent distribution of these lesions helps to make the distinction between these pathologies. Of note, the degree of central restricted diffusion is greater in COVID-19 lesions when compared with findings of ADEM seen secondary to other viral infections. Lesions are also reported in the corpus callosum, basal ganglia, brain stem, and cerebellum.[59,69] Enhancement may be associated with these lesions, as well as multiple microhemorrhages visualized on GRE/SWI imaging.[71] Upon follow-up imaging after the acute episode, lesions may

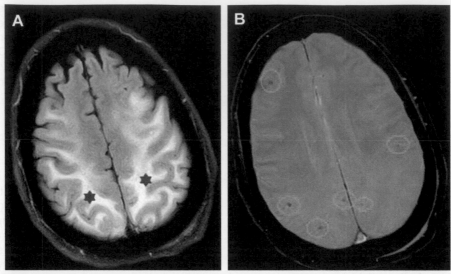

Fig. 4. 64-year-old man with ongoing COVID-19 pneumonia requiring intubation developed rhythmic jerking and status epilepticus. MRI FLAIR sequence (*A*) demonstrated extensive symmetric cerebral edema with a parieto-occipital dominance (*stars*) and scattered small foci of recent hemorrhage on the GRE sequence (*circles*) (*B*). Findings were consistent with a posterior reversible syndrome-like leukoencephalopathy with hemorrhage.

demonstrate more confluence on T2/FLAIR as well as development of cavitation and volume loss.[72]

More severe manifestations have also been described with imaging findings similar to AHLE.

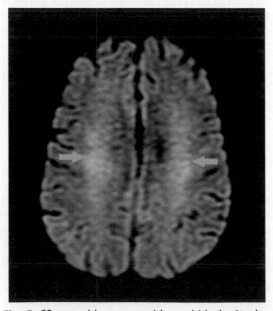

Fig. 5. 60-year-old woman with morbid obesity, hypertension, and asthma admitted with COVID-19 with hospital course complicated by acute renal failure requiring hemodialysis, respiratory failure, and flaccid quadriparesis. Brain MRI axial diffusion sequence showed restricted diffusion in the centrum semiovale bilaterally (*arrows*). Findings likely reflect a combination of hypoxia and critical illness-related encephalopathy.

A case report of a patient with severe acute respiratory syndrome and altered mental status described more central expansile T2/FLAIR hyperintensity involving the basal ganglia and thalami. There was more frank evidence of hemorrhage than seen in less severe ADEM-like cases. Predominantly peripheral enhancement was also seen.[73]

The underlying pathologic mechanism shares some similarity to the PRES-like syndrome, including suspected ACE-2-related endothelial dysfunction. Cytokine storms with elevated bloodstream cytokines and interleukins may also play a central role.[72] On pathology, a range of lesions are identified, including those that share features of ADEM and AHLE.[64] It may be that acute leukoencephalopathy in the setting of COVID-19 represents a spectrum of disorders rather than 1 entity.

NEUROPATHIES
Anosmia/Dysgeusia

Sudden onset and persistent alterations of taste and smell have been frequently reported in the setting of COVID-19 respiratory illness. In fact, loss of smell is reported as a helpful symptom in initial diagnosis of COVID-19. Several case reports and case series describe abnormal imaging findings in the anterior cranial fossa/olfactory bulbs seen in the early stages of infection (Fig. 6). An initial case report described T2/FLAIR signal abnormality in the gyrus rectus and olfactory bulbs at 3 days following presentation. At 28 days, the cortical edema had resolved, and atrophy was

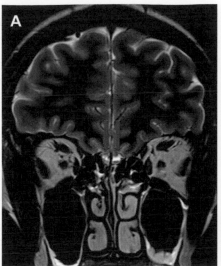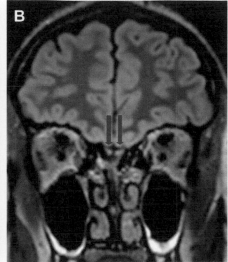

Fig. 6. 37-year-old man suffered from anosmia following COVID-19 infection with loss of smell worse on the right side. Coronal T2-weighted (A) and FLAIR (B) MR images 6 months after infection showed atrophy and hyperintensity of the olfactory bulbs bilaterally (arrows), worse on the right side.

demonstrated in the olfactory bulbs.[74] A follow-up case series identified intrinsic T1 hyperintensity and possible enhancement in the olfactory bulbs in 5 patients. Earlier work has shown central nervous system involvement via olfactory bulb invasion in experimental mouse models. This phenomenon has also been described in other viral infections.[75] More recent case series evaluating patients with persistent anosmia at least 1 month after presentation described variable findings of volume loss, morphologic change, and signal abnormality.[76] The pathologic mechanism is not yet completely understood. One possibility is injury of olfactory epithelial cells bearing ACE-2 receptors. Direct nerve invasion with retrograde tracking along the olfactory pathway has also been suggested, as seen in herpes simplex virus (HSV) infections; however, it remains unproven.[76]

Other Cranial Neuropathies

Other cranial neuropathies have been observed in COVID-19, such as palsy of the facial nerve[77–79] and abducens nerve.[77] These manifestations can occur as the initial symptom or develop more subacutely, usually up to 2 weeks from the initial onset of COVID-19 symptoms. Patients typically present with mild or absent respiratory or constitutional symptoms.

Characteristic imaging features include short-T1 inversion recovery (STIR) hyperintensity with gadolinium enhancements of the affected cranial nerve. Diffusion restriction may also be observed.[77] In facial nerve palsies, enhancement of the facial nerve may actually be normal and reflect anatomy, such as the circumneural venous plexus.[77] However, presence of asymmetric enhancement and correlation with clinical symptoms can increase confidence that the enhancement is actually pathologic.

As with olfactory neuropathies, the pathogenesis of these other cranial neuropathies is not well understood, but may be similar to that of neurotropic viruses, such as HSV and varicella zoster virus (VZV), in which direct viral invasion of the nerve can lead to axonal spread and subsequent inflammation and demyelination.[80] Immune-mediated injury of the nerve from proinflammatory cytokines may additionally play a role.[77]

SUMMARY

COVID-19 infections are associated with a myriad of acute neuroradiological features, many of which necessitate careful and prompt diagnoses. Cerebrovascular disease is a predominant complication of COVID-19 infection, attributing to the prothrombotic environment engendered by the SARS-COV-2 virus. Acute and subacute strokes, the most common neuroradiological findings, share typical features, including multiterritorial distributions, involvement of atypical vessels, and prevalence among younger patients. Appearances of intracerebral hemorrhages are more variable, although predilection for the cerebral hemispheres and corpus callosum are salient features. COVID-19-related leukoencephalopathies share similar imaging patterns with white matter diseases observed in other infections, such as PRES, ADEM, and AHLE. Acute cranial nerve neuropathies, such as anosmia and dysgeusia, can present with pathologic enhancement and nerve atrophy. Radiologists and clinicians alike should be aware of the typical neuroimaging features of COVID-19 infections as these findings can play a significant role in patient management and treatment outcomes.

CLINICS CARE POINTS

- Given that neurological manifestations in COVID-19 patients can be associated with poor prognosis, radiologists and clinicians should have a lower threshold to pursue neuroimaging in these patients
- Promptly recognizing characteristic imaging features of COVID-19-related strokes and intracranial hemorrhages can allow for earlier intervention and improved patient outcomes

DISCLOSURE

The authors have nothing to disclose.

REFERENCES

1. COVID-19 Map. Coronavirus Resource Center - John Hopkins University n.d.. Available at: https://coronavirus.jhu.edu/map.html. Accessed September 9, 2021.
2. Vogrig A, Gigli GL, Bnà C, et al. Stroke in patients with COVID-19: Clinical and neuroimaging characteristics. Neurosci Lett 2021;743:135564.
3. Helms J, Kremer S, Merdji H, et al. Neurologic features in severe SARS-CoV-2 Infection. N Engl J Med 2020;382:2268–70.
4. Mao L, Jin H, Wang M, et al. Neurologic manifestations of hospitalized patients with coronavirus disease 2019 in Wuhan, China. JAMA Neurol 2020;77:683–90.
5. Chou SH-Y, Beghi E, Helbok R, et al. Global incidence of neurological manifestations among patients hospitalized with COVID-19-a report for the GCS-NeuroCOVID consortium and the ENERGY consortium. JAMA Netw Open 2021;4:e2112131.
6. Yaghi S, Ishida K, Torres J, et al. SARS-CoV-2 and stroke in a New York healthcare system. Stroke 2020;51:2002–11.
7. Gulko E, Oleksk ML, Gomes W, et al. MRI brain findings in 126 patients with COVID-19: initial observations from a descriptive literature review. AJNR Am J Neuroradiol 2020;41:2199–203.
8. Jain R, Young M, Dogra S, et al. COVID-19 related neuroimaging findings: a signal of thromboembolic complications and a strong prognostic marker of poor patient outcome. J Neurol Sci 2020;414:116923.
9. Ntaios G, Michel P, Georgiopoulos G, et al. Characteristics and outcomes in patients with COVID-19 and acute ischemic stroke: the Global COVID-19 stroke registry. Stroke 2020;51:e254–8.
10. Belani P, Schefflein J, Kihira S, et al. COVID-19 is an independent risk factor for acute ischemic stroke. AJNR Am J Neuroradiol 2020;41:1361–4.
11. Katz JM, Libman RB, Wang JJ, et al. Cerebrovascular complications of COVID-19. Stroke 2020;51:e227–31.
12. John S, Kesav P, Mifsud VA, et al. Characteristics of large-vessel occlusion associated with COVID-19 and ischemic stroke. AJNR Am J Neuroradiol 2020;41:2263–8.
13. Radmanesh A, Raz E, Zan E, et al. Brain imaging use and findings in COVID-19: A single academic center experience in the epicenter of disease in the United States. AJNR Am J Neuroradiol 2020;41:1179–83.
14. Yoon BC, Buch K, Lang M, et al. Clinical and neuroimaging correlation in patients with COVID-19. AJNR Am J Neuroradiol 2020;41:1791–6.
15. Kaesmacher J, Mosimann PJ, Giarrusso M, et al. Multivessel occlusion in patients subjected to thrombectomy: prevalence, associated factors, and clinical implications. Stroke 2018;49:1355–62.
16. Umapathi T, Kor AC, Venketasubramanian N, et al. Large artery ischaemic stroke in severe acute respiratory syndrome (SARS). J Neurol 2014;251:1227–31.
17. Katz JM, Libman RB, Wang JJ, et al. COVID-19 severity and stroke: correlation of imaging and laboratory markers. AJNR Am J Neuroradiol 2021;42:257–61.
18. Hernández-Fernández F, Sandoval Valencia H, Barbella-Aponte RA, et al. Cerebrovascular disease in patients with COVID-19: neuroimaging, histological and clinical description. Brain 2020;143:3089–103.
19. Kihira S, Schefflein J, Mahmoudi K, et al. Association of coronavirus disease (COVID-19) with large vessel occlusion strokes: a case-control study. AJR Am J Roentgenol 2021;216:150–6.
20. Rennert RC, Wali AR, Steinberg JA, et al. Epidemiology, natural history, and clinical presentation of large vessel ischemic stroke. Neurosurgery 2019;85:S4–8.
21. Beyrouti R, Adams ME, Benjamin L, et al. Characteristics of ischaemic stroke associated with

COVID-19. J Neurol Neurosurg Psychiatry 2020;91: 889–91.

22. Franceschi AM, Arora R, Wilson R, et al. Neurovascular complications in COVID-19 infection: case series. AJNR Am J Neuroradiol 2020;41:1632–40.

23. Morassi M, Bagatto D, Cobelli M, et al. Stroke in patients with SARS-CoV-2 infection: case series. J Neurol 2020;267:2185–92.

24. Majidi S, Fifi JT, Ladner TR, et al. Emergent large vessel occlusion stroke during New York City's COVID-19 outbreak. Stroke 2020;51:2656–63.

25. Cavallieri F, Marti A, Fasano A, et al. Prothrombotic state induced by COVID-19 infection as trigger for stroke in young patients: a dangerous association. eNeurologicalSci 2020;20:100247.

26. Fridman S, Bullrich MB, Jimenez-Ruiz A, et al. Stroke risk, phenotypes, and death in COVID-19. Neurology 2020;95:e3373–85.

27. Mohamud AY, Griffith B, Rehman M, et al. Intraluminal carotid artery thrombus in COVID-19: another danger of cytokine storm? AJNR Am J Neuroradiol 2020;41:1677–82.

28. Esenwa C, Cheng NT, Lipsitz E, et al. COVID-19-Associated carotid atherothrombosis and stroke. AJNR Am J Neuroradiol 2020;41:1993. –5.

29. Siegler JE, Cardona P, Arenillas JF, et al. Cerebrovascular events and outcomes in hospitalized patients with COVID-19: the SVIN COVID-19 Multinational Registry. Int J Stroke 2021;16(4):437 47.

30. Cavalcanti DD, Raz E, Shapiro M, et al. Cerebral venous thrombosis associated with COVID-19. AJNR Am J Neuroradiol 2020;41:1370–6.

31. Gonçalves B, Righy C, Kurtz P. Thrombotic and hemorrhagic neurological complications in critically ill COVID-19 patients. Neurocrit Care 2020;33: 587–90.

32. Kihira S, Schefflein J, Pawha P, et al. Neurovascular complications that can be seen in COVID-19 patients. Clin Imaging 2021;69:280–4.

33. Chougar L, Mathon B, Weiss N, et al. Atypical deep cerebral vein thrombosis with hemorrhagic venous infarction in a patient positive for COVID-19. AJNR Am J Neuroradiol 2020;41:1377–9.

34. Poillon G, Obadia M, Perrin M, et al. Cerebral venous thrombosis associated with COVID-19 infection: causality or coincidence? J Neuroradiol 2021; 48:121–4.

35. Hughes C, Nichols T, Pike M, et al. Cerebral venous sinus thrombosis as a presentation of COVID-19. Eur J Case Rep Intern Med 2020;7:001691.

36. Patel P, Khandelwal P, Gupta G, et al. COVID-19 and cervical artery dissection- A causative association? J Stroke Cerebrovasc Dis 2020;29:105047.

37. Morassi M, Bigni B, Cobelli M, et al. Bilateral carotid artery dissection in a SARS-CoV-2 infected patient: causality or coincidence? J Neurol 2020;267: 2812–4.

38. Romero-Sánchez CM, Díaz-Maroto I, Fernández-Díaz E, et al. Neurologic manifestations in hospitalized patients with COVID-19: the ALBACOVID registry. Neurology 2020;95:e1060–70.

39. Gasso LF, Maneiro Melon NM, Cebada FS, et al. Multivessel spontaneous coronary artery dissection presenting in a patient with severe acute SARS-CoV-2 respiratory infection. Eur Heart J 2020;41: 3100–1.

40. Fukuhara S, Rosati CM, El-Dalati S. Acute type A aortic dissection during the COVID-19 outbreak. Ann Thorac Surg 2020;110:e405–7.

41. Dixon L, Coughlan C, Karunaratne K, et al. Immunosuppression for intracranial vasculitis associated with SARS-CoV-2: therapeutic implications for COVID-19 cerebrovascular pathology. J Neurol Neurosurg Psychiatry 2020. https://doi.org/10.1136/jnnp-2020-324291.

42. Gulko E, Overby P, Ali S, et al. Vessel wall enhancement and focal cerebral arteriopathy in a pediatric patient with acute infarct and COVID-19 infection. AJNR Am J Neuroradiol 2020;41:2348–50.

43. Mirzaee SMM, Gonçalves FG, Mohammadifard M, et al. Focal cerebral arteriopathy in a pediatric patient with COVID-19. Radiology 2020;297:E274–5.

44. Kihira S, Morgenstern PF, Raynes H, et al. Fatal cerebral infarct in a child with COVID-19. PediatrRadiol 2020;50:1479–80.

45. Sharifi-Razavi A, Karimi N, Rouhani N. COVID-19 and intracerebral haemorrhage: causative or coincidental? New Microbes New Infect 2020;35:100669.

46. Dogra S, Jain R, Cao M, et al. Hemorrhagic stroke and anticoagulation in COVID-19. J Stroke Cerebrovasc Dis 2020;29:104984.

47. Daci R, Kennelly M, Ferris A, et al. Bilateral basal ganglia hemorrhage in a patient with confirmed COVID-19. AJNR Am J Neuroradiol 2020;41:1797–9.

48. Al Saiegh F, Ghosh R, Leibold A, et al. Status of SARS-CoV-2 in cerebrospinal fluid of patients with COVID-19 and stroke. J Neurol Neurosurg Psychiatry 2020;91:846–8.

49. Savić D, Alsheikh TM, Alhaj AK, et al. Ruptured cerebral pseudoaneurysm in an adolescent as an early onset of COVID-19 infection: case report. Acta Neurochir 2020;162:2725–9.

50. Dakay K, Kaur G, Gulko E, et al. Reversible cerebral vasoconstriction syndrome and dissection in the setting of COVID-19 infection. J Stroke Cerebrovasc Dis 2020;29:105011.

51. Franceschi AM, Ahmed O, Giliberto L, et al. Hemorrhagic posterior reversible encephalopathy syndrome as a manifestation of COVID-19 infection. AJNR Am J Neuroradiol 2020;41:1173–6.

52. Doo FX, Kassim G, Lefton DR, et al. Rare presentations of COVID-19: PRES-like leukoencephalopathy and carotid thrombosis. Clin Imaging 2021;69: 94–101.

53. Polimeni A, Leo I, Spaccarotella C, et al. Differences in coagulopathy indices in patients with severe versus non-severe COVID-19: a meta-analysis of 35 studies and 6427 patients. Sci Rep 2021;11. https://doi.org/10.1038/s41598-021-89967-x.

54. Nicholson P, Alshafai L, Krings T. Neuroimaging findings in patients with COVID-19. AJNR Am J Neuroradiol 2020;41:1380–3.

55. Lin E, Lantos JE, Strauss SB, et al. Brain imaging of patients with COVID-19: Findings at an academic institution during the height of the outbreak in New York City. AJNR Am J Neuroradiol 2020;41:2001–8.

56. Wee NK, Fan EB, Lee KCH, et al. CT fluid-blood levels in COVID-19 intracranial hemorrhage. AJNR Am J Neuroradiol 2020;41:E76–7.

57. Masur J, Freeman CW, Mohan S. A double-edged sword: neurologic complications and mortality in extracorporeal membrane oxygenation therapy for COVID-19–related severe acute respiratory distress syndrome at a tertiary care center. AJNR Am J Neuroradiol 2020;41:2009–11.

58. Kowalewski M, Fina D, Słomka A, et al. COVID-19 and ECMO: the interplay between coagulation and inflammation—a narrative review. Crit Care 2020; 24:205.

59. Sachs JR, Gibbs KW, Swor DE, et al. COVID-19–associated Leukoencephalopathy. Radiology 2020; 296:E184–5.

60. Riech S, Kallenberg K, Moerer O, et al. The pattern of brain microhemorrhages after severe lung failure resembles the one seen in high-altitude cerebral edema. Crit Care Med 2015;43:e386–9.

61. Breit H, Jhaveri M, John S. Concomitant delayed posthypoxic leukoencephalopathy and critical illness microbleeds. Neurol Clin Pract 2018;8:e31–3.

62. Kallenberg K, Dehnert C, Dörfler A, et al. Microhemorrhages in nonfatal high-altitude cerebral edema. J Cereb Blood Flow Metab 2008;28:1635–42.

63. Fanou EM, Coutinho JM, Shannon P, et al. Critical illness–associated cerebral microbleeds. Stroke 2017;48:1085–7.

64. Reichard RR, Kashani KB, Boire NA, et al. Neuropathology of COVID-19: a spectrum of vascular and acute disseminated encephalomyelitis (ADEM)-like pathology. Acta Neuropathol 2020;140:1–6.

65. D'Amore F, Vinacci G, Agosti E, et al. Pressing issues in COVID-19: probable cause to seize SARS-CoV-2 for its preferential involvement of posterior circulation manifesting as severe posterior reversible encephalopathy syndrome and posterior strokes. AJNR Am J Neuroradiol 2020;41:1800–3.

66. Conte G, Avignone S, Carbonara M, et al. COVID-19–associated PRES–like encephalopathy with perivascular gadolinium enhancement. AJNR Am J Neuroradiol 2020. https://doi.org/10.3174/ajnr.A6762.

67. Kishfy L, Casasola M, Banankhah P, et al. Posterior reversible encephalopathy syndrome (PRES) as a neurological association in severe COVID-19. J Neurol Sci 2020;414:116943.

68. Rogg J, Baker A, Tung G. Posterior reversible encephalopathy syndrome (PRES): another imaging manifestation of COVID-19. InterdiscipNeurosurg 2020;22:100808.

69. Kihira S, Delman BN, Belani P, et al. Imaging features of acute encephalopathy in patients with COVID-19: A Case Series. AJNR Am J Neuroradiol 2020;41:1804–8.

70. Lang M, Buch K, Li MD, et al. Leukoencephalopathy associated with severe COVID-19 infection: sequela of hypoxemia? AJNR Am J Neuroradiol 2020;41:1641–5.

71. Kandemirli SG, Dogan L, Sarikaya ZT, et al. Brain MRI findings in patients in the intensive care unit with COVID-19 infection. Radiology 2020;297:E232–5.

72. Agarwal S, Conway J, Nguyen V, et al. Serial imaging of virus-associated necrotizing disseminated acute leukoencephalopathy (VANDAL) in COVID-19. AJNR Am J Neuroradiol 2021;42:279–84.

73. Poyiadji N, Shahin G, Noujaim D, et al. COVID-19–associated acute hemorrhagic necrotizing encephalopathy: imaging features. Radiology 2020;296:E119–20.

74. Politi LS, Salsano E, Grimaldi M. Magnetic resonance imaging alteration of the brain in a patient with coronavirus disease 2019 (COVID-19) and anosmia. JAMA Neurol 2020;77:1028–9.

75. Aragão MFVV, Aragão MFV, Leal MC, et al. Anosmia in COVID-19 associated with injury to the olfactory bulbs evident on MRI. AJNR Am J Neuroradiol 2020. https://doi.org/10.3174/ajnr.a6675.

76. Kandemirli SG, Altundag A, Yildirim D, et al. Olfactory bulb MRI and paranasal sinus CT findings in persistent COVID-19 anosmia. Acad Radiol 2021;28:28–35.

77. Corrêa DG, Hygino da Cruz LC Jr, Lopes FCR, et al. Magnetic resonance imaging features of COVID-19-related cranial nerve lesions. J Neurovirol 2021;27:171–7.

78. Goh Y, Beh DLL, Makmur A, et al. Pearls & oysters: facial nerve palsy in COVID-19 infection. Neurology 2020;95:364–7.

79. Lima MA, Silva MTT, Soares CN, et al. Peripheral facial nerve palsy associated with COVID-19. J Neurovirol 2020;26:941–4.

80. Eviston TJ, Croxson GR, Kennedy PGE, et al. Bell's palsy: aetiology, clinical features and multidisciplinary care. J Neurol Neurosurg Psychiatry 2015;86:1356–61.

Coronavirus Disease
Subacute to Chronic Neuroimaging Findings

Monique A. Mogensen, MD[a],*, Christopher G. Filippi, MD[b]

KEYWORDS

• Coronavirus disease • Severe acute respiratory syndrome coronavirus 2 • Neuroimaging
• Postcoronavirus syndrome

KEY POINTS

- Several neuroimaging findings are associated with coronavirus disease 2019 (COVID-19) in the subacute to chronic phase of illness including leukoencephalopathy, microhemorrhages, hypoxic-ischemic injury, and posterior reversible encephalopathy syndrome (PRES).
- Postinfectious immune-mediated syndromes such as acute disseminated encephalomyelitis (ADEM) and Guillain-Barre syndrome (GBS) may be associated with COVID-19, typically in the subacute phase.
- COVID-19-related PRES and ADEM are more commonly associated with intraparenchymal hemorrhage or microhemorrhage than non-COVID-19-related PRES or ADEM, which may be secondary to underlying coagulopathies or vascular endothelial dysfunction.
- Several neurologic and psychiatric symptoms are associated with post-COVID syndrome, and the role of imaging in diagnosis and prognosis remains unclear.

INTRODUCTION

In December of 2019, a novel coronavirus, now known as severe acute respiratory syndrome coronavirus 2 (SARS-CoV-2) emerged from Wuhan, China, causing an illness known as coronavirus disease 2019 (COVID-19).[1] The virus spread worldwide in 2020 creating a global pandemic. As of Aug. 31, 2021, the World Health Organization (WHO) tallied 216,867,420 cases and 4,507,837 deaths worldwide.[2]

Although COVID-19 primarily manifests as a respiratory illness, neurologic involvement is well documented.[3,4] Initial articles reported neurologic complications in 36% (78 of 214) of COVID-19 patients, including dizziness (16.8%), headache (13.1%), and impaired consciousness (7.5%), all

relatively nonspecific.[5] In a later large prospective study, neurologic disorders were diagnosed in 13.5% of hospitalized COVID-19 patients and were associated with increased risk of in-hospital mortality and decreased likelihood of discharge home.[6]

PATHOGENESIS OF NEUROLOGIC INVOLVEMENT BY CORONAVIRUS DISEASE

Multiple theories are proposed for SARS-CoV-2 involvement in the central nervous system (CNS). The systemic immune response to SARS-CoV-2 results in an inflammatory state that can progress to an exaggerated, uncontrolled response known as a cytokine storm mediated by proinflammatory cytokines, which induce endothelial cell dysfunction,

[a] Department of Radiology, University of Washington School of Medicine, 1959 Northeast Pacific Street, Seattle, WA 98195, USA; [b] Department of Radiology, Tufts University School of Medicine, 800 Washington Street, Boston, MA 02111, USA
* Corresponding author.
E-mail address: mogensen@uw.edu

Neuroimag Clin N Am 33 (2023) 69–82
https://doi.org/10.1016/j.nic.2022.07.004
1052-5149/23/© 2022 Elsevier Inc. All rights reserved.

neuroimaging.theclinics.com

vascular damage, and activation of the coagulation cascade resulting in hypercoagulability.[7–9]

Endothelial cell dysfunction may also occur by direct viral interactions with the vascular endothelium via the angiotensin converting enzyme-2 (ACE-2) receptor.[10] The ACE-2 receptor is the obligate receptor for the spike protein of the SARS-CoV-2 virus. This ubiquitous receptor is found throughout the body, including within endothelial cells of arteries and veins and within glial cells and brainstem nuclei.[11] SARS-CoV-2 particles have been found in brain capillary endothelium and adjacent neuronal cells supporting a hematogenous route of neurotropic viral entry into the CNS.[12]

Direct invasion of the CNS by SARS-CoV-2 via neuronal retrograde spread from nasal mucosa to the olfactory bulb has been proposed and is supported by symptoms of anosmia and several autopsy series showing positive SARS-CoV-2 polymerase chain reaction (PCR) signals in the olfactory bulb.[13–17] Lastly, the virus may infect circulating immune cells, which then act as Trojan horses, carrying the virus across the blood-brain-barrier (BBB), facilitating CNS disease.[13] Cerebrospinal fluid (CSF)-confirmed SARS-CoV-2 associated with viral encephalitis has been reported,[18] but more commonly CSF and autopsy samples test negative, suggesting that direct CNS involvement by SARS-CoV-2 is unlikely.[6]

NEUROIMAGING FEATURES IN SUBACUTE TO CHRONIC CORONAVIRUS DISEASE

Regardless of time course since COVID-19 onset, most neuroimaging studies in COVID-19 patients show normal or nonspecific findings.[19,20] One study that imaged 242 patients in the acute to subacute phase of illness (<2 weeks) showed that the most common imaging finding was nonspecific white matter (WM) microangiopathy (55.4%).[20] Early reports on the neuroimaging findings in subacute and chronic COVID-19 infection centered on patients requiring mechanical ventilation in the intensive care unit (ICU) with delayed awakening after sedation. In 1 study, 44% (12 of 27) of COVID-19 ICU patients with neurologic symptoms had positive MRI scans, most showing abnormal cortical or WM signal; the remaining examinations were normal.[19]

Early literature during the acute crisis of a worldwide pandemic was rapidly published, often with incomplete data. Radiologists used clinical information and pattern recognition of well-described radiological entities to assign a diagnostic label or infer pathophysiology of the COVID-19 associated neuroimaging features. This method was both valuable and subject to diagnostic error. Heterogeneity of imaging protocols and treatments in ICU settings also made it difficult to compare imaging findings. Despite these challenges, some common neuroimaging features have emerged in the ICU setting and the subacute to chronic phases of COVID-19 (Table 1). Neuroimaging findings including leukoencephalopathy, microhemorrhages, posterior reversible encephalopathy syndrome (PRES), and hypoxic-ischemic injury are reported and may be the result of an immune response or complications from prolonged illness and treatments. Postinfectious autoimmune manifestations are also reported after the acute COVID-19 infection, including acute disseminated encephalomyelitis (ADEM) and Guillain-Barré syndrome (GBS).[9] Despite overlap between imaging findings, particularly in the ICU setting, recognizing more typical features of each disorder can help the radiologist suggest the most likely diagnosis with implications on treatment and prognosis.

Leukoencephalopathy with or without microhemorrhage

WM changes with or without microhemorrhages can occur in critically ill COVID-19 patients requiring mechanical ventilation and long ICU stays, and are typically detected by imaging later in the hospitalization course.[19,21,22] One study reporting on 35 patients with cerebral leukoencephalopathy and/or microbleeds found patients with these findings had longer hospitalizations, required longer ventilator support, were more severely thrombocytopenic, and had higher D-dimer values.[22]

MRI findings typically show abnormal symmetric and confluent T2-hyperintensity extending from the precentral gyrus through the centrum semiovale and corona radiata, with relative sparing of subcortical and callosal WM that may be more conspicuous on diffusion weighted imaging (DWI) (Fig. 1).[21,22] Associated microhemorrhages vary from a few to innumerable, are predominantly punctate, and involve the subcortical WM and/or corpus collosum, particularly the splenium (Fig. 2). Inconsistently reported or obtained, CSF samples are typically negative for SARS-CoV-2 PCR assay.[19,21]

Previous studies published before the pandemic documented diffuse leukoencephalopathy with or without microhemorrhages along the corticomedullary junction and in the corpus callosum in critically ill ICU patients.[23,24] Studies of mountain climbers with high-altitude cerebral edema also show similar patterns of WM edema, albeit reversible, with callosal involvement followed by accrual

Table 1
Neuroimaging findings in subacute to chronic coronavirus disease infection

Clinical Syndrome	Imaging Findings (Computed Tomography or MRI)	Proposed Pathogenesis
Leukoencephalopathy with or without microhemorrhages	• Symmetric, confluent T2-hyperintensity in cerebral WM with increased conspicuity on DWI extending from precentral gyrus through cerebral WM along corticospinal tracts sparing subcortical and callosal WM • Associated microhemorrhages usually punctate in subcortical WM and corpus collosum (splenium most common)	• Hypoxemia • Endothelial cell dysfunction via immune-mediated cytokine storm or direct viral interactions
PRES	• Symmetric subcortical WM vasogenic edema in parietal-occipital distribution • COVID-19-related PRES more commonly associated with micro- and/or macrohemorrhages	• Endothelial cell dysfunction via immune-mediated cytokine storm or direct viral interaction • Comorbidities and treatment-related complications
Hypoxic-ischemic injury	• Mild: cortical diffusion restriction in border zone distribution • Moderate to severe: restricted diffusion of entire cerebral cortex, hippocampus, basal ganglia, and/or thalamus	Hypoxia from cardiac arrest or profound hypotension
• ADEM • AHLE	• T2-hyperintense lesions in deep WM > corpus collosum and subcortical WM with arc enhancement along leading edge • Lesions may be larger in AHLE • AHLE and COVID-19-related ADEM more likely to have hemorrhagic foci; deep gray matter (GM) involvement is less common • ± spinal cord involvement	Autoimmune-mediated
GBS	• Spinal nerve root and spinal leptomeningeal enhancement • Cranial nerve and brainstem leptomeningeal enhancement	Autoimmune-mediated
MIS-C	• Reversible discrete, ovoid, T2-hyperintense foci with variable diffusion restriction in splenium of corpus callosum most common	Postinfectious immune dysregulation

of microhemorrhages in the subcortical WM and corpus callosum on follow-up MRI.[25]

Despite these apparently divergent narratives of disease, hypoxemia is a common factor, suggesting a similar etiology either related to hypoxemia itself or hypoxic-induced hydrostatic or chemical changes leading to breakdown of the BBB with subsequent microhemorrhages.[23,24] BBB disruption from endothelial damage caused by interactions of SARS-CoV-2 spike proteins with capillary endothelial cells or an exaggerated immune response may also occur,[1,26] since cytokine

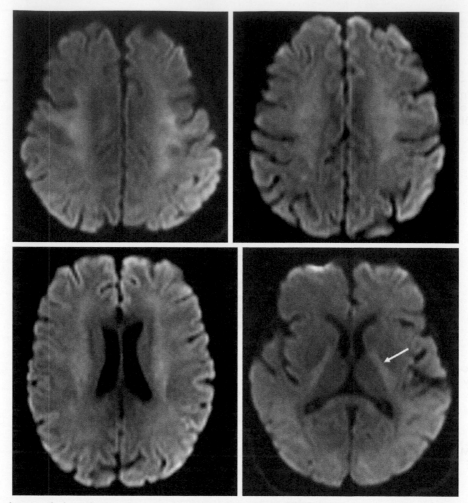

Fig. 1. Leukoencephalopathy in a 67-year-old patient with chronic COVID-19 and encephalopathy. Multiple axial diffusion-weighted images through the brain show symmetric and confluent hyperintensity extending along the corticospinal tracts through the centrum semiovale, corona radiata, and posterior limb of the internal capsule (*white arrow*) with relative sparing of subcortical WM.

release and tissue damage are enhanced in hypoxic conditions.[13]

Another potential explanation for diffuse leukoencephalopathy is a delayed posthypoxic leukoencephalopathy (DPHL) that can develop in ICU patients, and has been reported in intubated patients with subacute COVID-19.[21,27] DPHL typically follows a biphasic course with a period of recovery after hypoxic-ischemic injury follow by neurologic deterioration with leukoencephalopathy on MRI (Fig. 3).[28,29]

Posterior reversible encephalopathy syndrome

PRES is a neurologic disorder presenting with headaches, seizures, and neurologic deficits.[30] Neuroimaging of classic PRES shows symmetric subcortical vasogenic edema in a parietal-

occipital distribution that reverses on follow-up imaging; however, atypical patterns can involve the frontotemporal lobes, basal ganglia, thalamus, and infratentorial brain.[31] Typical risk factors for PRES include hypertension, renal failure, immunosuppressive agents, cytotoxic drugs, (pre)eclampsia, and sepsis.

PRES has been reported in COVID-19 patients, often coexisting with similar risk factors and respiratory distress requiring intensive care (Fig. 4).[32–34] In a retrospective study on COVID-19 patients with neuroimaging (n = 278), the prevalence of PRES was 1.1%.[32] The onset of PRES varies, but most cases occur more than 2 weeks after hospitalization for COVID-19.[34]

The cause of COVID-19-related PRES is unclear, but likely involves endothelial cell dysfunction.[33] In a postmortem MRI virtual autopsy study on COVID-19 patients, findings included

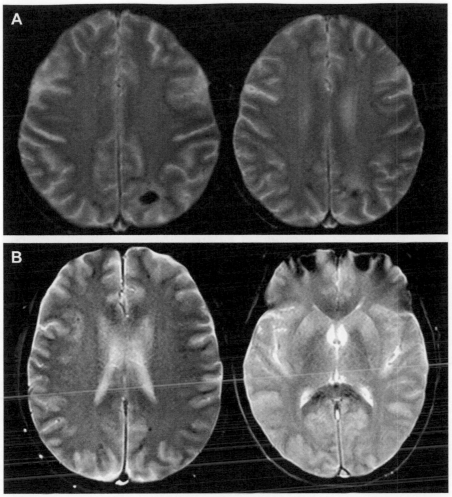

Fig. 2. Leukoencephalopathy with microhemorrhages in 2 COVID-19 patients with encephalopathy and chronic (>3 weeks) ICU stays on mechanical ventilation. Axial T2-weighted images (*A*) in an elderly patient show diffuse WM hyperintensity with hypointense microhemorrhages along the corticomedullary junction bilaterally. Axial susceptibility weighted images (*B*) in a different elderly patient showing punctate foci of susceptibility compatible with microhemorrhages along the corticomedullary junction and within the genu and splenium of the corpus collosum.

subcortical micro- and macrobleeds and cortico-subcortical edema reminiscent of PRES, for which viral-induced endothelial damage either by direct infection or by a systemic cytokine storm was postulated.[35]

Many reported cases of COVID-19-related PRES show evidence of subcortical or callosal micro- and/or macrohemorrhages on MRI susceptibility weighted sequences (**Fig. 5**).[32–34,36,37] Classic PRES is associated with hemorrhages in only about 15% to 30% of patients, suggesting that hemorrhage may be more common in COVID-19-related PRES.[31,38] Coagulopathy from cytokine storm and antithrombotic therapy in combination with endothelial cell dysfunction may increase the risk of developing hemorrhage in COVID-19-related

PRES, necessitating early cessation or reversal of antithrombotic therapy.[33] Approximately 70% to 90% of patients with PRES have clinical recovery with resolution of vasogenic edema on neuroimaging.[34] To date, the literature does not suggest that COVID-19-related PRES has a worse prognosis, but further studies are needed to substantiate this claim. Imaging resolution of vasogenic edema and the parieto-occipital distribution can help differentiate PRES from other leukoencephalopathies associated with COVID-19.

Hypoxic-ischemic injury

Hypoxic-ischemic brain injury is usually caused by an acute event such as cardiac arrest or profound hypotension[39] and can be seen as a presenting or

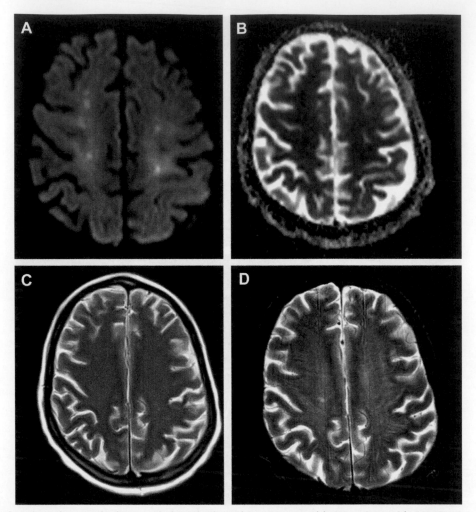

Fig. 3. Delayed posthypoxic leukoencephalopathy (DPHL) in a 71-year-old ICU patient with COVID-19. Initial MRI early in hospitalization prior to intubation with axial DWI (*A*), axial ADC (*B*), and axial T2-weighted (*C*) images showing punctate foci of diffusion restriction compatible with acute infarcts in the centrum semiovale with otherwise normal-appearing WM. Follow-up MRI during the fifth week of hospitalization after prolonged intubation with an axial T2-weighted image (*D*) shows diffuse, symmetric abnormal T2-hyperintensity bilaterally in the centrum semiovale consistent with DPHL.

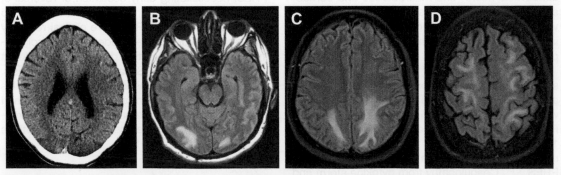

Fig. 4. Posterior reversible encephalopathy syndrome in a 67-year-old patient with subacute COVID-19 infection, hypertension, and diabetes. Axial noncontrast CT (*A*) demonstrates bilateral, symmetric parieto-occipital hypodensities, and axial FLAIR MRI images show relatively symmetric subcortical WM hyperintensities in the parieto-occipital (*B*, *C*) and frontal (*D*) WM.

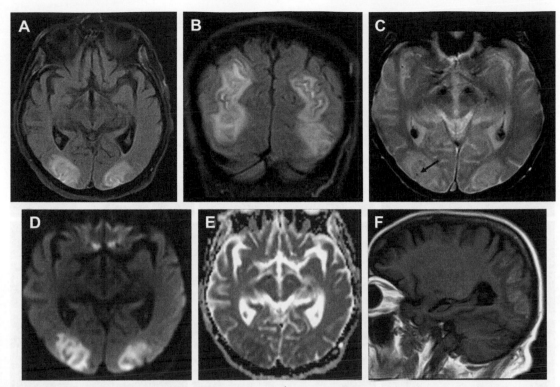

Fig. 5. Posterior reversible encephalopathy syndrome in an ICU patient with subacute to chronic COVID-19 infection and labile hypertension. MRI of the brain shows symmetric abnormal T2-hyperintensity in the parieto-occipital subcortical WM on axial (A) and coronal (B) FLAIR images with associated punctate susceptibility consistent with microhemorrhage on an axial SWI (black arrow, C). Axial DWI (D) and ADC image (E) show reduced diffusivity in the same region. On sagittal T1-weighted imaging (F), there is associated parieto-occipital gyral hyperintensity that may reflect cortical laminar necrosis.

delayed complication of COVID-19 infection. In 1 large study, hypoxic-ischemic injury was more common after hospital admission for COVID-19 and among critically ill patients with respiratory distress, sepsis, acute renal failure, hypoxia, and hypotension.[6]

In milder cases of hypoperfusion or hypo-oxygenation, diffuse hypoxic-ischemic injury shows cortical diffusion restriction on MRI in a border zone distribution (Fig. 6).[40] After a moderate-to-severe hypoxic-ischemic insult, bilateral, symmetric diffuse abnormal signal in the entire cerebral cortex, cerebellum, hippocampus, basal ganglia, and thalamus may be observed.[24,40] Overall, the prognosis is poor, with a high mortality rate and severe neurologic or cognitive deficits in survivors of prolonged and profound hypoxia.[39]

Neuroinflammatory syndromes

Acute disseminated encephalomyelitis and acute hemorrhagic leukoencephalitis

ADEM is a rare immune-mediated demyelinating disorder with delayed neurologic deficits including encephalopathy.[41] ADEM is typically a monophasic illness thought to be secondary to cross-reactivity in immunity to viral antigens and is more common in children and adolescents.[41]

ADEM and its severe variant, acute hemorrhagic leukoencephalitis (AHLE), have been reported after COVID-19 infection, with 80% of cases occurring in adult patients.[42] One study reported a mean interval between onset of COVID-19 and ADEM symptoms of 24.7 days (range 0 to 214 days).[42]

On neuroimaging, classic ADEM typically shows T2-hyperintense lesions of varying sizes in the bilateral supratentorial or infratentorial WM, with variable involvement of the deep gray matter, thalami, and brainstem.[41] Lesions often demonstrate ring or arc contrast enhancement along the leading edge of inflammation. In COVID-19-related ADEM, the deep WM was most frequently involved, followed by the corpus collosum and subcortical WM; contrast enhancement was reported in 89% of cases (Fig. 7).[42] Deep gray matter was less frequently involved compared with classic ADEM. In about one-third of classic ADEM cases, there is spinal cord involvement, which was also noted in COVID-19-related cases.[43,44] One study reported that 42% of

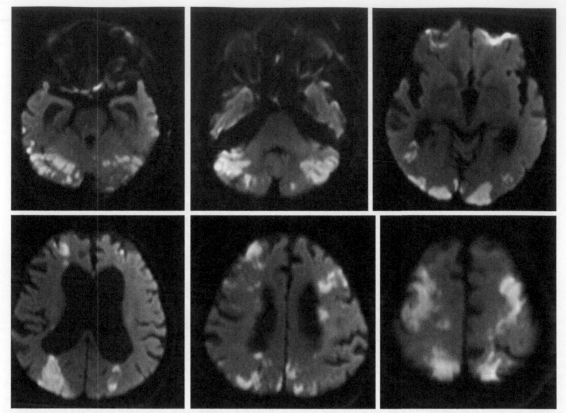

Fig. 6. Hypoxic-ischemic injury in an elderly COVID-19 patient. Multiple axial diffusion-weighted images through the brain show bilateral, symmetric-appearing areas of restricted diffusion compatible with acute infarcts in a border zone distribution suggestive of hypoperfusion.

patients (18 of 43) with COVID-19-related ADEM and AHLE had evidence of intracranial hemorrhage on neuroimaging, which is significantly higher than that seen with classic ADEM.[44] Like COVID-19-related PRES, COVID-19-related ADEM may be more susceptible to hemorrhagic changes because of underlying coagulopathies or endothelial dysfunction.

Of note, almost two-thirds of COVID-19 patients who developed ADEM or AHLE needed intensive care for the antecedent infection.[44] Unlike classic ADEM, the morbidity associated with COVID-19-related ADEM and AHLE was high even with standard treatments, and mortality ranged from 10% to 32%, suggesting it is a relatively poor prognostic marker.[42,44]

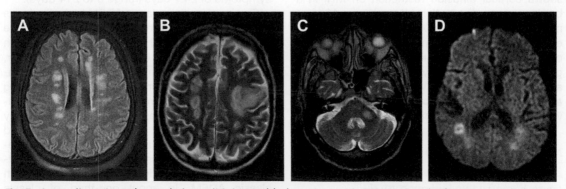

Fig. 7. Acute disseminated encephalomyelitis in an elderly patient with COVID-19 and subacute encephalopathy. Noncontrast MRI of the brain with axial FLAIR (A) and T2-weighted (B, C) images show ovoid and ring-like hyperintense lesions in the periventricular WM and left brachium pontis most compatible with demyelinating lesions, with several posterior lesions demonstrating restricted diffusion on axial DWI (D).

Guillain-Barré syndrome

An association of GBS with SARS-CoV-2 infection is recognized, with the overall prevalence of GBS in the COVID-19 population (approximately 15 cases per 100,000 population) exceeding the general population (approximately 2 cases per 100,000 population).[45] GBS includes a spectrum of immune-mediated polyneuropathies with multiple subtypes triggered by multiple different viral and bacterial infections.[46]

A systematic review of 73 patients with COVID-19 and GBS from 52 publications reported that most cases resembled the classic acute inflammatory demyelinating polyradiculopathy (AIDP) subtype.[47] In nearly all patients (n = 68), symptoms of GBS developed after COVID-19 symptoms (median = 14 days). A subsequent systematic review reporting on 109 patients similarly found that COVID-19-related GBS most commonly presents as the AIDP subtype, often with facial palsy.[48] Another large systematic review and meta-analysis reported patients with COVID-19 (n = 136,746) had increased odds for demyelinating GBS subtypes (odds ratio [OR] 3.27, 95% confidence interval [CI]:1.32–8.09) with olfactory or cranial nerve involvement in 41.4% and 42.8%, respectively.[45]

Brain and spinal MRI in COVID-19-related GBS can show cranial nerve enhancement, brainstem leptomeningeal enhancement, or spinal nerve root or cord leptomeningeal enhancement (Fig. 8).[47] CSF SARS-CoV-2 PCR assay is typically negative, and most patients (>70%) have a good prognosis after treatment with intravenous immunoglobulin comparable to noninfected contemporary or historical GBS controls.[45,47]

The CSF results, response to treatment, and approximate 2-week latency between COVID-19 symptoms and onset of GBS all suggest a postinfectious autoimmune-mediated mechanism. However, further studies are needed to determine the association and pathophysiological mechanism of GBS in COVID-19 patients.[46,48] The causal association between COVID-19 and GBS is controversial. Retrospective epidemiologic data and a prospective cohort study from the United Kingdom did not support any significant causal association between COVID-19 and GBS.[49]

CORONAVIRUS DISEASE NEUROLOGIC INVOLVEMENT IN CHILDREN AND ADOLESCENTS

Children and adolescents are mostly spared severe COVID-19 infection; however, when they are hospitalized, 1 multicenter cohort estimated 22% (365/1695) have neurologic involvement.[50]

Another recent large study found that among hospitalized children and adolescents (n = 1334), neurologic or psychiatric manifestations are common (3.8 cases per 100), with most patients presenting after their acute COVID-19 illness had resolved.[51]

Neurologic symptoms in these young patients are often attributed to a parainfectious or postinfectious immune-mediated disorder such as ADEM. Nevertheless, some patients also present with a novel inflammatory process termed multisystem inflammatory syndrome in children (MIS-C).[51] The most common neurologic symptom in patients with MIS-C is encephalopathy, typically occurring weeks after SARS-CoV-2 infection. In 1 study, two-thirds of MIS-C patients with neurologic symptoms (17 of 23 patients) had abnormal brain imaging, most commonly showing reversible splenial lesions in the corpus collosum.[51] Splenial lesions in this patient population appear as ovoid, T2-hyperintense foci with variable restricted diffusion, sometimes extending into adjacent WM.[52]

Patients with MIS-C were more likely to require supportive care in the ICU than pediatric patients with other COVID-19-related neurologic diseases; however, early outcomes were similar, with death being uncommon and disability in approximately one-third of patients.[51] Future studies are needed to determine long-term neurocognitive outcomes in children.

POSTCORONAVIRUS SYNDROME: LONG HAULERS

There is increasing evidence of distinct, chronic manifestations of COVID-19 infection that affect multiple organ systems.[53] Chronic or long-term COVID-19 symptoms have been referred to as postacute sequelae of SARS-COV-2 (PASC), post-COVID syndrome, or long COVID. People suffering with chronic COVID-19 symptoms are sometimes called long haulers. An exact medical definition of post-COVID syndrome is evolving. Recent literature suggests a couple of definitions: (a) subacute or ongoing COVID-19 infection including symptoms or abnormalities 4 to 12 weeks beyond acute COVID-19 infection and/or (b) chronic or post-COVID syndrome in which symptoms or abnormalities persist beyond 12 weeks of acute COVID-19 infection not attributable to another diagnosis.[53]

Post-COVID syndrome symptoms include fatigue, brain fog (cognitive impairment), headache, numbness/tingling, dysgeusia, anosmia, and myalgias.[53-55] Neuropsychiatric symptoms have also been reported in up to 30% to 40% of COVID-19 survivors including anxiety, depression,

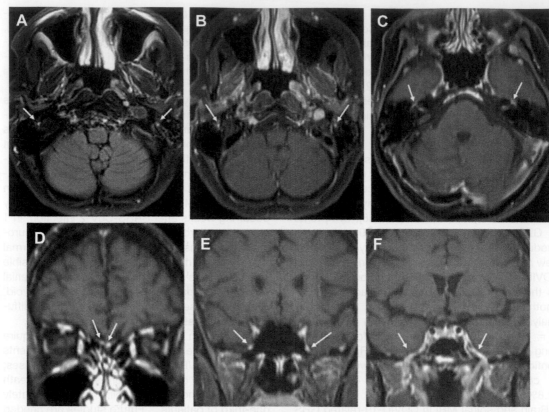

Fig. 8. Acute motor and sensory axonal neuropathy (AMSAN) subtype of Guillain-Barré syndrome in a 63-year-old patient who recovered from COVID-19 respiratory illness 3 weeks prior and then developed facial palsy, difficulty swallowing, and ascending numbness. MRI of the brain with axial postgadolinium FLAIR (*A*) and postgadolinium T1-weighted (*B, C*) images through the skull base show abnormal enhancement of the mastoid (*arrows, A, B*) canalicular, labyrinthine, and tympanic segments (*arrows, C*) of the facial nerves bilaterally. Coronal T1-weighted postgadolinium images show abnormal enhancement along the bilateral olfactory (*arrows, D*), V2 (*arrows, E*) and V3 (*arrows, F*) segments of the trigeminal nerves.

sleep disturbances, and post-traumatic stress disorder, which is similar to that reported with other coronaviruses.[53,55,56] Chronic neuropsychiatric sequelae have also been reported with other less common types of viral encephalitis.[57]

A study of 62,354 COVID-19 survivors showed a significantly higher likelihood of a new psychiatric diagnosis compared to controls, including anxiety and mood disorders, sleep disturbances, and dementia in the elderly.[58] In a retrospective cohort study of 236,379 COVID-19 survivors, the incidence of a neurologic or psychiatric diagnosis 6 months following the acute infection was 33.6%, with 12.8% receiving such a diagnosis for the first time.[59] For patients with severe COVID-19 infection prompting ICU admission, risks were greater, with 46.4% receiving a neurologic or psychiatric diagnosis 6 months following the acute infection and 25.8% receiving such a diagnosis for the first time.[59] In another study of 18 patients with mild-to-moderate COVID-19 infection nearly 3 months following recovery,

over 75% had problems with memory, attention, and concentration, suggesting that even with milder infections, long-term cognitive deficits are a potential sequela.[60]

Confounding the post-COVID syndrome discussion is that many of the known complications of COVID-19 infection such as stroke, hypoxic-ischemic injury, and leukoencephalopathy leave surviving patients with long-term neurologic deficits that may manifest as lingering symptoms.[53] It remains puzzling that post-COVID syndrome affects patients across the entire spectrum of disease severity from the relatively asymptomatic to ICU patients. One study involving over 4000 COVID-19 survivors reported that age greater than 70, more than 5 symptoms during the acute illness, presence of comorbidities, and female sex were associated with higher risk of development of post-COVID syndrome.[61]

Potential pathophysiologic mechanisms of post-COVID syndrome are similar to those proposed for COVID-19 CNS involvement.[53] Stefano

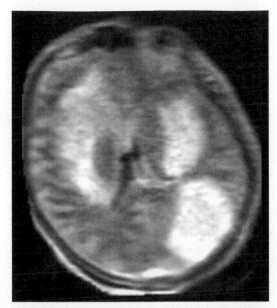

Fig. 9. Ultralow field (0.064 Tesla) portable MRI in an ICU patient with COVID-19. Axial T2-weighted image shows areas of bilateral infarction. Portable MRI was used as a triage tool in the height of the pandemic particularly in chronically intubated patients.

and colleagues[62] also postulated that cerebral hypoxia causes neuronal cell metabolic derangement and mitochondrial dysfunction, leading to cognitive impairment. Others proposed that post-COVID syndrome symptoms overlap with those of myalgic encephalomyelitis/chronic fatigue syndrome such that there may commonality in terms of pathophysiology.[54]

There is also imaging evidence of limbic structural brain changes in patients with cognitive decline after milder COVID-19 infection not requiring hospitalization. A longitudinal imaging study utilized the UK Biobank to compare brain MRIs from individuals before and after COVID-19 infection to well-matched controls and demonstrated a greater reduction in gray matter thickness in the orbitofrontal cortex and parahippocampal gyrus, as well as greater changes in mean diffusivity in areas functionally connected to the olfactory cortex.[63]

As of this writing, it is not clear how long the symptoms reported with post-COVID syndrome will last, nor is it clear what role imaging may play in diagnosis or prognosis. Advanced neuroimaging such as diffusion tensor imaging (DTI), cerebral fluorodeoxyglucose (FDG)-positron emission tomography (PET), and perfusion imaging may lead to better understanding of how COVID-19 impacts neuroconnectivity and function.[64–67]

CHALLENGES AND LIMITATIONS

Early in the COVID-19 pandemic, neuroimaging was performed on only the sickest patients because of the contagious nature of SARS-CoV-2. Safety concerns around transportation to imaging suites and the repeated use of imaging equipment, coupled with the inherent challenges of scanning patients on mechanical ventilation, limit the complete understanding of the prevalence of subacute to chronic neuroimaging findings in COVID-19 patients. One potential alternative for critically ill patients in the ICU setting is the use of a low-field (0.064-T) portable MRI at bedside (**Fig. 9**).[68] One study obtained neuroimaging in 20 patients with COVID-19 on ventilation using portable, low-field MRI at bedside and observed positive neuroimaging findings in 40% of patients.[68] Imaging critically ill SARS-CoV-2 patients with encephalopathy is challenging but should be considered given the potential to inform treatment planning and prognosis.

Determining the etiology or causality of chronic CNS complications in COVID-19 infection is challenging given the novel nature of the disease, emergence of novel variants, a complex clinical course, particularly in ICU patients, and polypharmacy from different treatment regimens. There remains a critical, unmet need for histopathology, CSF-specific markers, and autopsy studies to establish with greater certainty the pathophysiology and long-term consequences of SARS-CoV-2 on the CNS. Collaborative and thoughtful future research efforts by radiologists will lead to greater understanding of the role of neuroimaging in evaluating COVID-19 CNS complications.

SUMMARY

COVID-19 is associated with subacute to chronic neurologic disorders related to immune system activation resulting in coagulopathy and cytokine storm with endothelial cell dysfunction that may lead to leukoencephalopathy, microhemorrhages, and PRES. Immune system activation may also manifest as autoimmune disorders such as ADEM and GBS. Comorbidities such as hypertension play a role in development of PRES, and complications from critical illness and prolonged ICU stays contribute to hypoxic-ischemic injury and leukoencephalopathy. Evidence for direct viral invasion of the CNS is minimal, but it may play a role in olfactory symptoms. Future imaging studies utilizing databases and advanced neuroimaging may help to establish the long-term consequences of SARS-CoV-2 on the CNS.

CLINICS CARE POINTS

- Neuroimaging findings of leukoencephalopathy and ADEM are relatively poor prognostic markers in COVID-19 patients.
- Prognosis of COVID-19-related and non-COVID-19-related PRES and GBS is similar.
- Currently, the role of imaging in Post-COVID syndrome remains unclear.

DISCLOSURE

The authors have nothing to disclose.

REFERENCES

1. Baig AM, Khaleeq A, Ali U, et al. Evidence of the COVID-19 virus targeting the CNS: tissue distribution, host-virus interaction, and proposed neurotropic mechanisms. ACS Chem Neurosci 2020; 11(7):995–8.
2. WHO Coronavirus (COVID-19) Dashboard. Available at: https://covid19.who.int. Accessed September 5, 2021.
3. Revzin MV, Raza S, Srivastava NC, et al. Multisystem imaging manifestations of COVID-19, part 2: from cardiac complications to pediatric manifestations. Radiographics 2020;40(7):1866–92.
4. Gulko E, Oleksk ML, Gomes W, et al. MRI brain findings in 126 patients with COVID-19: initial observations from a descriptive literature review. AJNR Am J Neuroradiol 2020;41(12):2199–203.
5. Mao L, Jin H, Wang M, et al. Neurologic manifestations of hospitalized patients with coronavirus disease 2019 in Wuhan, China. JAMA Neurol 2020; 77(6):683.
6. Frontera JA, Sabadia S, Lalchan R, et al. A prospective study of neurologic disorders in hospitalized patients with COVID-19 in New York City. Neurology 2021;96(4):e575.
7. Ragab D, Salah Eldin H, Taeimah M, et al. The COVID-19 cytokine storm; what we know so far. Front Immunol 2020;11:1446.
8. Katz JM, Libman RB, Wang JJ, et al. COVID-19 severity and stroke: correlation of imaging and laboratory markers. Am J Neuroradiol 2021;42(2):257–61.
9. Moonis G, Filippi CG, Kirsch CFE, et al. The spectrum of neuroimaging findings on CT and MRI in adults with coronavirus disease (COVID-19). AJR Am J Roentgenol 2020. https://doi.org/10.2214/AJR.20.24839.
10. Varga Z, Flammer AJ, Steiger P, et al. Endothelial cell infection and endotheliitis in COVID-19. Lancet Lond Engl 2020;395(10234):1417–8.
11. Xia H, Lazartigues E. Angiotensin-converting enzyme 2 in the brain: properties and future directions. J Neurochem 2008;107(6):1482–94.
12. Paniz-Mondolfi A, Bryce C, Grimes Z, et al. Central nervous system involvement by severe acute respiratory syndrome coronavirus-2 (SARS-CoV-2). J Med Virol 2020;92(7):699–702.
13. Li Z, Liu T, Yang N, et al. Neurological manifestations of patients with COVID-19: potential routes of SARS-CoV-2 neuroinvasion from the periphery to the brain. Front Med 2020;14(5):533–41.
14. Serrano GE, Walker JE, Arce R, et al. Mapping of SARS-CoV-2 brain invasion and histopathology in COVID-19 disease. medRxiv 2021. https://doi.org/10.1101/2021.02.15.21251511.
15. Deigendesch N, Sironi L, Kutza M, et al. Correlates of critical illness-related encephalopathy predominate postmortem COVID-19 neuropathology. Acta Neuropathol (Berl) 2020;140(4):583–6.
16. Meinhardt J, Radke J, Dittmayer C, et al. Olfactory transmucosal SARS-CoV-2 invasion as a port of central nervous system entry in individuals with COVID-19. Nat Neurosci 2021;24(2):168–75.
17. Solomon IH, Normandin E, Bhattacharyya S, et al. Neuropathological features of COVID-19. N Engl J Med 2020;383(10):989–92.
18. Moriguchi T, Harii N, Goto J, et al. A first case of meningitis/encephalitis associated with SARS-Coronavirus-2. Int J Infect Dis 2020;94:55–8.
19. Kandemirli SG, Dogan L, Sarikaya ZT, et al. Brain MRI findings in patients in the intensive care unit with COVID-19 infection. Radiology 2020;297(1):E232–5.
20. Radmanesh A, Raz E, Zan E, et al. Brain imaging use and findings in COVID-19: a single academic center experience in the epicenter of disease in the United States. AJNR Am J Neuroradiol 2020; 41(7):1179–83.
21. Radmanesh A, Derman A, Lui YW, et al. COVID-19-associated diffuse leukoencephalopathy and microhemorrhages. Radiology 2020;297(1):E223–7.
22. Agarwal S, Jain R, Dogra S, et al. Cerebral microbleeds and leukoencephalopathy in critically ill patients with COVID-19. Stroke 2020;51(9):2649–55.
23. Fanou EM, Coutinho JM, Shannon P, et al. Critical illness-associated cerebral microbleeds. Stroke 2017;48(4):1085–7.
24. Muttikkal TJE, Wintermark M. MRI patterns of global hypoxic-ischemic injury in adults. J Neuroradiol J Neuroradiol 2013;40(3):164–71.
25. Hackett PH, Yarnell PR, Weiland DA, et al. Acute and evolving MRI of high-altitude cerebral edema: microbleeds, edema, and pathophysiology. AJNR Am J Neuroradiol 2019;40(3):464–9.
26. Mehta P, McAuley DF, Brown M, et al. COVID-19: consider cytokine storm syndromes and immunosuppression. Lancet 2020;395(10229):1033–4.

27. Lang M, Buch K, Li MD, et al. Leukoencephalopathy associated with severe COVID-19 infection: sequela of hypoxemia? AJNR Am J Neuroradiol 2020;41(9): 1641–5.

28. Zamora CA, Nauen D, Hynecek R, et al. Delayed posthypoxic leukoencephalopathy: a case series and review of the literature. Brain Behav 2015;5(8): e00364.

29. Beeskow AB, Oberstadt M, Saur D, et al. Delayed post-hypoxic leukoencephalopathy (DPHL)-an uncommon variant of hypoxic brain damage in adults. Front Neurol 2018;9:708.

30. Fischer M, Schmutzhard E. Posterior reversible encephalopathy syndrome. J Neurol 2017;264(8): 1608–16.

31. Liman TG, Bohner G, Heuschmann PU, et al. The clinical and radiological spectrum of posterior reversible encephalopathy syndrome: the retrospective Berlin PRES study. J Neurol 2012;259(1): 155–64.

32. Lin E, Lantos JE, Strauss SB, et al. Brain imaging of patients with COVID-19: findings at an academic institution during the height of the outbreak in New York City. AJNR Am J Neuroradiol 2020;41(11): 2001–8.

33. Motolese F, Ferrante M, Rossi M, et al. Posterior reversible encephalopathy syndrome and brain haemorrhage as COVID-19 complication: a review of the available literature. J Neurol 2021;1–8. https://doi.org/10.1007/s00415-021-10709-0.

34. Anand P, Lau KHV, Chung DY, et al. Posterior reversible encephalopathy syndrome in patients with coronavirus disease 2019: two cases and a review of the literature. J Stroke Cerebrovasc Dis 2020;29(11): 105212.

35. Coolen T, Lolli V, Sadeghi N, et al. Early postmortem brain MRI findings in COVID-19 non-survivors. Neurology 2020;95(14):e2016–27.

36. Dias DA, de Brito LA, Neves L de O, et al. Hemorrhagic PRES: an unusual neurologic manifestation in two COVID-19 patients. Arq Neuropsiquiatr 2020;78:739–40.

37. Franceschi AM, Ahmed O, Giliberto L, et al. Hemorrhagic posterior reversible encephalopathy syndrome as a manifestation of COVID-19 infection. Am J Neuroradiol 2020;41(7):1173–6.

38. Hefzy HM, Bartynski WS, Boardman JF, et al. Hemorrhage in posterior reversible encephalopathy syndrome: imaging and clinical features. AJNR Am J Neuroradiol 2009;30(7):1371–9.

39. Howard RS, Holmes PA, Koutroumanidis MA. Hypoxic-ischaemic brain injury. Pract Neurol 2011; 11(1):4–18.

40. White ML, Zhang Y, Helvey JT, et al. Anatomical patterns and correlated MRI findings of non-perinatal hypoxic-ischaemic encephalopathy. Br J Radiol 2013;86(1021):20120464.

41. Pohl D, Alper G, Van Haren K, et al. Acute disseminated encephalomyelitis: updates on an inflammatory CNS syndrome. Neurology 2016;87(9):S38–45.

42. Wang Y, Wang Y, Huo L, et al. SARS-CoV-2-associated acute disseminated encephalomyelitis: a systematic review of the literature. J Neurol 2021;1–22. https://doi.org/10.1007/s00415-021-10771-8.

43. Paterson RW, Brown RL, Benjamin L, et al. The emerging spectrum of COVID-19 neurology: clinical, radiological and laboratory findings. Brain 2020; 143(10):3104–20.

44. Manzano GS, McEntire CRS, Martinez-Lage M, et al. Acute disseminated encephalomyelitis and acute hemorrhagic leukoencephalitis following COVID-19: systematic review and meta-synthesis. Neurol Neuroimmunol Neuroinflammation 2021;8(6):e1080.

45. Palaiodimou L, Stefanou M, Katsanos AH, et al. Prevalence, clinical characteristics and outcomes of Guillain–Barré syndrome spectrum associated with COVID-19: a systematic review and meta-analysis. Eur J Neurol 2021. https://doi.org/10.1111/ene. 14860.

46. Agosti E, Giorgianni A, D'Amore F, et al. Is Guillain-Barrè syndrome triggered by SARS-CoV-2? Case report and literature review. Neurol Sci 2021;42(2): 607–12.

47. Abu-Rumeileh S, Abdelhak A, Foschi M, et al. Guillain–Barré syndrome spectrum associated with COVID-19: an up-to-date systematic review of 73 cases. J Neurol 2021;268(4):1133–70.

48. Aladawi M, Elfil M, Abu-Esheh B, et al. Guillain-Barre syndrome as a complication of COVID-19: a systematic review. Can J Neurol Sci J Can Sci Neurol 1-11. doi:10.1017/cjn.2021.102.

49. Keddie S, Pakpoor J, Mousele C, et al. Epidemiological and cohort study finds no association between COVID-19 and Guillain-Barré syndrome. Brain 2020;awaa433. https://doi.org/10.1093/brain/awaa433.

50. LaRovere KL, Riggs BJ, Poussaint TY, et al. Neurologic involvement in children and adolescents hospitalized in the United States for COVID-19 or multisystem inflammatory syndrome. JAMA Neurol 2021;78(5):536–47.

51. Ray STJ, Abdel-Mannan O, Sa M, et al. Neurological manifestations of SARS-CoV-2 infection in hospitalised children and adolescents in the UK: a prospective national cohort study. Lancet Child Adolesc Health 2021;5(9):631–41.

52. Lindan CE, Mankad K, Ram D, et al. Neuroimaging manifestations in children with SARS-CoV-2 infection: a multinational, multicentre collaborative study. Lancet Child Adolesc Health 2021;5(3):167–77.

53. Nalbandian A, Sehgal K, Gupta A, et al. Post-acute COVID-19 syndrome. Nat Med 2021;27(4):601–15.

54. Graham EL, Clark JR, Orban ZS, et al. Persistent neurologic symptoms and cognitive dysfunction in

non-hospitalized COVID-19 "long haulers. Ann Clin Transl Neurol 2021;8(5):1073–85.

55. Huang C, Huang L, Wang Y, et al. 6-month consequences of COVID-19 in patients discharged from hospital: a cohort study. Lancet 2021;397(10270): 220–32. https://doi.org/10.1016/S0140-6736(20) 32656-8.

56. Rogers JP, Chesney E, Oliver D, et al. Psychiatric and neuropsychiatric presentations associated with severe coronavirus infections: a systematic review and meta-analysis with comparison to the COVID-19 pandemic. Lancet Psychiatry 2020;7(7):611–27.

57. Ng BY, Lim CCT, Yeoh A, et al. Neuropsychiatric sequelae of Nipah virus encephalitis. J Neuropsychiatry Clin Neurosci 2004;16(4):500–4.

58. Taquet M, Luciano S, Geddes JR, et al. Bidirectional associations between COVID-19 and psychiatric disorder: retrospective cohort studies of 62 354 COVID-19 cases in the USA. Lancet Psychiatry 2021;8(2):130–40.

59. Taquet M, Geddes JR, Husain M, et al. 6-month neurological and psychiatric outcomes in 236 379 survivors of COVID-19: a retrospective cohort study using electronic health records. Lancet Psychiatry 2021;8(5):416–27.

60. Mazza MG, De Lorenzo R, Conte C, et al. Anxiety and depression in COVID-19 survivors: role of inflammatory and clinical predictors. Brain Behav Immun 2020;89:594–600.

61. Sudre CH, Murray B, Varsavsky T, et al. Attributes and predictors of long COVID. Nat Med 2021; 27(4):626–31.

62. Stefano GB, Ptacek R, Ptackova H, et al. Selective neuronal mitochondrial targeting in SARS-CoV-2 infection affects cognitive processes to induce 'brain fog' and results in behavioral changes that favor viral survival. Med Sci Monit Int Med J Exp Clin Res 2021;27:e930886-1–930886-4.

63. Douaud G, Lee S, Alfaro-Almagro F, et al. SARS-CoV-2 is associated with changes in brain structure in UK Biobank. Nature 2022;1–17. https://doi.org/10. 1038/s41586-022-04569-5.

64. Hugon J, Msika EF, Queneau M, et al. Long COVID: cognitive complaints (brain fog) and dysfunction of the cingulate cortex. J Neurol 2021;1–3. https://doi. org/10.1007/s00415-021-10655-x.

65. Blazhenets G, Schroeter N, Bormann T, et al. Altered regional cerebral function and its association with cognitive impairment in COVID-19: A prospective FDG PET study. J Nucl Med 2021;62(Suppl 1):41.

66. Lu Y, Li X, Geng D, et al. Cerebral micro-structural changes in COVID-19 Patients – an MRI-based 3-month follow-up study. EClinicalMedicine 2020;25. https://doi.org/10.1016/j.eclinm.2020.100484.

67. Qin Y, Wu J, Chen T, et al. Long-term microstructure and cerebral blood flow changes in patients recovered from COVID-19 without neurological manifestations. J Clin Invest 2021;131(8):147329.

68. Sheth KN, Mazurek MH, Yuen MM, et al. Assessment of brain injury using portable, low-field magnetic resonance imaging at the bedside of critically ill patients. JAMA Neurol 2021;78(1):41–7.

Imaging of Uncommon Bacterial, Rickettsia, Spirochete, and Fungal Infections

Jitender Saini, MBBS, MD[a],*, Shilpa S. Sankhe, MD, DNB[b],
Aleum Lee, MD, PhD[c]

KEYWORDS

• Bacterial infections • Rickettsia • Spirochetes • Fungal infections • Aspergillosis • Mucormycosis

KEY POINTS

• Cerebral abscess and meningitis are frequent manifestations of bacterial and fungal infection, with distinct imaging findings.
• Uncommon bacterial organisms and fungal infections may show preferential anatomic involvement and unique patterns of disease spread, resulting in specific imaging manifestations that could serve as imaging hallmarks aiding in the accurate diagnosis of these organisms.
• Rickettsia infections are associated with a variety of imaging appearances, including scattered foci of white matter lesions.
• Borrelia infection is characterized by scattered white matter lesions and cranial neuritis, whereas neurosyphilis manifestations depend on the stage of the disease, with imaging phenotypes ranging from granulomatous meningitis, gummas, vascular changes, and ischemic lesions as well as brain parenchymal and spinal cord signal abnormalities.

INTRODUCTION

The imaging evaluation of patients with a suspected central nervous system (CNS) infection typically includes a computed tomography (CT) scan, which is usually performed in emergency room. MR imaging has higher sensitivity and specificity for detecting brain parenchymal and meningeal abnormalities, with added information provided by MR diffusion-weighted imaging (DWI) and MR spectroscopy (MRS). Bacterial infections of the CNS usually manifest as meningitis, encephalitis, ventriculitis, cerebral abscess, subdural, and epidural empyema.[1] Most of the bacterial organisms follow these patterns of CNS involvement and show similar stereotypical imaging features as described in Article 2: "Imaging Patterns of Meningitis, Ventriculitis, Cerebritis and Abscess." Nevertheless, certain bacteria such as brucella, spirochetes, rickettsia, and actinomycosis may exhibit atypical neuroimaging patterns that can aid in their identification. CNS fungal infections are infrequent and are usually seen in patients with underlying predisposing conditions. Common fungal infections may show characteristic imaging findings that can help in early diagnosis and thereby expedite the initiation of specific antifungal therapy. In this article, the

[a] Department of Neuroimaging and Interventional Radiology, Faculty Block, 3rd Floor, National institute of Mental health and Neurosciences, Hosur Road, Near Bangalore Milk Dairy, Bangalore, Karnataka 560029, India; [b] Department of Radiology, King Edward Memorial Hospital, Parel, Mumbai 400012, India; [c] Department of Radiology, Soon Chun Hyang University Hospital, 170 Jomaruro, Bucheonsi, Gyunggido, Bucheon 14584, Republic of Korea
* Corresponding author.
E-mail address: jsaini76@gmail.com

Neuroimag Clin N Am 33 (2023) 83–103
https://doi.org/10.1016/j.nic.2022.07.005
1052-5149/23/© 2022 Elsevier Inc. All rights reserved.

authors review imaging features of atypical bacterial and common fungal infections affecting brain.

Bacterial Infections

Many uncommon bacterial infections tend to have a restricted geographic distribution, propensity to cause granulomatous disease, or preferentially involve specific anatomic structures such as the brainstem, cranial nerves, dura, or blood vessels, resulting in atypical but distinct neuroimaging patterns. Knowledge of these imaging findings can assist in establishing the correct diagnosis, recommending appropriate laboratory investigations and starting recommended therapy. Most importantly, many of these can be treated using antibiotics that are readily available.

Neurobrucellosis

Neurobrucellosis is a chronic granulomatous multisystemic infection caused by an intracellular bacterium of the genus Brucella and is commonly detected in people engaged in animal husbandry and agriculture.[2] Human transmission occurs through direct contact or consumption of infected milk products. The organism enters the circulation via the local reticuloendothelial system and subsequently circulates throughout the body including the meninges and CNS.[3,4]

Imaging: Cranial imaging findings include inflammatory lesions such as meningitis, brain abscess, granulomas, white matter (WM) lesions, and stroke (Table 1). Meningeal enhancement may be associated with cranial nerve thickening and enhancement, most commonly affecting the vestibulocochlear nerve.[5] Other cranial nerves including the optic nerve and optic chiasma may also be affected. Granulomas appear as focal nodular enhancing brain lesions, whereas Brucella abscess demonstrates imaging findings similar to those of other bacterial abscesses.[3,6] There could be focal or diffuse demyelinating WM lesions that may look like multiple sclerosis lesions. Larger, confluent WM lesions involving arcuate fibers or periventricular regions have been reported[2,5] (Fig. 1). Infectious vasculitis may appear as lacunar infarcts in the perforator territories or large territorial infarcts.[7] Microaneurysm rupture–related hemorrhage can be seen in patients with Brucella endocarditis.[3]

Neuromelioidosis

Neuromelioidosis is caused by *Burkholderia pseudomallei*, which is a gram-negative aerobic bacillus found in the soil and water in the tropics and enters the human body via skin abrasions, inhalation, and ingestion.[8] Important risk factors for

Table 1
Summary of clinical and imaging findings in neurobrucellosis

Organism	Brucella melitensis, Brucella abortus, Brucella suis, Brucella canis
Transmission	Consumption of unpasteurized animal milk products, contact with infected animal and animal parts, inhalation of aerosolized particles
Neurologic forms of disease	1. Meningitis, meningoencephalitis, encephalitis, brain abscess, vascular disease, and demyelination. 2. Pseudotumor cerebri 3. Peripheral neuropathy and radiculopathy 4. Spinal arachnoiditis, epidural empyema, and spondylodiscitis
Imaging findings	1. Normal study 2. Meningeal enhancement 3. Nodular enhancing granulomatous parenchymal lesions 4. Cerebral abscess with imaging features similar to other bacterial abscesses 5. Discrete WM signal changes appearing hyperintense on T2W/FLAIR images 6. Vascular manifestations include lacunar infarcts, venous thrombosis, and hemorrhages. Mycotic aneurysms may be seen

Abbreviation: T2W/FLAIR, T2-weighted/fluid-attenuated inversion recovery.

melioidosis include diabetes mellitus and immunosuppression.[8] It mainly infects the lungs, skin, and genitourinary system. CNS infection is uncommon, manifesting as encephalitis, brain abscesses, cranial nerve palsies, and myelitis[9–11] (Table 2).

Imaging: Multiple, small enhancing lesions or clusters of well-formed abscesses may be seen in the cerebral parenchyma. Lesions may be seen spreading along the commissural and projection WM tracts. Cranial nerve enhancement, particularly along the fifth nerve may be seen[9] (Fig. 2). Other findings include isolated leptomeningeal disease, focal extradural collection, and overlying bone infection.[9,10] A list of CNS infections that may be associated with cranial nerve enhancement is enumerated in Box 1.[12]

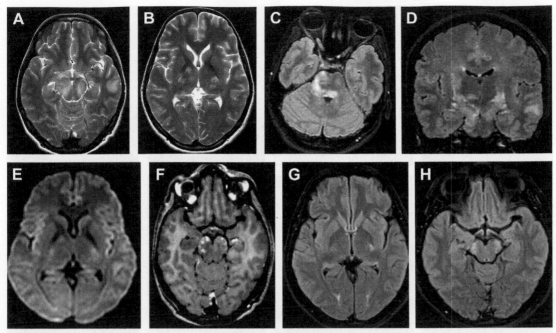

Fig. 1. Neurobrucellosis. There is increased signal in bilateral thalami, internal capsule, cerebral peduncles, and pons on T2-weighted/FLAIR images (*A–D*). Diffusion study is normal (*E*). Contrast study (*F*) shows patchy enhancement in the cerebral peduncle lesions. Follow-up imaging after treatment (*G, H*) shows partial resolution of abnormalities. FLAIR, fluid attenuated inversion recovery.

Actinomycosis infection of central nervous system

Actinomycosis is a chronic suppurative disease caused by Actinomyces species that are gram-positive, anaerobic bacteria that colonize the mouth, colon, and vagina. Infection follows mucosal injury caused by local trauma, resulting in a suppurative, granulomatous inflammatory soft tissue lesion with dense fibrosis.[13] CNS infection can occur through hematogenous route or by direct extension from the cervicofacial region. Disease manifestations are summarized in Table 3.

Imaging: Chronic meningitis in actinomycosis resembles tubercular meningitis, and cerebrospinal fluid (CSF) findings are also similar in both conditions. Pachymeningeal masslike lesions resembling en-plaque tuberculoma or meningioma may also be seen; these lesions may be identified by permeative bone destruction and an abundance of soft tissue (Fig. 3). Actinomycosis

Table 2	
Summary of clinical and imaging findings in neuromelioidosis	
Organism	***Burkholderia pseudomallei***
Transmission	Ingestion or inhalation of contaminated materials Direct inoculation through skin abrasions or injury
Neurologic forms of disease	Meningitis, *meningoencephalitis,* encephalitis, abscess, cranial neuritis
Imaging findings	1. Normal study 2. Leptomeningeal and rarely dural enhancement. 3. Multiple cerebral abscesses extending along major WM (corticospinal tract and corpus callosum). Contiguous disease changes seen involving brainstem and cerebellum. 5. Cranial nerve (CN) enhancement and thickening (most commonly fifth CN). 6. Skull vault osteomyelitis, spinal cord abscess, and epidural collections

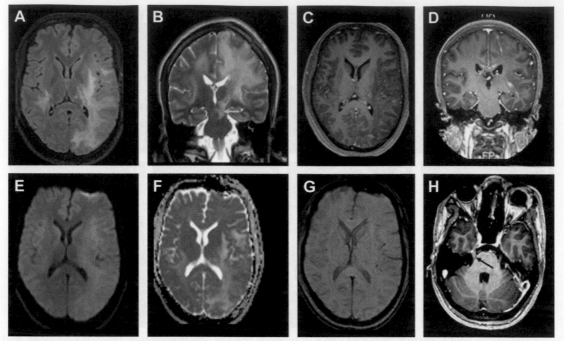

Fig. 2. Neuromelioidosis. Multiple ill-defined lesions in WM and corpus callosum. Lesions seem hyperintense on FLAIR (*A*) and T2-weighted images (*B*), with ill-defined patchy, nodular, and linear enhancement on T1-weighted (T1W) image (*C, D*). Abnormalities extend along corticospinal tract (*green arrow*) and across corpus callosum (*blue arrow*) and show increased signal on both DWI and ADC maps (*E, F*). SWI shows no evidence of susceptibility (*G*). Right trigeminal nerve seems thickened and shows enhancement on postcontrast T1W images (*black arrow, H*).

abscess can be seen in the thalamus and gangliocapsular region and shows imaging findings similar to other pyogenic abscesses. Infrequently, focal nodular or ring enhancing lesions may be observed in the brain parenchyma.[13–15]

Nocardiosis

Nocardiosis is a rare CNS infection caused by the gram-positive, aerobic, branching filamentous bacteria *Nocardia asteroides* and *Nocardia farcinica*. They are ubiquitous in the soil and dust seen throughout the world. Infection is contracted via

inhalation or direct inoculation and spreads to the brain via the hematogenous route. Predisposing risk factors include steroid use, malignancy, chronic lung disease, and transplant. In addition, Nocardia can also cause isolated CNS infections.[16,17] CNS manifestations include cerebral abscess, meningitis, and ventriculitis.

Imaging: Nocardia abscesses are often multiple and show typical imaging findings such as ring enhancement and restricted diffusion. Multiple enhancing rims and irregular multilobulated appearance on neuroimaging are valuable diagnostic clues for Nocardia abscess (Fig. 4). It can also cause numerous small microabscesses in the brain mimicking tuberculosis.[18] Spectroscopy shows lipid peak and absent amino acid resonances and small or absent lactate. Nocardia being an aerobe does not show succinate and acetate peaks that are typically observed in anaerobic abscess.[19] Meningitis is a less frequent manifestation of Nocardiosis.[20]

Whipple disease

Whipple disease is a rare infection caused by the gram-positive bacillus *Tropheryma whipplei*, which is commonly found in soil and water, particularly in sewage. Transmission primarily occurs

---

Box 1
Infections associated with cranial nerve enhancement

Bacterial: Tuberculosis, syphilis, leprosy, mycoplasma, neuroborreliosis, brucella, *Burkholderia pseudomallei infection*, and pyogenic meningitis

Viral: Herpes simplex virus type 1, cytomegalovirus, and varicella zoster

Fungal: Cryptococcus   neoformans, mucormycosis

Parasitic: Neuroschistosomiasis

Table 3
Clinical and imaging findings in actinomycosis

Organism	*Actinomyces israelii* (Common Organism)
Transmission	Hematogenous spread, direct extension from cervicofacial infection, direct inoculation
Clinical findings	Chronic disease with mass like features, presence of sinus tract, and cervicofacial infection are features that suggest possible actinomycosis
Imaging findings	1. Meningitis 2. Pachymeningitis with large mass like lesions spread across tissue boundaries, involving overlying bone and scalp tissues 3. Cerebral abscess commonly seen in frontal and temporal lobes 4. Extra-axial empyema 5. Skull vault osteomyelitis 6. Actinomycetoma

through the feco-oral route and infrequently via droplets. CNS infection is associated with cognitive decline, hypothalamic dysfunction, and neuro-ophthalmic manifestations.[21,22] Diagnosis is based on CSF polymerase chain reaction or bowel biopsy.

Imaging: Brain imaging findings are usually nonspecific. Commonly described neuroimaging findings include T2-weighted (T2W)/fluid attenuated inversion recovery (FLAIR) hyperintensity involving hypothalamus, thalamus, brainstem, medial temporal lobes, and corticospinal tracts

(Fig. 5). These lesions are often ill-defined and do not cause mass effect or show enhancement. Nonetheless, nodular or rim enhancing lesions have also been described[23] (Fig. 6).

Listeriosis

Listeria monocytogenes is an anerobic intracellular bacterial pathogen that grows at low temperatures in stored meats and milk products.[24,25] Risk factors include chronic illness, extremes of age, diabetes, and immunosuppressive medication. The infection spreads to the CNS via either

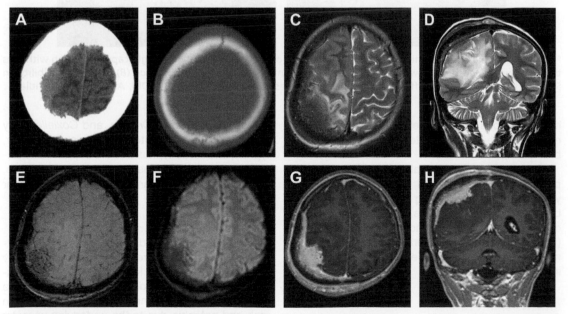

Fig. 3. Actinomycosis. Axial CT (*A*, *B*) shows right side calvarial bone thickening and sclerosis with abnormal soft tissue. T2-weighted MR images (*C*, *D*) confirming scalp and bony changes and hypointense dural-based mass. Lesion shows multiple tiny foci of susceptibility on SWI (*E*), no diffusion restriction (*F*), and strong homogeneous enhancement (*G*, *H*) mimicking en-plaque meningioma or tuberculoma.

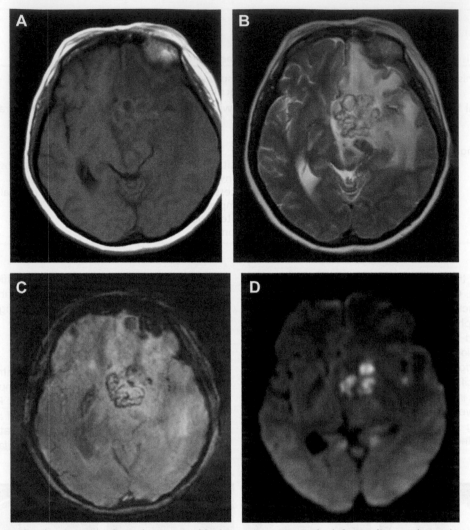

Fig. 4. Nocardia abscess. Multiple coalescing ringlike lesions are seen in the left gangliocapsular region with rims that are hyperintense on T1-weighted image (*A*), hypointense on T2-weighted image (*B*), with susceptibility on SWI (*C*); there is restricted diffusion on DWI (*D*). (*Courtesy* of Sarbesh Tiwari, MD, DM, AIIMS Jodhpur, India.)

hematogenous route (cerebral hemispheres) or retrograde neurogenic route (trigeminal nerves to brainstem).[25,26]

Imaging: Rhombencephalitis is a characteristic pattern typically observed in immunocompetent young patients manifesting as poorly marginated brainstem signal changes, which may exhibit contrast enhancement and diffusion restriction (**Fig. 7**). Meningitis, cerebritis, and cerebral abscess are other manifestations of Listeria infection.[25,27,28]

Rickettsial Infections

The rickettsia are genetically related, intracellular gram-negative bacteria[29] transmitted to humans by ticks, mites, lice, or fleas and include the genera

Rickettsiae, Ehrlichia, Orientia, and *Coxiella.* They are broadly classified into 3 groups: spotted fever, typhus, and scrub typhus and are capable of multiplying within the endothelial cells of blood vessels, causing vasculitis and increased vascular permeability.[30]

Spotted fever rickettsioses

Rocky Mountain spotted fever, caused by *Rickettsia rickettsii*, has been reclassified more generally as a spotted fever rickettsiosis, as many tick-borne rickettsia are serologically indistinguishable and cause a febrile illness with associated skin rash and petechia due to the underlying vascular injury. CNS infection may be caused by hematogenous spread during the systemic phase of the disease.[30,31]

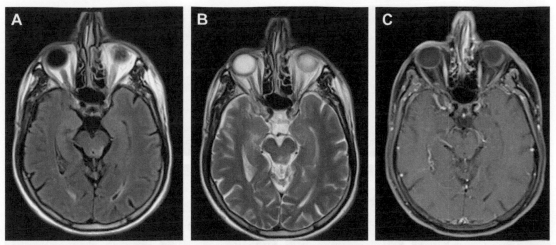

Fig. 5. Whipple disease. Axial T2-weighted (*A*) and FLAIR images (*B*) showing ill-defined focal area of signal changes in the midbrain. No abnormal enhancement is seen on contrast-enhanced study (*C*). (*Courtesy* of Girish Bathla, MD, University of Iowa Hospitals and Clinic, Iowa City, IA.)

Imaging: Imaging could be normal or may show cerebral edema, meningeal enhancement, lacunar infarcts, and enlarged perivascular spaces.[32] Other reported findings include multifocal punctate diffusion restricting T2 hyperintense lesions described as "starry sky" sign, features of vasculitis,[33] focal splenial hyperintensity,[34] and features of raised intracranial pressure.[34] **Box 2** summarises conditions that may result in the "starry sky" appearance on imaging.[35]

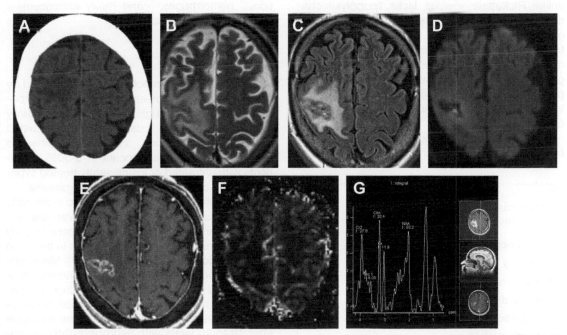

Fig. 6. Whipple disease in a patient with history of Crohn disease and seizure. Axial noncontrast head CT (*A*) shows ill-defined hypoattenuation in the right frontal lobe, with corresponding T2 prolongation (*B, C*), without associated restricted diffusion (*D*), but with heterogenous curvilinear peripheral postcontrast enhancement (*E*). Lesion shows low rCBV on perfusion study (*F*), and short TE (30 ms) MRS (*G*) shows slightly elevated choline to creatine ratio and presence of lipid/lactate. rCBV, relative cerebral blood volume. (*Courtesy* of Suyash Mohan, MD, PDCC, Hospital of the University of Pennsylvania, Philadelphia, PA.)

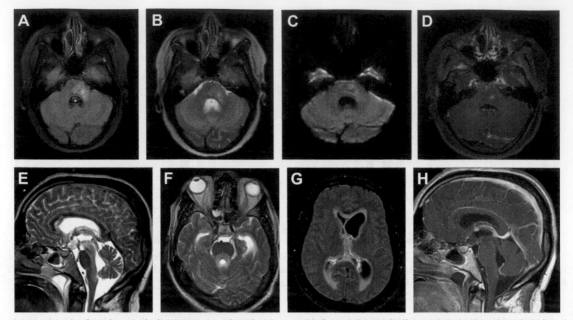

Fig. 7. Listeria rhombencephalitis. Patient 1 (*A–D*): pons and left middle cerebellar peduncle showing ill-defined hyperintensity on T2-weighted/FLAIR images (*A, B*), subtle hyperintensity on DWI (*C*), and enhancement on post-contrast study (*D*). Patient 2 (*E–H*): increased signal seen in the dorsal medulla, pons, and midbrain (*E, F*) with hydrocephalus and ventriculitis (*G*) but no enhancement after contrast injection (*H*). (*Courtesy* of Sarbesh Tiwari, MD, DM, AIIMS Jodhpur, India.)

Scrub typhus

Orientia tsutsugamushi causes scrub typhus and, unlike Rickettsia species, lacks lipopolysaccharide in its cell wall. It affects highly vascular organs such as the liver, lungs, and brain by targeting the endothelial cells.[29,31,36] It is a common vector-borne infection in the Asia Pacific region transmitted by mites. Upto two third of patients with severe infection may develop symptomatic CNS disease commonly due to meningitis or encephalitis.[37]

Imaging: Imaging findings range from normal[37] to meningeal enhancement, generalized cerebral

edema,[38] and signal changes in WM and basal ganglia.[39] Lesions may show diffusion restriction,[40] hemorrhages,[38] and rarely enhancement on contrast study (**Fig. 8**).[38,39]

Spirochetes

Neurosyphilis

Syphilis is a chronic infectious disease caused by the gram-negative, coil-shaped spirochete *Treponema pallidum*. Although it is primarily a sexually transmitted infection, it can rarely be transmitted by blood transfusions and from mother to newborn. Neurosyphilis occurs in 5-30% of patients with untreated or insufficiently treated syphilis and can occur at any stage of the disease.[41]

Neurosyphilis may be asymptomatic in the early stages or manifest as meningeal and vascular disease and uncommonly as chronic parenchymal disease presenting as general paresis in the brain and tabes dorsalis in the spinal cord.[42] Meningitis is usually seen within 2 years of the primary infection and presents as headache, meningeal signs, and cranial nerve dysfunction. Vascular neurosyphilis manifests after 5 to 10 years, general paresis after 10 to 20 years with neuropsychiatric symptoms, and tabes dorsalis after 20 to 30 years with spinal cord symptoms[41,42] (**Table 4**).

Imaging: Imaging findings in syphilitic meningitis include meningeal enhancement, cranial nerve enhancement (most commonly affecting the

---

Box 2
Differential diagnosis for "starry sky" appearance on MR imaging

1. Neurocysticercosis
2. Miliary tuberculosis
3. Rickettsial infection
4. Lyme disease
5. Cryptococcal infection
6. Septic emboli

From Crapp, S., Harrar, D., Strother, M., Wushensky, C., & Pruthi, S. (2011). Rocky Mountain spotted fever: "starry sky" appearance with diffusion-weighted imaging in a child. Pediatric Radiology, 42(4), 499–502.

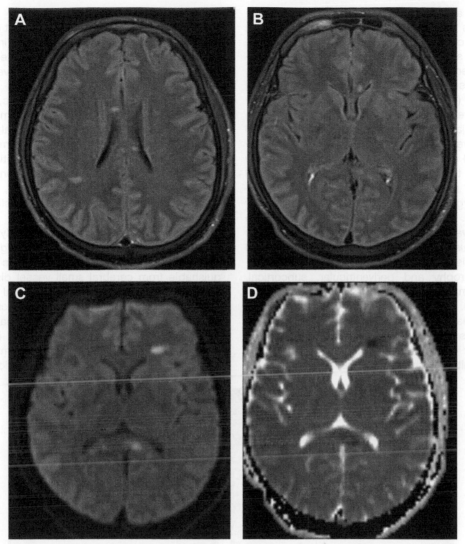

Fig. 8. Scrub typhus. Multifocal WM lesions seen on T2W and FLAIR (*A*, *B*) and DWI. DWI (*C*) showing increased signal intensity in the lesions with corresponding hypointensity on ADC maps (*D*).

Table 4
Neurologic and corresponding imaging features of neurosyphilis

Neurologic Disease	Imaging Findings
1. Asymptomatic with CSF abnormalities	1. Normal
2. Syphilitic meningitis and cranial nerve palsy	2. Meningitis, hydrocephalus, cranial nerve enhancement
3. Meningovascular syphilis: meningeal symptoms with ischemic manifestations due to involvement of large-, medium-, and small-sized vessels	3. Syphilitic gummas are meningeal-based ring or nodular enhancing lesions Lacunar infarcts (in the basal ganglia, thalamus, and brainstem regions). MRA may show vascular narrowing or occlusion. Vessel wall imaging may show vessel wall enhancement.
4. Parenchymatous syphilis: encephalitis, psychiatric symptoms, or general paresis and myelopathy or Tabes dorsalis	4. Cortical atrophy, ventricular prominence, and WM hyperintensities

seventh and eighth cranial nerves), and hydro-cephalus[32,41,43] (see Table 4). Syphilitic gumma is a rare chronic granulomatous form of meningo-vascular syphilis that develops years after the pri-mary infection and is seen as poorly vascularized, meninges-based enhancing mass with perilesional edema[25] (Fig. 9). Adjacent brain parenchyma may be involved by the direct extension of inflammation from adjacent pia or from small parenchymal blood vessels. Vascular syphilis is typically detected as infarcts in the middle cerebral artery territory, thalami, and brainstem along with focal vascular narrowing and occlusions of medium- and large-sized arteries on angiography[43] (Fig. 10). Vessel wall imaging may demonstrate vessel wall enhancement indistinguishable from other causes of vasculitis.[25] Chronic parenchymal disease is characterized by diffuse or frontotem-poral atrophy and periventricular, subcortical, and temporal region WM signal changes[41] (Fig. 11). Susceptibility weighted imaging (SWI) may reveal cortical iron deposition.[44] Tabes dorsa-lis shows an abnormal spinal cord signal in the posterior column. In addition, lytic lesions of the skull vault and orbital periostitis may be seen.

Neuroborreliosis

Lyme neuroborreliosis (LNB) is the most common tick-borne zoonotic disease and is an inflamma-tory disorder caused by the spirochete *Borrelia burgdorferi*.[45,46] Lyme disease has 3 overlapping stages—early localized, early, and late dissemi-nated stages—and can cause neurologic, cardiac, chronic skin, or articular disease. LNB manifesta-tions include meningoradiculitis, cranial neuritis, plexopathy, mononeuritis multiplex, lymphocytic meningitis, and infrequently, encephalitis. Facial palsy is a common clinical presentation of early LNB. Chronic meningitis, encephalitis, myelitis, and cerebral vasculitis are late manifestations of LNB.[45]

Imaging: Imaging studies are usually normal. MR abnormalities include nonenhancing subcor-tical and/or periventricular WM lesions indistin-guishable from cerebral small vessel disease or multiple sclerosis lesions.[47,48] Atypical imaging features include masslike appearance or hemor-rhagic encephalitis.[47,48] Meningeal enhancement is uncommon, although cranial nerves, including facial nerves and spinal nerve roots may show enhancement[48] (Fig. 12). Neuroborreliosis may

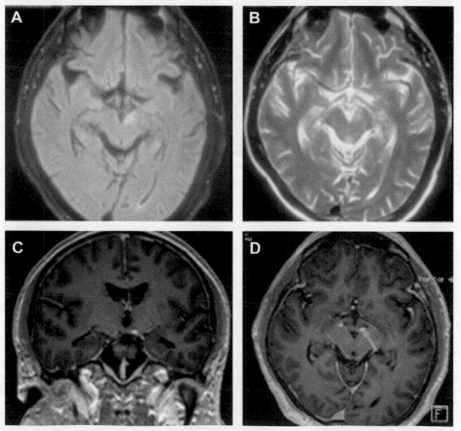

Fig. 9. Syphilitic gumma. Axial FLAIR (*A*) and T2-weighted images (*B*) showing focal hyperintense signal in the left cerebral peduncle. Postcontrast study shows 2 small meningeal-based enhancing lesions (*arrow; C, D*).

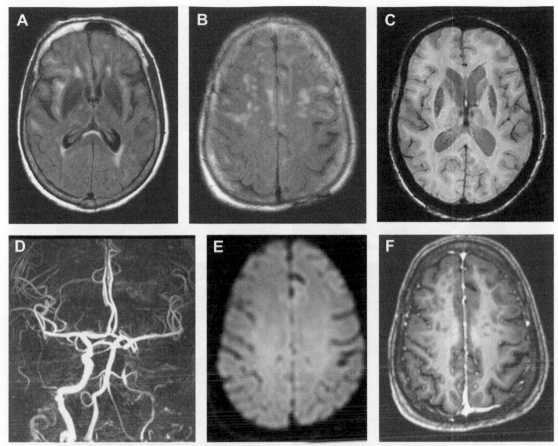

Fig. 10. Neurosyphilis. Scattered WM hyperintensities seen predominantly in the frontal and parietal WM on FLAIR images (*A, B*) with hypointense signal in bilateral basal ganglia structures on both FLAIR and SWI (*C*). MRA shows left ICA occlusion (*D*), no signal change seen on DWI (*E*), and no enhancement of lesions seen on contrast study (*F*). ICA, internal carotid artery.

be associated with vasculitis, ischemic strokes, intracerebral hemorrhage, or subarachnoid hemorrhage (SAH). Angiography may show multifocal narrowing and poststenotic dilatation of the medium- and large-calibre cerebral vessels.[49]

Fungal Infections

Fungal infections are rare cause of meningitis, meningoencephalitis, cerebritis, or abscess formation. In conjunction with clinical symptoms, knowledge of the underlying predisposing condition, and laboratory investigations, radiological patterns can suggest the correct diagnosis and help in initiating definitive treatment.[50,51]

Aspergillosis
Aspergillus species are common spore-forming septated, branching saprophytic fungi with worldwide distribution.[50,52] Aspergillus fumigatus commonly infect lungs and can spread to the brain through hematogenous route. Other routes are

through contiguous spread from the paranasal sinuses and rarely direct inoculation. It causes meningitis, granulomatous lesions, cerebritis, cerebral abscess, and cerebrovascular manifestations. It is frequently seen in immunocompromised hosts or patients with underlying lung disease[52,53] (Table 5).

Imaging: Focal cerebritis typically appears as a heterogeneous lesion with surrounding edema and exhibits variable enhancement on postcontrast imaging. Lesions frequently show areas of T2 shortening, either due to hemorrhages or due to the accumulation of various paramagnetic elements by the fungal hyphae. Cerebral abscess shows ring enhancement and restricted diffusion.[50,51,54] Granulomatous disease is characterized by chronic masslike lesions affecting the brain parenchyma, meninges, or both with the involvement of adjacent skull base, paranasal sinuses, and orbits. These lesions seem isodense or hyperdense on plain CT, show isointense to

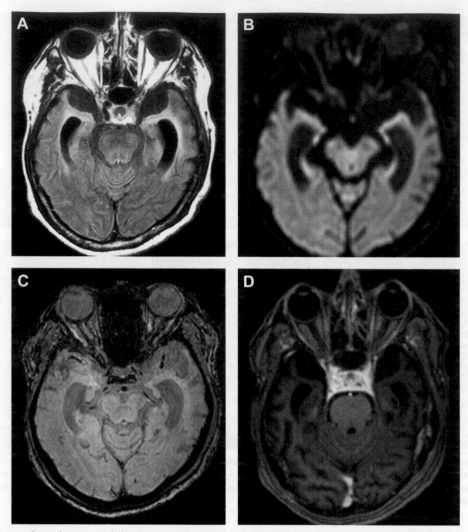

Fig. 11. Parenchymal neurosyphilis. Symmetric medial temporal signal changes noted on FLAIR images (*A*) with severe focal atrophy and ventricular dilatation. Lesion shows no abnormality on DWI (*B*), SWI images (*C*), and no enhancement on contrast-enhanced T1W images (*D*).

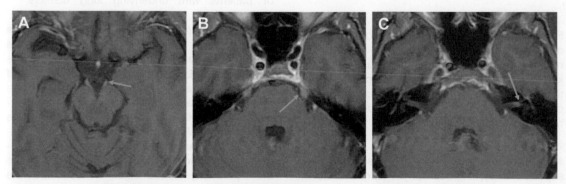

Fig. 12. Lyme neuroborreliosis. Postcontrast Axial T1W images showing enhancement of third nerve (*arrow*, *A*), fifth nerve (*B*), and seventh and eighth nerves (*C*) bilaterally. (*Courtesy* of Rajiv Mangla, MD, Upstate University Hospital, Syracuse, NY.)

Table 5
Predisposing conditions and imaging findings in central nervous system Aspergillosis

Predisposing conditions	Neutropenia, steroids use, chronic granulomatous disease, advanced HIV infection, leukaemia, severe liver disease, influenza infection, and extra corporeal membrane oxygenation therapy

Imaging findings	1. Meningitis
	2. Cerebritis and cerebral abscess
	3. Granuloma
	4. Rhinocerebral aspergillosis
	5. Cerebrovascular abnormalities
	  a. Infarcts
	  b. Aneurysm and subarachnoid hemorrhage
	  c. Rarely cerebral venous sinus thrombosis

Abbreviation: HIV, human immunodeficiency virus.

hypointense signal on T1-weighted images, characteristically hypointense signal on T2W images and moderate homogenous enhancement[64,65] (Fig. 13).

Rhinocerebral form of Aspergillus infection is characterized by contiguous disease spread involving sinuses, meninges, and the brain, with thickened enhancing dura and cerebral parenchymal signal changes due to cerebritis, abscess, or granuloma formation[50,51,54] (Fig. 14). Vascular involvement is less common and involves vessels in the vicinity of the skull base due to direct spread, forming large fusiform aneurysms. Distal cerebral vessels may show small mycotic aneurysms due to hematogenous spread of infection.[51,54,56] Fungal arteritis involving small perforating arteries of the brain and occasionally large vessels at the skull base may cause vessel occlusion and infarction.[50,51,54]

Mucormycosis

Mucormycosis (MCR) is caused by fungi of the order Mucorales and family Mucoraceae, with *Rhizopus* species being the most implicated organism. They are widely present in environment, and CNS infection occurs either via hematogenous spread from the primary site in the lung or through direct spread from the paranasal sinuses and orbit. Many cases of MCR were documented during the COVID-19 pandemic, particularly in India (which already has the highest prepandemic burden of MCR in the world), probably associated with poorly controlled diabetes mellitus, other comorbidities, and corticosteroids used to treat COVID-19.[57] Rhinocerebral MCR, isolated CNS infection, infarcts, and rarely hemorrhages have been described[50–52] (Table 6).

Imaging: MR imaging is the preferred imaging modality. Sinonasal MCR is characterized by thickened mucosa, "black turbinate" sign, absent mucosal contrast enhancement, and the presence of restricted diffusion in the affected mucosa on DWI.[58] Angioinvasive hyphae cause vascular thrombosis in the mucosal tissue and turbinates, resulting in gangrenous changes that are seen as foci of nonenhancing mucosal tissue on MR imaging, producing the so-called black turbinate sign. Although direct invasion from the ethmoid sinus is common, transosseous spread without bone destruction also occurs; imaging findings include fat stranding, focal abscess formation, proptosis, and posterior globe tenting. In addition, MCR may also cause optic nerve thickening, enhancement, and optic nerve infarction (Fig. 15). There may be thickening and enhancement of the cranial nerves, often seen involving the trigeminal nerve, optic nerves, and seventh and eighth nerve complex. Rarely, it can spread retrogradely and involve the cranial nerve nuclei, which may show signal alteration and contrast enhancement. Contiguous spread with meningeal thickening and enhancement as well as frontal or temporal lobe signal changes may be present. Typical manifestations of empyema and intracerebral abscess may be seen.[59]

Septic emboli may initially cause bland infarcts in the cortical, subcortical, and gangliocapsular regions, followed by direct parenchymal invasion by fungal elements, causing cerebritis and later abscess formation.[60] These lesions may show restricted diffusion on DWI and hemorrhage on gradient echo/SWI. Fungal abscesses as compared with bacterial abscesses are often multiple and deep seated, may show higher apparent diffusion coefficient (ADC) values, peripheral zone of diffusion restriction, heterogenous T2 signal, and show intracavitary projections on T1W and T2W images.[61,62] Fungal invasion of large- and medium-sized vessels near the base of skull causes ischemic stroke. Similarly, cavernous sinus and ophthalmic vein thrombosis can occur due to venous invasion and spread of infection. Rarely, angioinvasion may lead to mycotic aneurysm formation, which may rupture and cause subarachnoid hemorrhage.[50,51,60,63]

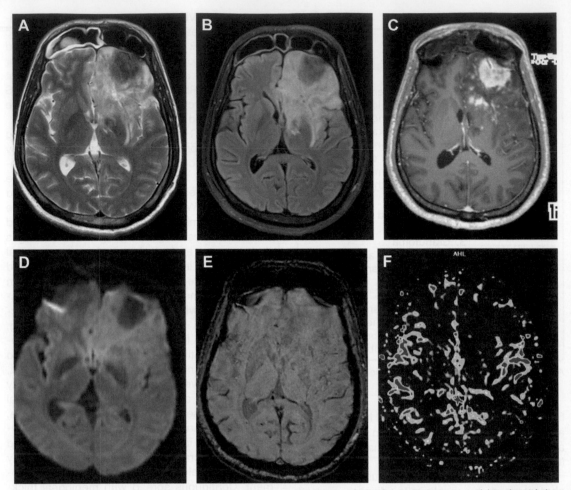

Fig. 13. Aspergilloma. A large left frontal lesion showing T2-weighted/FLAIR hypointense signal (*A*, *B*), with heterogeneously hyperintense edema in the adjoining brain parenchyma. Contrast study (*C*) shows strong homogenous enhancement of the lesion with adjoining brain parenchyma showing patchy enhancement. Lesion shows low signal on DWI (*D*), no susceptibility on SWI (*E*), and low CBF in perfusion study (*F*).

Bony erosions are more frequent in fungal infections as compared with bacterial infections. Aspergillus infection shows a higher incidence of sinocranial extension, whereas mucor has greater incidence of sino-orbital and cranial disease. Aspergillus infections more commonly show dural-based lesions, whereas mucor shows a higher propensity to cause cerebritis and cerebral abscess. Vascular complications and infarctions are more common in mucor infection.[58]

Cryptococcosis

Cryptococcus neoformans, a yeast-like encapsulated fungus commonly found in soil, is the commonest mycotic infection affecting the CNS. It commonly affects immunocompromised individuals, although infection can also be seen in immunocompetent individuals. Cryptococcus causes a

latent respiratory infection, which then spreads to the CNS through hematogenous route.[50,52]

Imaging: Brain infection can manifest as meningitis, enlarged Virchow-Robin spaces, or cryptococcoma. Meningitis may appear as nodular enhancement involving the basal cisterns region. Enlarged perivascular spaces (due to the accumulation of mucoid gelatinous material produced by fungus) can be seen in the basal ganglia, thalamus, brainstem, and cerebral WM. They appear hyperintense on T2W images, hypointense on T1W images, and usually do not enhance and show facilitated diffusion on DWI.[50] Meningitis may be complicated by hydrocephalus and rarely lacunar infarcts, which are frequently present in the basal ganglia, thalamus, and cerebral WM.[64] High signal intensity lesions in the periventricular distribution may be seen on T2W/FLAIR images.[65] Cryptococcomas

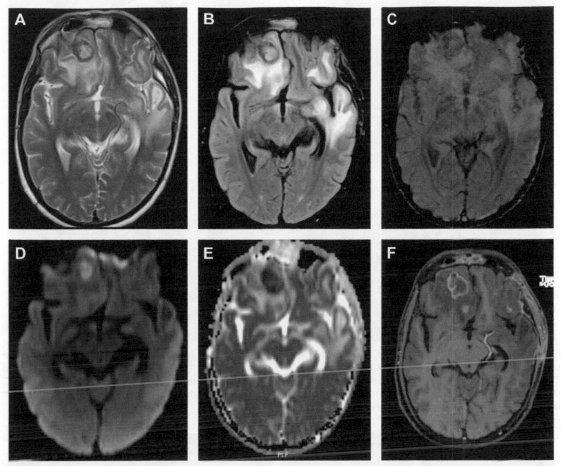

Fig. 14. Aspergillus abscess. Right frontal lobe showing a mass with hyperintense center and hypointense rim and perilesional edema on FLAIR/T2-weighted image (A, B). It shows no hemorrhage on SWI (C), central restricted diffusion (D, E), and peripheral enhancement on contrast study. Multiple other small enhancing lesions are also seen (F).

are the result of fungal invasion of brain parenchyma and appear hyperintense on T2W/FLAIR images and hypointense on T1W images with marginal enhancement[66,67] (Fig. 16). Other imaging findings include choroid plexitis and intraventricular and parenchymal cysts (Table 7). MRS reveals a trehalose peak at 3.4 and 5.2 ppm, which is a useful diagnostic marker of focal cryptococcus lesions.[68]

Table 6
Predisposing conditions and imaging findings in central nervous system mucormycosis

Predisposing conditions	Neutropenia, steroids use, diabetes especially diabetic ketoacidosis, deferoxamine treatment, solid organ transplant, stem cell transplantation, patients receiving antifungal prophylaxis such as itraconazole or voriconazole, SARS-COV-2 infection

Imaging findings	1. Rhinocerebral mucormycosis
	2. Cerebritis and cerebral abscess
	3. Cranial nerve enhancement suggesting perineural spread
	4. Cerebrovascular abnormalities
	    a. Arterial vascular occlusions and stenosis
	    b. Infarcts
	    c. Aneurysm and subarachnoid hemorrhage
	    d. Venous thrombosis commonly affecting cavernous sinus

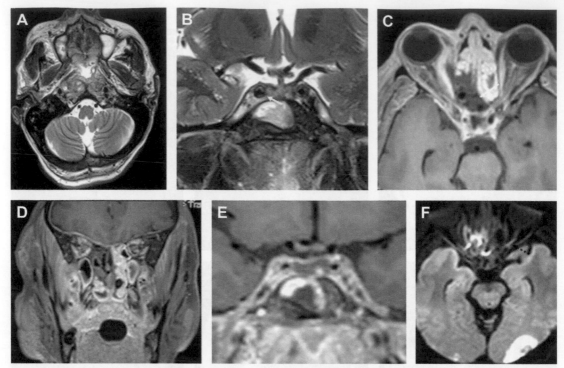

Fig. 15. Post-COVID 19 mucormycosis. T2-weighted images (*A, B*) showing heterogeneously increased signal from skull base osteomyelitis, bilateral ICA narrowing with luminal irregularity (*yellow arrow*) (*B*). Contrast-enhanced T1-weighted images (*C–E*) showing necrosis of ethmoidal mucosa (*black arrow*) and nonenhancing turbinates (*C, D*), dural thickening, and heterogeneous enhancement. On DWI, posterior watershed infarcts with left optic nerve hyperintensity (*black arrow*) are seen (*F*).

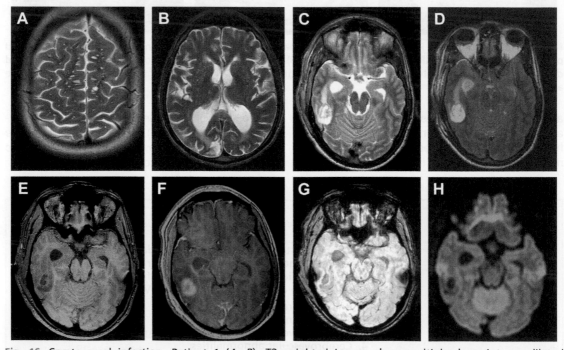

Fig. 16. Cryptococcal infection. Patient 1 (*A, B*): T2-weighted images show multiple, hyperintense dilated Virchow-Robin perivascular spaces in bilateral frontal lobe white matter. (*A, B*) Patient 2 (*C–H*) with right temporal cystic lesion with perilesional edema that is hyperintense on T2-weighted/FLAIR images (*C, D*) and hypointense on T1-weighted images (*E*) showing enhancement after contrast injection (*F*). There is no hemorrhage on SWI (*G*) or diffusion restriction (*H*).

Table 7
Predisposing conditions and imaging findings in central nervous system cryptococcal infection

Predisposing conditions	Hematologic malignancies, glucocorticoid therapy, advanced HIV infection with low CD4+ T-lymphocyte count. *Cryptococcus gatti* infection is often seen in immunocompetent subjects

Imaging Findings	1. Meningitis
	2. Uncommonly hydrocephalus and ventricular cysts
	3. Choroid plexitis
	4. Lacunar infarcts
	5. Parenchymal disease
	   a. Enlarged VR spaces
	   b. Periventricular WM signal changes
	   c. Cryptococcomas
	   d. Parenchymal cysts

Abbreviation: VR, Virchow-Robin.

Candidiasis

Candida albicans is a small, round to oval, thin-walled yeast fungal commensal in the oral cavity and gastrointestinal tract.[69] When immune mechanisms are compromised, Candida species proliferate, leading to the development of invasive Candidiasis.[51] Patients with neutropenia, diabetes, AIDS with low CD4 count, extensive

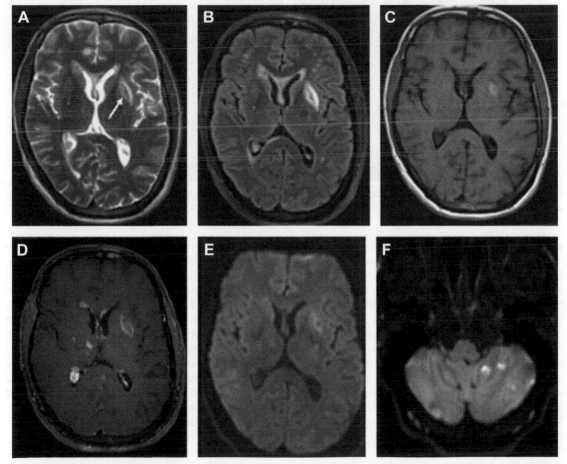

Fig. 17. Candidiasis. Multiple lesions in right thalamus, basal ganglia, and posterior fossa that are small, appearing hyperintense on T2-weighted/FLAIR images (*A, B*), isointense on T1-weighted images (*C*), and show nodular enhancement on contrast study (*D*) and hyperintensity on DWI (*E, F*). In addition, left striatal subacute infarct (*arrow*) is seen with ventriculitis and right side choroid plexitis.

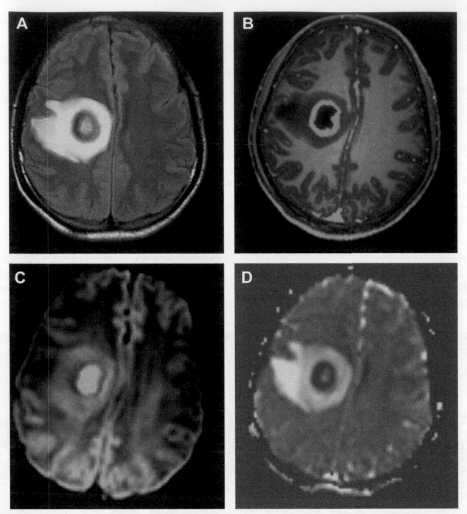

Fig. 18. *Cladophialophora bantiana* cerebral abscess: a large right frontal lobe mass with thick hypointense rim on FLAIR (*A*) that shows enhancement on contrast study (*B*) and restricted diffusion on DWI and ADC (*C, D*).

wounds, burns, indwelling catheters, and hematologic malignancies; premature infants; and the transplant recipients are at risk for invasive candidiasis and fungemia. CNS infection occurs in patients with disseminated Candidiasis and following neurosurgical procedures.[70]

Imaging: Cerebral microabscesses are the most common manifestation that are seen as ill-defined lesions with punctate nodular enhancement on postcontrast study (Fig. 17). They show variable signal on T2W images, hemorrhage, diffusion restriction, and enhancement on contrast study. Meningitis, vasculitis with basal ganglia infarction, and rarely aneurysm formation with SAH may be seen.[51,70]

Cladophialophora bantiana

Pheohyphomycosis refers to a group of fungi with melanin in its cell wall. *Cladophialophora bantiana*

is the most common cause of CNS pheohyphomycosis, with most of the cases described from Asia, especially India. It is universally present in the soil and decaying organic matter and is a highly neurotropic fungus that causes brain abscess and affects both immunocompetent and immunocompromised individuals. The infection spreads to brain via the hematogenous route.[71] Abscesses caused by *C bantiana* are typically found in the frontal lobe, and they may be single or multiple. On MR imaging, an abscess caused by *C bantiana* exhibits ring enhancement and central restricted diffusion[72] (Fig. 18).

SUMMARY

Neuroimaging abnormalities provide extremely useful diagnostic information, and knowledge of the spectrum of imaging manifestations of uncommon bacterial organisms and fungal infections can assist in narrowing the differential diagnosis, thereby avoiding invasive diagnostic procedures and facilitating early initiation of appropriate therapy. Knowledge of underlying predisposing conditions and the geographic distribution of different organism is useful for suggesting the correct diagnosis.

CLINICS CARE POINTS

- In addition to common manifestations such as meningitis and brain abscess, uncommon bacterial infections may exhibit uncommon imaging patterns.

- These imaging characteristics may be attributable to the involvement of specific brain structures such as the brainstem in Listeria infection, cranial neuritis in brucellosis, borrelia and neurosyphilis, corticospinal tracts in neuromelioidosis, and temporal WM in parenchymal neurosyphilis.

- Infection may spread along WM tracts in neuromelioidosis, across tissue planes in Actinomycosis, into the orbits, sinuses, meninges, and brain in mucormycosis and aspergillosis.

- Meningeal-based masslike lesions may be seen in patients with actinomycosis and aspergillosis.

- Lesions dispersed throughout the WM can indicate Rickettsia infection.

- Brain abscesses with peripheral rim of diffusion restriction, intracavitary projections, and angioinvasive disease may indicate a fungal infection.

DISCLOSURE

The authors have nothing to disclose.

REFERENCES

1. Larry Jameson J, Fauci AS, Kasper DL, et al. Harrison's principles of internal medicine. 20th edition. New York: McGraw-Hill Professional Publishing; 2018.
2. Zheng N, Wang W, Zhang J-T, et al. Neurobrucellosis. Int J Neurosci 2018;128:55–62.
3. Kizilkilic O, Calli C. Neurobrucellosis. Neuroimaging Clin N Am 2011;21:927–37.
4. Pappas G, Akritidis N, Bosilkovski M, et al. Brucellosis. N Engl J Med 2005;352:2325–36.
5. Erdem H, Senbayrak S, Meriç K, et al. Cranial imaging findings in neurobrucellosis: results of Istanbul-3 study. Infection 2016;44:623–31.
6. Al-Sous MW, Bohlega S, Al-Kawi MZ, et al. Neurobrucellosis: clinical and neuroimaging correlation. AJNR Am J Neuroradiol 2004;25:395–401.
7. Turkoglu SA, Halicioglu S, Sirmatel F, et al. Vasculitis and neurobrucellosis: Evaluation of nine cases using radiologic findings. Brain Behav 2018;8:e00947.
8. Wiersinga WJ, van der Poll T, White NJ, et al. Melioidosis: insights into the pathogenicity of Burkholderia pseudomallei. Nat Rev Microbiol 2006;4:272–82.
9. Hsu CC-T, Singh D, Kwan G, et al. Neuromelioidosis: Craniospinal MRI Findings in *Burkholderia pseudomallei* Infection: Craniospinal MRI Findings in B. pseuodomallei. J Neuroimaging 2016;26:75–82.
10. Muthusamy KA, Waran V, Puthucheary SD. Spectra of central nervous system melioidosis. J Clin Neurosci 2007;14:1213–5.
11. Norton R, Aquilina C, Deuble M. Neurologic Melioidosis. Am J Trop Med Hyg 2013;89:535–9.
12. Saremi F, Helmy M, Farzin S, et al. MRI of Cranial Nerve Enhancement. Am J Roentgenol 2005;185:1487–97.
13. Heo SH, Shin SS, Kim JW, et al. Imaging of Actinomycosis in Various Organs: A Comprehensive Review. RadioGraphics 2014;34:19–33.
14. Mohindra S, Savardekar A, Rane S. Intracranial actinomycosis: Varied clinical and radiologic presentations in two cases. Neurol India 2012;60:325.
15. Ravindra N, Sadashiva N, Mahadevan A, et al. Central Nervous System Actinomycosis—A Clinicoradiologic and Histopathologic Analysis. World Neurosurg 2018;116:e362–70.
16. Anagnostou T, Arvanitis M, Kourkoumpetis TK, et al. Nocardiosis of the Central Nervous System: Experience From a General Hospital and Review of 84 Cases From the Literature. Medicine (Baltimore) 2014;93:19–32.
17. Corti ME, Villafañe Fioti ME. Nocardiosis: a review. Int J Infect Dis 2003;7:243–50.
18. Tanaka H, Kiko K, Watanabe Y, et al. Miliary cerebrospinal lesions caused by Nocardia beijingensis in an immunocompetent patient. IDCases 2020;20:e00737.
19. Sartoretti E, Sartoretti T, Gutzwiller A, et al. Advanced multimodality MR imaging of a cerebral nocardiosis abscess in an immunocompetent patient with a focus on Amide Proton Transfer weighted imaging. Bjrcase Rep 2020;6:20190122.
20. Ambrosioni J, Lew D, Garbino J. Nocardiosis: Updated Clinical Review and Experience at a Tertiary Center. Infection 2010;38:89–97.
21. Anderson M. Neurology of Whipple's disease. J Neurol Neurosurg Psychiatry 2000;68:2–5.
22. Louis ED, Lynch T, Kaufmann P, et al. Diagnostic guidelines in central nervous system Whipple's disease. Ann Neurol 1996;40:561–8.

23. Black DF, Aksamit AJ, Morris JM. MR Imaging of Central Nervous System Whipple Disease: A 15-Year Review. Am J Neuroradiol 2010;31:1493–7.

24. Allerberger F, Wagner M. Listeriosis: a resurgent foodborne infection. Clin Microbiol Infect 2010;16:16–23.

25. do Carmo RL, Alves Simão AK, do Amaral LLF, et al. Neuroimaging of Emergent and Reemergent Infections. RadioGraphics 2019;39:1649–71.

26. Hsu CC-T, Singh D, Watkins TW, et al. Serial magnetic resonance imaging findings of intracerebral spread of listeria utilising subcortical U-fibres and the extreme capsule. Neuroradiol J 2016;29:425–30.

27. Arslan F, Ertan G, Emecen AN, et al. Clinical Presentation and Cranial MRI Findings of Listeria monocytogenes Encephalitis: A Literature Review of Case Series. Neurologist 2018;23:198–203.

28. Bortolussi R. Listeriosis: a primer. Can Med Assoc J 2008;179:795–7.

29. Fisher J, Card G, Soong L. Neuroinflammation associated with scrub typhus and spotted fever group rickettsioses. PLoS Negl Trop Dis 2020;14:e0008675.

30. Chen LF, Sexton DJ. What's New in Rocky Mountain Spotted Fever? Infect Dis Clin North Am 2008;22:415–32.

31. Sekeyová Z, Danchenko M, Filipčík P, et al. Rickettsial infections of the central nervous system. PLoS Negl Trop Dis 2019;13:e0007469.

32. Akgoz A, Mukundan S, Lee TC. Imaging of Rickettsial, Spirochetal, and Parasitic Infections. Neuroimaging Clin N Am 2012;22:633–57.

33. Bradshaw MJ, Byrge KC, Ivey KS, et al. Meningoencephalitis due to Spotted Fever Rickettsioses, Including Rocky Mountain Spotted Fever. Clin Infect Dis 2020;71:188–95.

34. Ooi ST, Moy WL. Abducens Nerve Palsy and Meningitis by Rickettsia typhi. Am J Trop Med Hyg 2015;92:620–4.

35. Crapp S, Harrar D, Strother M, et al. Rocky Mountain spotted fever: 'starry sky' appearance with diffusion-weighted imaging in a child. Pediatr Radiol 2012;42:499–502.

36. Banerjee A, Kulkarni S. Orientia tsutsugamushi: The dangerous yet neglected foe from the East. Int J Med Microbiol 2021;311:151467.

37. Misra UK, Kalita J, Mani VE. Neurological manifestations of scrub typhus. J Neurol Neurosurg Psychiatry 2015;86:761–6.

38. Sood AK, Chauhan L, Gupta H. CNS Manifestations in Orientia tsutsugamushi Disease (Scrub Typhus) in North India. Indian J Pediatr 2016;83:634–9.

39. Yum KS, Na S-J, Lee KO, et al. Scrub typhus meningo-encephalitis with focal neurologic signs and associated brain MRI abnormal findings: Literature review. Clin Neurol Neurosurg 2011;113:250–3.

40. Bhoil R, Kumar S, Sood RG, et al. Cerebellitis as an atypical manifestation of scrub typhus. Neurology 2016;86:2113–4.

41. Nagappa M, Sinha S, Taly AB, et al. Neurosyphilis: MRI features and their phenotypic correlation in a cohort of 35 patients from a tertiary care university hospital. Neuroradiology 2013;55:379–88.

42. Hook EW. Syphilis. Lancet 2017;389:1550–7.

43. Brightbill TC, Ihmeidan IH, Post MJ, et al. Neurosyphilis in HIV-positive and HIV-negative patients: neuroimaging findings. AJNR Am J Neuroradiol 1995;16:703–11.

44. Pesaresi I, Sabato M, Doria R, et al. Susceptibility-weighted imaging in parenchymal neurosyphilis: identification of a new MRI finding. Sex Transm Infect 2015;91:489–92.

45. Koedel U, Fingerle V, Pfister H-W. Lyme neuroborreliosis—epidemiology, diagnosis and management. Nat Rev Neurol 2015;11:446–56.

46. Stanek G, Wormser GP, Gray J, et al. Lyme borreliosis. Lancet Lond Engl 2012;379:461–73.

47. Agarwal R, Sze G. Neuro-Lyme Disease: MR Imaging Findings. Radiology 2009;253:167–73.

48. Garkowski A, Łebkowska U, Kubas B, et al. Imaging of Lyme Neuroborreliosis: A Pictorial Review. Open Forum Infect Dis 2020;7:ofaa370.

49. Garkowski A, Zajkowska J, Zajkowska A, et al. Cerebrovascular Manifestations of Lyme Neuroborreliosis—A Systematic Review of Published Cases. Front Neurol 2017;8:146.

50. Gupta R, Jain K, Mittal S, et al. Imaging features of central nervous system fungal infections. Neurol India 2007;55:241.

51. Mathur M, Johnson CE, Sze G. Fungal Infections of the Central Nervous System. Neuroimaging Clin N Am 2012;22:609–32.

52. Murthy JMK, Sundaram C. Fungal infections of the central nervous system. Handbook Clin Neurol 2014;121:1383–401.

53. Meena DS, Kumar D, Bohra GK, et al. Clinical manifestations, diagnosis, and treatment outcome of CNS aspergillosis: A systematic review of 235 cases. Infect Dis Now 2021. https://doi.org/10.1016/j.idnow.2021.04.002.

54. Saini J, Gupta AK, Jolapara MB, et al. Imaging Findings in Intracranial Aspergillus Infection in Immunocompetent Patients. World Neurosurg 2010;74:661–70.

55. Naik V, Ahmed FU, Gupta A, et al. Intracranial Fungal Granulomas: A Single Institutional Clinicopathologic Study of 66 Patients and Review of the Literature. World Neurosurg 2015;83:1166–72.

56. Marzolf G, Sabou M, Lannes B, et al. Magnetic Resonance Imaging of Cerebral Aspergillosis: Imaging and Pathological Correlations. PLoS One 2016;11:e0152475.

57. John TM, Jacob CN, Kontoyiannis DP. When Uncontrolled Diabetes Mellitus and Severe COVID-19

Converge: The Perfect Storm for Mucormycosis. J Fungi 2021;7:298.

58. Bhalla DS, Bhalla A, Manchanda S. Can imaging suggest the aetiology in skull base osteomyelitis? A systematic literature review. Pol J Radiol 2021; 86:309–21.

59. Pai V, Sansi R, Kharche R, et al. Rhino-orbito-cerebral Mucormycosis: Pictorial Review. Insights Imaging 2021;12:167.

60. Lersy F, Royer-Leblond J, Lhermitte B, et al. Cerebral mucormycosis: neuroimaging findings and histopathological correlation. J Neurol 2022. https:// doi.org/10.1007/s00415-021-10701-8.

61. Luthra G, Parihar A, Nath K, et al. Comparative Evaluation of Fungal, Tubercular, and Pyogenic Brain Abscesses with Conventional and Diffusion MR Imaging and Proton MR Spectroscopy. Am J Neuroradiol 2007;28:1332–8.

62. Mueller-Mang C, Castillo M, Mang TG, et al. Fungal versus bacterial brain abscesses: Is diffusion-weighted MR imaging a useful tool in the differential diagnosis? Neuroradiology 2007;49:651–7.

63. Aribandi M, McCoy VA, Bazan C. Imaging Features of Invasive and Noninvasive Fungal Sinusitis: A Review. RadioGraphics 2007;27:1283–96.

64. Mishra AK, Arvind VH, Muliyil D, et al. Cerebrovascular injury in cryptococcal meningitis. Int J Stroke 2018;13:57–65.

65. Lee W-J, Ryu YJ, Moon J, et al. Enlarged periventricular space and periventricular lesion extension on

baseline brain MRI predicts poor neurological outcomes in cryptococcus meningoencephalitis. Sci Rep 2021;11:6446.

66. Ho T-L, Lee H-J, Lee K-W, et al. Diffusion-weighted and conventional magnetic resonance imaging in cerebral cryptococcoma. Acta Radiol 2005;46:411–4.

67. Uppar A, Raj ARP, Konar S, et al. Intracranial Cryptococcoma—Clinicopathologic Correlation and Surgical Outcome: A Single-Institution Experience. World Neurosurg 2018;115:e349–59.

68. Vanherp L, Poelmans J, Weerasekera A, et al. Trehalose as quantitative biomarker for in vivo diagnosis and treatment follow-up in cryptococcomas. Transl Res 2021;230:111–22.

69. Starkey J, Moritani T, Kirby P. MRI of CNS Fungal Infections: Review of Aspergillosis to Histoplasmosis and Everything in Between. Clin Neuroradiol 2014; 24:217–30.

70. Chaussade H, Cazals X, Desoubeaux G, et al. Central nervous system candidiasis beyond neonates: Lessons from a nationwide study. Med Mycol 2021;59:266–77.

71. Chakrabarti A, Kaur H, Rudramurthy SM, et al. Brain abscess due to *Cladophialophora bantiana* : a review of 124 cases. Med Mycol 2016;54:111–9.

72. Ahmad M, Jacobs D, Wu H, et al. Cladophialophora Bantiana: A Rare Intracerebral Fungal Abscess—Case Series and Review of Literature. Surg J 2017; 03.e62–8.

Central Nervous System Mycobacterium Infection
Tuberculosis and Beyond

Mina Park, MD, PhD[a],*, Rakesh K. Gupta, MD[b]

KEYWORDS

- Tuberculosis • Central nervous system • Mycobacterium • MR imaging • Computed tomography
- Infection

KEY POINTS

- Tuberculosis is the most common mycobacterial infection of central nervous system (CNS) and a global concern in endemic areas, especially among patients living with HIV.
- Leptomeningitis is the most common tuberculosis, with predominant basal meningeal enhancement, hydrocephalus, and cerebral infarction.
- Tuberculomas have four stages, namely non-caseating granuloma, caseating granuloma, caseating granuloma with central liquefaction, and calcified granuloma, each having typical image features.
- Nontuberculous mycobacteria involvement of the CNS, which occurs in disseminated disease, usually presenting as meningitis or meningoencephalitis, is rare but should not be overlooked because of high mortality rates.
- Leprosy is a chronic granulomatous disease with extremely rare CNS involvement.

INTRODUCTION TO MYCOBACTERIUM

There are more than 100 species of mycobacteria, which are small, rod-shaped, acid-fast bacilli. Three groups are important for central nervous system (CNS) infection: (1) *Mycobacterium tuberculosis*, (2) *Mycobacterium leprae*, and (3) a distinct group called nontuberculous mycobacteria (NTM).[1] Among them, *M tuberculosis* is responsible for most mycobacterial infections of the CNS, whereas NTM rarely infects the CNS. Leprosy usually involves the peripheral nervous system, with CNS involvement being extremely rare (Fig. 1).

TUBERCULOSIS

Tuberculosis (TB) is a contagious infectious disease caused by *M tuberculosis* and is the leading cause of death from a single infectious agent, estimated to infect a quarter of the world's population.[2] According to the World Health Organization, eight endemic countries account for two-thirds of the global TB infections: India, Indonesia, China, the Philippines, Pakistan, Nigeria, Bangladesh, and South Africa.[2] The risk factors for CNS TB infection include human immunodeficiency virus (HIV) infection, malnutrition, concomitant malignancy, and the use of

[a] Department of Radiology, Gangnam Severance Hospital, Yonsei University College of Medicine, 20 Eonjuro 63-gil, Gangnam-gu, Seoul, South Korea; [b] Department of Radiology, Fortis Memorial Research Institute, Sector - 44, Opposite HUDA City Centre, Gurugram, Haryana, India 122002
* Corresponding author.
E-mail address: to.minapark@yuhs.ac

Neuroimag Clin N Am 33 (2023) 105–124
https://doi.org/10.1016/j.nic.2022.07.006
1052-5149/23/© 2022 Elsevier Inc. All rights reserved.

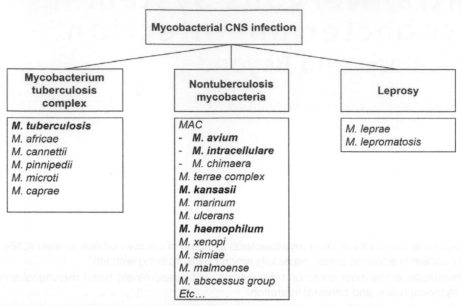

Fig. 1. Mycobacterial species associated with CNS infection.

immunosuppressive drugs; there has been a TB resurgence in nonendemic countries in recent years.[3–6] Moreover, several studies in developed countries have reported that patients born outside of developed countries are overrepresented among CNS TB patients.[7] Therefore, radiologists should be aware of the high incidence of TB and its diagnosis should be suspected with an understanding of the geographic information of pandemic areas and the patient's immune status.

Primarily affecting the respiratory system, TB spreads through the air via droplets containing tubercle bacilli that are released through coughing.[8] Although TB typically manifests as pulmonary infection, it can also affect other body parts, including the CNS. The route of disease spread to the CNS is hematogenous, usually from pulmonary TB. Classically, the rupture of a subpial or subependymal tubercle (known as a rich focus) from hematogenous spread, results in the bacilli entering the subarachnoid space.[9] Because of the lack of defensive white blood cells in the cerebrospinal fluid (CSF), TB can spread rapidly, especially in the basal cisterns.[10]

It may be hard to distinguish acute TB from other infections, and mycobacterium takes a long time to grow in laboratory culture. However, CSF findings can help rule out other pathogens. Typical laboratory results that suggest TB are lymphocytic pleocytosis, low glucose level, high protein level, and high adenosine deaminase level (Table 1).[11] Identification of bacilli often requires examination of large volumes of fluid from repeated lumbar punctures. Commercial kits for detecting M

tuberculosis using genetic amplification technology can also be used: although CSF culture is often negative, polymerase chain reaction assay is positive in 60% to 90% of samples.[12,13] CNS involvement by TB can present either as a diffuse form (leptomeningitis) or as a localized form (tuberculoma, abscess, or cerebritis) (Table 2).

CRANIAL TUBERCULOSIS
Tuberculous Meningitis

TB leptomeningitis is the most common type of TB affecting the CNS. An inflammatory reaction with a

Table 1	
Typical abnormal laboratory results of CNS TB	
CSF analysis	Lymphocytic pleocytosis (50–500 cell/mm^3) High protein level (0.5–3.0 g/L) Low glucose level ($\leq$45 mg/dL or $\leq$40%–50% of serum glucose) High lactate level (5.0–10.0 mmol/L) High adenosine deaminase level ($\geq$8 u/L)
CSF culture	Identification of AFB on stain and culture
CSF PCR	TB PCR positive (amplification of the MPB64 gene or IS6110)

Abbreviation: PCR, polymerase chain reaction.

Table 2
Types of CNS TB involvement

Location	Common	Less Common	Complications	Others
Intracranial	• Leptomeningitis • Vasculitis • Tuberculoma • Abscess	• Cerebritis • Miliary TB • Pachymeningitis • Ventriculitis	• Hydrocephalus • Acute infarction • Cranial nerve palsy	• Tuberculous encephalopathy • Paradoxic response
Intraspinal	• Spondylitis • Myelitis	• Meningitis • Intramedullary tuberculoma		• Longitudinally extensive transverse myelitis

variable admixture of exudative, proliferative, and necrotizing components in the subarachnoid cisterns is typical.[10] High viscosity and high-protein exudates are commonly found in the basal cisterns in TB leptomeningitis, and this may cause communicating hydrocephalus by obstructing CSF circulation.[10] The clinical symptoms include prodromal headache, fever, vomiting, and neck stiffness, followed by vomiting, confusion, and focal neurologic signs.[14] Evidence of concomitant extrameningeal TB is present in about three-fourths of cases.[15] In many cases, however, there is no clinical or historical clues to suggest TB. Radiologically, meningeal involvement is most pronounced at the basal cistern with involvement of the suprasellar/chiasmatic region, ambient cistern, and interpeduncular fossa.

Neuroimaging shows a thick basal meningeal enhancement, hydrocephalus, and small parenchymal infarctions, which are highly specific for TB meningitis (Table 3).[10,16] Computed tomography (CT) often presents with nonspecific hydrocephalus and isodense to mildly hyperdense basal and sulcal cisterns may be seen. On MR imaging, abnormal basal CSF exudates show T1 isointense signal intensity to the brain parenchyma. Fluid-attenuated inversion recovery (FLAIR) images show increased signal intensity in the sulci and cisterns when there is high CSF protein concentration.[17,18] After contrast injection,

characteristic thick leptomeningeal enhancement is seen, predominantly in the basal cisterns; this can be the only imaging finding of TB CNS infection (Fig. 2).[19] Basal enhancement reflects microabscess formation and intense inflammation in the basal meninges and may indicate poor outcome.[20] In the evaluation of leptomeningitis, contrast-enhanced FLAIR sequence may show high sensitivity for detecting meningeal enhancement (Fig. 3).[21,22]

Basal enhancement in TB leptomeningitis may present differently in patients with and without HIV, with positive meningeal enhancement or enhanced meningeal nodules more frequently observed on contrast-enhanced CT scan in patients with HIV than in patients without HIV.[23,24] However, some studies have shown little or no meningeal enhancement or basal exudates on CT or MR imaging in patients with HIV, with the suggested mechanism including an impaired immunologic response.[17] However, the diagnostic sensitivity and specificity of various imaging features for TB leptomeningitis are undefined. Furthermore, approximately 30% of individuals at an early stage in TB leptomeningitis may have normal brain CT findings, and around 15% have normal brain MR imaging findings.[14]

Hydrocephalus is the most common complication of TB leptomeningitis, and may indicate poor prognosis with high morbidity and mortality.[25] In

Table 3
Summary of TB leptomeningitis

	Clinical Symptoms	Imaging Finding	Recommended Protocols
Leptomeningitis	Prodromal headache, fever, vomiting and neck stiffness, vomiting, confusion	• Thick basal meningeal enhancement • Hydrocephalus • Small parenchymal infarctions • Cranial nerve enhancement/thickening	Precontrast/postcontrast-enhanced T1 and FLAIR images

Abbreviation: FLAIR, fluid-attenuated inversion recovery.

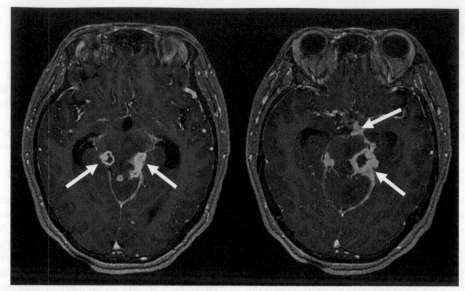

Fig. 2. Tuberculous meningitis. Axial T1-weighted postcontrast MR imaging shows thick nodular meningeal enhancement at the basal cisterns with abscess formation (*arrows*).

addition to the dilatation of lateral ventricles, periventricular T2 hyperintensity may be seen on MR imaging as a sign of transependymal edema (Fig. 4).[10] Although hydrocephalus may also occur transiently in bacterial meningitis, radiologists should consider the possibility of a TB cause whenever hydrocephalus is prominent.[26]

Cranial nerve involvement is reported in 17% to 40% of TB meningitis, especially cranial nerve (CN) II, III, IV, VI, and VII, considering their proximal location in the basal cistern. It occurs because of ischemic changes in the nerve or entrapment of the nerve in the basal exudates.[27] Clinically,

multiple cranial nerve palsies may occur; MR imaging shows diffuse thickening and enhancement of the involved cranial nerve, usually in their cisternal segments (Fig. 5).[28]

Cerebral Infarction and Vasculitis

Cerebral infarction is reported in 28% to 45% of patients with TB leptomeningitis.[29-31] The inflammatory exudate in the basal cistern can involve the perivascular space and adventitia of the perforator vessels, progressing to panarteritis of the vessel wall with secondary occlusion.[32,33]

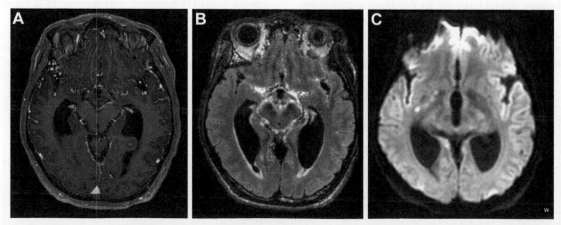

Fig. 3. Tuberculous meningitis. Axial T1-weighted postcontrast MR imaging shows subtle faint meningeal enhancement at the basal cisterns with hydrocephalus (*A*). Corresponding axial postcontrast FLAIR image shows much more prominent basal cisternal enhancement (*B*). A tiny acute infarction at the right lateral basal ganglia is also noted on diffusion-weighted imaging (DWI) (*C*).

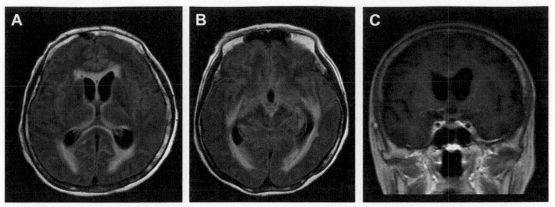

Fig. 4. Tuberculous meningitis with secondary hydrocephalus. An axial FLAIR image shows the diffuse dilatation of the bilateral lateral ventricle with periventricular hyperintensity from transependymal edema (*A, B*). Axial T1-weighted postcontrast MR imaging shows basal cisternal enhancement (*C*).

Vascular involvement of TB leptomeningitis may cause secondary vasculitis.[27,29,34] TB vasculitis may cause secondary cerebral infarction and most of the infarcts are found as small, multiple, and bilateral lesions in the basal ganglia, thalamus, and internal capsule, where the vascular territories of the basal perforators originate from the M1 segment of middle cerebral artery and from the basilar artery.[31] MR imaging patterns of acute infarction in TB typically exhibit multiple, bilateral diffusion restrictive, FLAIR high signal intense lesions, located often in the basal ganglia and the anterior thalamus (Fig. 6).[27,35,36]

On angiography, irregular beaded narrowing of the supraclinoid internal carotid artery and pericallosal artery, and a delayed circulation in the middle cerebral vein with a reduced collateral circulation are reported (Table 4).[37] Magnetic resonance angiography (MRA) may also demonstrate abnormalities, commonly in the middle cerebral artery and the posterior cerebral artery.[38,39] Patients with baseline MRA abnormalities may have a greater chance of developing infarctions than those with normal MRA results. The recently introduced high-resolution vessel wall imaging has demonstrated contrast enhancement in the involved arterial wall with predominant nodular and smooth enhancement (Fig. 7).[40]

Tuberculoma

Tuberculomas occur because of conglomeration and coalescence of microgranulomas, and are the second most common CNS manifestations of

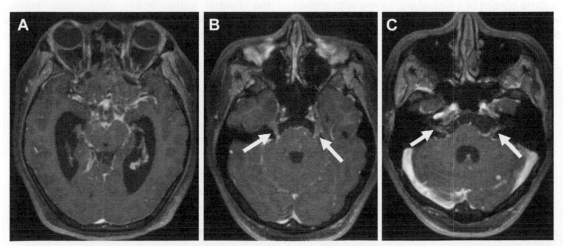

Fig. 5. Tuberculous meningitis with cranial nerve involvement. Axial T1-weighted postcontrast MR images show thick basal cisternal enhancement with hydrocephalus (*A*), diffuse thick enhancement along the cranial nerve V (*B*), and VII/VIII complexes (*arrows*) (*C*).

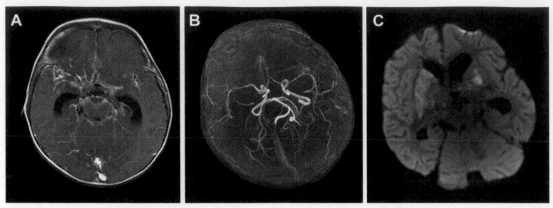

Fig. 6. Tuberculous meningitis with secondary acute infarction. Axial T1-weighted postcontrast MR imaging shows extensive enhancement in the basal cisterns (*A*). On time-of-flight MR angiography, there is luminal irregularity in the bilateral middle cerebral artery (MCA) (*B*). Axial DWI shows multifocal acute infarctions in the bilateral basal ganglia and thalamus (*C*).

TB after leptomenigitis.[10,35] They are mostly found at the gray matter and white matter junction as the hematogenous spreading microbes are captured in the distal arteries (Fig. 8).[10] A small number of tuberculomas can also gain entry into the brain parenchyma via the perivascular space around small penetrating arteries, from direct extension of leptomeningitis.[10,32] Tuberculomas are more common in children and are predominantly located in the infratentorial region, whereas in adults they tend to be predominantly supratentorial.[41] Tuberculomas can vary in size, but most are small, and the miliary nodules are often a few millimeters in diameter (discussed later). Tuberculomas typically pass through four different stages: (1) noncaseating granuloma, (2) solid caseating granuloma, (3) caseating granuloma with central liquefaction, and (4) calcified granuloma. Pathologically, tuberculoma consist of a typical granuloma with epithelioid cells, Langerhans giant cells, a peripheral rim of lymphocytes surrounding central caseous

necrosis, followed by liquefaction.[42] Tuberculomas may resolve completely, or form calcified granulomas.

Imaging findings of tuberculomas depend on their stage (Table 5). Noncaseating tuberculomas typically present as homogeneously enhancing nodular lesions with low signal on T1-weighted images and high signal intensity on T2-weighted images, usually surrounded by vasogenic edema (Fig. 9).[10,35] Solid caseating tuberculoma showed ring enhancement with central heterogeneous enhancement with hypointensity/isointensity on T1-weighted images (Fig. 10).[10,35] Sold caseating granulomas may show slightly hypointense T2 signal intensity because of the paramagnetic free radicals released from the inflammatory cells, with a combination of fibrosis and gliosis.[43,44] When caseating granuloma show liquefaction, the central enhancement disappears, leaving irregular, thick ring enhancement with central hyperintensity on T2-weighted images,[35] and

Table 4
Summary of TB vasculitis

	Clinical Symptoms	Imaging Finding	Recommended Protocols
Vasculitis	Focal neurologic signs	• Small, multiple acute infarction in the basal ganglia, thalamus, and internal capsule • Irregular beaded narrowing of distal ICA, proximal MCA, and ACA • Nodular and smooth vessel wall enhancement	DWIs, intracranial TOF MRA or CTA, high-resolution vessel wall MR imaging

Abbreviations: ACA, anterior cerebral artery; CTA, CT angiography; DWI, diffusion-weighted imaging; ICA, internal carotid artery; MCA, middle cerebral artery; MRA, magnetic resonance angiography; TOF, time of flight.

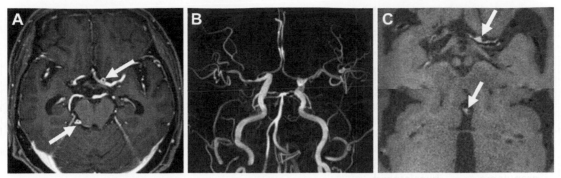

Fig. 7. Tuberculous meningitis with secondary vasculitis. Axial T1-weighted postcontrast MR imaging shows a few rim-enhancing nodular lesions in the basal cisterns (*arrows*) (*A*). Irregular narrowing of the bilateral anterior cerebral artery (ACA), middle cerebral artery (MCA), and posterior cerebral artery (PCA) is seen on MRA (*B*). High-resolution vessel wall imaging (*C*) reveals nodular thick enhancement along the left MCA and bilateral ACA (*arrows*).

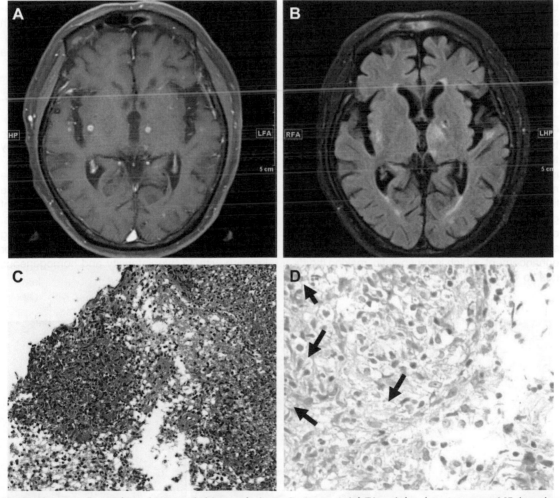

Fig. 8. Noncaseating tuberculoma with histopathologic findings. Axial T1-weighted postcontrast MR imaging and unenhanced FLAIR MR imaging show several rim-enhancing lesions in the right basal ganglia, left thalamus, and bilateral temporo-occipital lobe (*A, B*). The lesions were surgically resected. (*C*) Granulomatous inflammation with necrosis and suppurative inflammation (hematoxylin-eosin, original magnification ×200). (*D*) Ziehl-Neelsen staining reveals a few acid-fast bacilli under higher magnification (*arrows*) (original magnification ×600).

Table 5
Stage of tuberculomas with histopathologic/MR imaging appearance

Stage	T1-Weighted/ T2-Weighted Images	Contrast-Enhancement	DWI
Noncaseating granuloma	T1: hypointense T2: hyperintense	Homogeneous enhancement	No diffusion restriction
Caseating granuloma	T1: isointense/ hypointense T2: hypointensity	Ring enhancement with central heterogeneous enhancement	No diffusion restriction
Caseating granuloma with central liquefaction	T1: isointense to hypointense T2: central hyperintensity	Ring enhancement	Diffusion restriction (+/−)
Calcified granuloma	T2: dark signal intensity Blooming artifact (+)	No enhancement	No diffusion restriction

restricted diffusion on diffusion-weighted imaging because of high viscosity; unlike pyogenic abscess, there is less edema (**Fig. 11**).[35] Magnetization transfer (MT) imaging has demonstrated higher MT ratio in the nonenhancing cores of TB than in abscesses, likely related to their higher cellularity.[45]

Tubercular Abscess

CNS involvement of TB may rarely present as a true pyogenic abscess; they can occur in less than 10% of patients with CNS TB.[46] TB abscess is characterized by cavity formation with central necrosis, containing more bacilli, macrophages, liquefied necrotic debris, and pus than caseating granuloma.[47] Imaging finding of TB abscess includes central T1 hypointensity and T2 hyperintensity with central diffusion restriction and rim enhancement, which is nonspecific, making it difficult to differentiate it from pyogenic abscesses.

Compared with TB granulomas, TB abscesses are larger in size, and show a multiloculated thin-walled lesion (**Fig. 12**, see also **Table 5**),[27,48] with a lower MT ratio than tuberculoma. MR spectroscopy may help in differential diagnosis, with a high lipid peak in TB abscess.[48]

Miliary Tuberculosis

Miliary TB are mostly seen in immunocompromised patients. They are usually accompanied by extracranial and meningeal involvement of TB.[49] Miliary TB show innumerable scattered foci in the brain parenchyma, predominantly located at the gray matter and white matter junction because of hematogenous spread, similar to tuberculomas. On MR imaging, numerous, small noncaseating granulomas are scattered at the gray-white matter junction with T2 hypointensity and homogeneous enhancement (**Fig. 13**).[50]

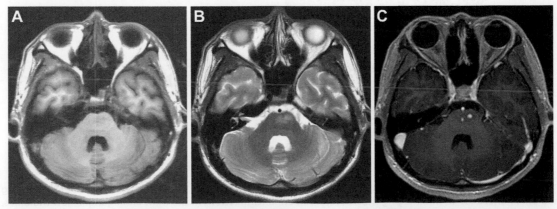

Fig. 9. Noncaseating tuberculoma. Axial T1-weighted MR imaging (A) shows a hypointense lesion in the ventral pons. Corresponding axial T2-weighted MR imaging (B) shows infiltrative high signal intensity, with homogeneous contrast enhancement on axial T1-weighted postcontrast MR imaging (C).

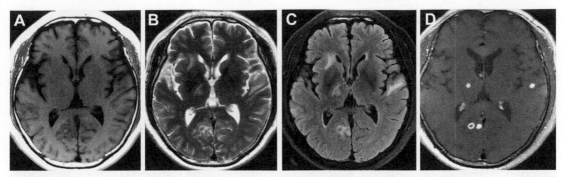

Fig. 10. Solid caseating tuberculoma. Multiple small nodular lesions are scattered in the right thalamus, right occipital lobe, and left frontal operculum. Axial T1-weighted MR imaging (*A*) shows hyposignal or isosignal intensity, whereas axial T2-weighted (*B*) and FLAIR (*C*) images shows central hyposignal intensity surrounded by high signal. There is solid or rim enhancement on axial T1-weighted postcontrast MR imaging (*D*).

Tuberculosis Cerebritis

TB cerebritis is a rare presentation involving focal brain parenchyma reported in patients without HIV infection, with or without concurrent leptomeningitis.[27] On MR imaging, parenchymal swelling with T1 hypointensities and T2 hyperintensities is noted with patchy contrast enhancement.[28] Histopathologically, it is composed of tubercular microgranulomata with scarce tubercular bacilli and without the associated caseous necrosis.

Tuberculosis Encephalopathy

TB encephalopathy is typically found in children with clinical symptoms of seizures and altered mental status.[42] It may be associated with type IV hypersensitivity, in which patients are reactive to a tuberculin protein.[37] Histopathologic examination reveals extensive white matter injury and perivascular demyelination, but without invasion by tuberculous bacilli. On imaging, TB encephalopathy presents severe unilateral or bilateral cerebral edema with T2 hyperintensity in the white matter without meningeal involvement (Fig. 14).[51] Diffuse contrast enhancement of the involved white matter may be observed.[52,53] Acute disseminated encephalomyelitis is an important differential diagnosis of TB encephalopathy.

Tuberculosis Pachymeningitis

Pachymeningitis in CNS TB is not commonly observed, and it usually occurs secondary to acute or chronic leptomeningitis. TB pachymeningitis is localized or in a diffuse form. On MR imaging, it is characterized by focal or diffuse dural thickening with prominent contrast enhancement and a FLAIR sequence may be helpful for detecting dural thickening.[54] Isolated TB pachymeningitis is difficult to differentiate from other types of pachymeningitis, such as

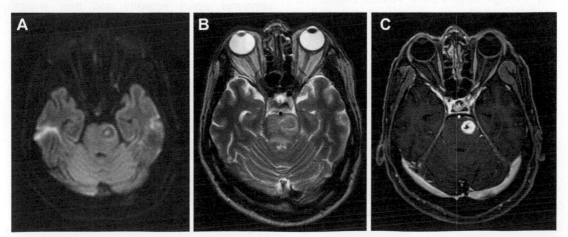

Fig. 11. Caseating granuloma with central necrosis. Axial DWI (*A*) shows a centrally diffusion-restrictive lesion in the left side pons with mixed T2 high signal intensity (*B*) and irregular thick rim enhancement (*C*).

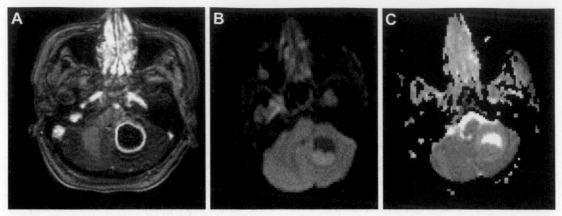

Fig. 12. Tuberculous abscess. A large, solitary abscess shows thin rim enhancement on axial T1-weighted postcontrast MR imaging (A) with central diffusion restriction on DWI (B, C).

neurosarcoid, neurosyphilis, and idiopathic hypertrophied pachymeningitis.[42]

Tuberculosis Ventriculitis

Subependymal TB focus may rupture into the ventricles or late-stage TB leptomeningitis can spread retrogradely to the ventricles. On MR imaging, CSF in the ventricles shows heterogeneous T1 signal intensity with diffuse thickening and enhancement along the ependymal lining (Fig. 15).[55] It is usually associated with hydrocephalus.

SPINAL TUBERCULOSIS
Tuberculosis Spondylitis

TB spondylitis is the most common presentation of skeletal infection of TB. TB spondylitis results from hematogenous spread of disease to the vertebral body through paravertebral venous plexus. TB spondylitis usually presents as multiple vertebral body involvement with intervertebral disk sparing in the early stage because mycobacteria are unable to degrade the collagenous annulus of the disk because of lack of proteolytic enzymes (Table 6).[56] TB spondylitis commonly shows paraspinal soft tissue extension and paravertebral abscess formation is also often detected.[28] There is a predilection of TB for the anterior vertebral body.[57] Severe complications of vertebral collapse resulting in kyphosis and cord compression is observed.[56]

Imaging findings of TB spondylitis show bone edema with low signal intensity on T1-weighted and hyperintense on T2-weighted/STIR images with contrast enhancement in its early stage (Fig. 16).[27] Later, extensive bony destruction of vertebral body becomes evident typically involving three or more vertebral levels of subligamental and paravertebral soft tissue enhancement or abscess formation (Fig. 17).[56,58] A well-defined paraspinal abnormal signal intensity and thin, smooth,

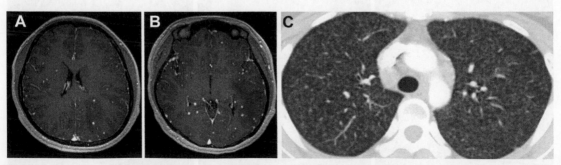

Fig. 13. Miliary TB. Axial T1-weighted postcontrast MR imaging show innumerable tiny enhancing foci scattered in the gray and white matter junction of the brain (A, B). Chest CT also shows diffuse miliary micronodules distributed throughout both lungs (C).

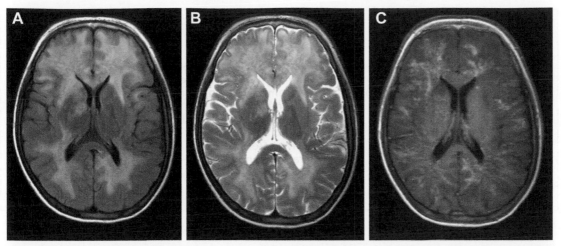

Fig. 14. Tuberculous encephalopathy. Axial FLAIR (A) and T2-weighted images (B) show severe symmetric diffuse white matter edema. Axial T1-weighted postcontrast MR imaging shows diffuse white matter contrast enhancement (C).

enhancing paraspinal and intraosseous abscess are also well-known imaging findings of TB spondylitis (Fig. 18).[58,59]

Tuberculosis Spinal Meningitis

Infrequently, TB causes spinal meningitis from cranial extension or from extension of adjacent TB spondylitis as a gelatinous granulomatous exudate that fills the subarachnoid space, causing focal spinal cord and nerve root inflammation.[10,35] In chronic cases, the exudate produces adhesions and fibrosis. Similar to cranial leptomeningitis, spinal meningitis can also cause local vasculitis and focal segmental infarction.[10,60] Imaging findings of spinal meningitis include spinal subarachnoid space loculations/obliteration, nerve root thickening or clumping, combined with irregular meningeal or nerve root enhancement (Fig. 19).[61] In the late stage of the disease, syringomyelia can occur

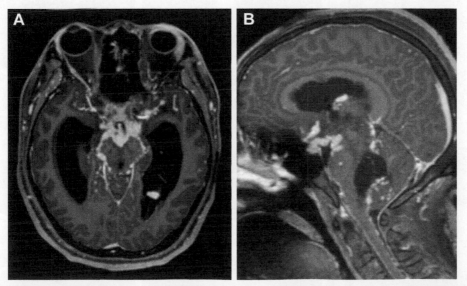

Fig. 15. Tuberculous ventriculitis and meningitis. Axial T1-weighted postcontrast MR imaging shows diffuse extensive thick enhancement of the basal cisterns that extends to the occipital horn of the left lateral ventricle and secondary hydrocephalus (A). Sagittal T1-weighted postcontrast MR imaging shows involvement of the suprasellar cistern, inferior ependymal lining of the fourth ventricle, and dorsal surface of the upper cervical spinal cord (B).

Table 6
Summary of TB spondylitis

	Clinical Symptoms	Imaging Finding	Recommended Protocols
Spondylitis	Back pain, stiffness, lower limb weakness, paraplegia	• 3 or more vertebral bodies involvement sparing intervertebral disks • Bone marrow edema with contrast enhancement (early phase) • Paraspinal and paravertebral soft tissue/abscess formation • Vertebral body collapse	Precontrast/postcontrast-enhanced T1 T2-weighted and fat suppressed T2-weighted

secondary to chronic arachnoiditis and appears as cystic central canal dilatation on MR imaging (Fig. 20).[10]

Tuberculosis Myelitis

TB myelitis is the second most common involvement of the spine, after spondylitis. In most cases, it appears in individuals younger than the age of 30, and involves intracranial TB. Clinical symptoms may vary from radicular pain to weakness. The thoracic spinal cord is most commonly affected, followed by lumbar and cervical cord. An affected spinal cord appears hyperintense on T2-weighted images and hypointense or isointense on T1-weighted images, with or without cord expansion.[61] Obliteration of spinal subarachnoid space, clumping nerve roots, and nodular intradural enhancement may be seen when meningitis is also present (Fig. 21).[62] Rarely, longitudinally extensive transverse myelitis as contiguous immune-mediated inflammatory lesion has been reported without pathologic evidence of active TB invasion of the spinal cord.[63,64]

Tuberculosis Intramedullary Tuberculoma

TB intramedullary spinal tuberculoma is a rare neurologic manifestation of TB and usually arises from hematogenous dissemination.[10] The most

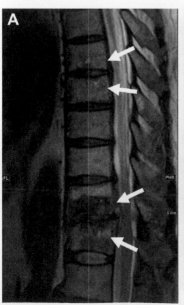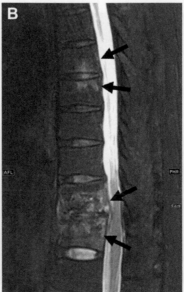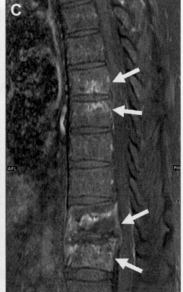

Fig. 16. Early stage of tuberculous spondylitis. Sagittal T2-weighted (*A*) and fat-suppressed T2-weighted MR imaging (*B*) show high signal bone marrow edema in the T7, T8, T11, and T12 vertebral bodies (*arrows*), skipping the intervertebral disks and intervening normal segments. (*C*) The lesions show enhancement on sagittal T1-weighted postcontrast MR imaging.

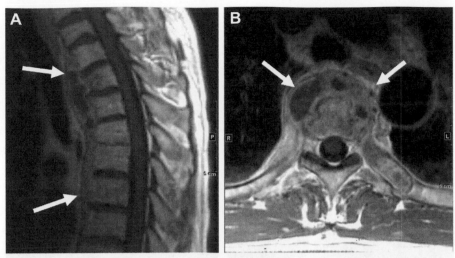

Fig. 17. Tuberculous spondylitis. Sagittal (A) and axial T1-weighted postcontrast MR imaging (B) show subligamentous extension of the enhancing prevertebral abscess (arrows) along the anterior longitudinal ligament at multiple vertebral levels.

common symptom is motor and sensory deficit, depending on the location of the lesion.[37,65,66] The MR imaging findings are similar to the characteristic appearance of intracranial tuberculomas, usually showing focal rim enhancement on postcontrast study.[67]

Paradoxic Reaction

Paradoxic reaction is defined as paradoxic clinical and/or radiologic deterioration after effective TB treatment initiation, and occurs because of excessive inflammatory response against mycobacterial antigens.[68,69] It is common in HIV-infected and HIV-uninfected patients with CNS TB and approximately one-third of patients with TB

leptomeningitis undergo paradoxic reaction.[69] Mycobacterial cell wall antigens are present in the affected brain tissues and trigger an exaggerated inflammatory reaction following treatment.[69] Patients exhibit aggravated clinical symptoms and imaging findings, such as basal cisternal enhancement, increased tuberculoma, development of infarctions, and worsening ventriculomegaly (Fig. 22).[69]

NONTUBERCULOUS MYCOBACTERIAL INFECTION

NTM are ubiquitous microorganisms that are widely distributed in water and soil.[70] CNS

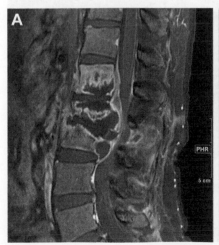
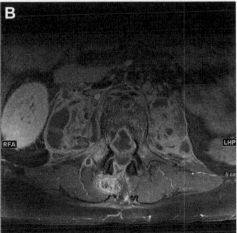

Fig. 18. Tuberculous spondylitis with abscess formation. Sagittal (A) and axial T1-weighted postcontrast MR imaging (B) show well-defined thin, rim-enhancing paraspinal, intraosseous, and epidural abscess with nonenhancing central cavity. There is also bilateral psoas abscess formation.

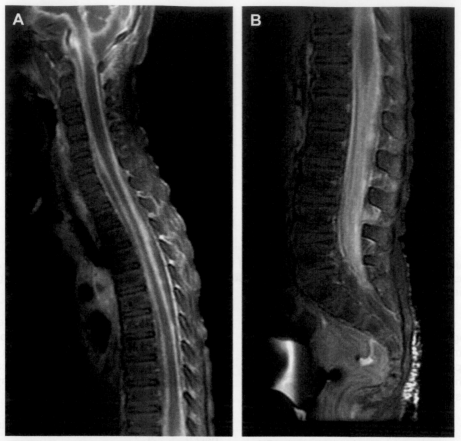

Fig. 19. Tuberculous spinal meningitis. Sagittal T1-weighted postcontrast (A,B) imaging shows extensive diffuse, thick meningeal and cauda equina enhancement.

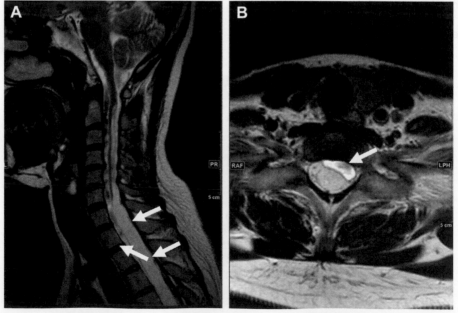

Fig. 20. Chronic arachnoiditis after remote TB spinal meningitis. Sagittal T2-weighted MR imaging (A) and axial T2-weighted MR imaging (B) show a syrinx formation in the cervicothoracic spinal cord with arachnoid cysts (arrows).

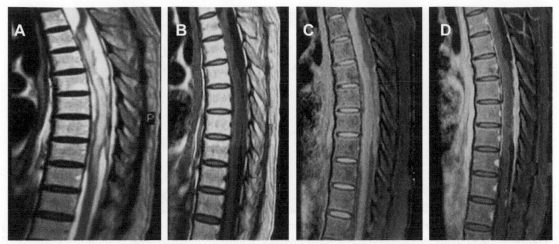

Fig. 21. Tuberculous myelitis. Sagittal T2-weighted MR imaging (A) and sagittal T1-weighted MR imaging (B) show diffuse cord swelling with T2 hyperintensity and T1 isointensity and ventral subarachnoid space obliteration. There is diffuse dural enhancement on sagittal T1-weighted postcontrast MR imaging (C, D).

infections caused by NTM are extremely rare, but there are increasing reports; high mortality is often associated with CNS involvement.[71] NTM usually infect immunosuppressed individuals, primarily those with HIV infection or transplant-associated immunosuppression, or those with hematologic malignancies.[70,72] CNS infection of NTM occurs in the settings of disseminated disease.[73] It usually presents as meningitis or meningoencephalitis.[74,75] The suggested mechanism of NTM-CNS infection is either through the hematogenous route because of high-grade bacteremia associated with disseminated NTM infections, or through direct inoculation, such as trauma, neurosurgery, and otolaryngologic infection.[1,76] Mycobacterium

avium is the most common species of NTM-CNS infection, followed by Mycobacterium fortuitum, Mycobacterium kansasii, and Mycobacterium abscessus. The clinical presentations of NTM-CNS infection vary from headache, fever, and vomiting to hemiplegia, seizures, and altered mental state.[76–78] Diagnosis of NTM-CNS infection may be challenging because of the nonspecific clinical features and rarity of the disease.

Imaging findings of NTM-CNS infection are not established because there are only a few reports of the disease. The common imaging manifestations include meningeal enhancement and/or cerebral involvement (Fig. 23).[79–81] However, radiologic features may not distinguish NTM

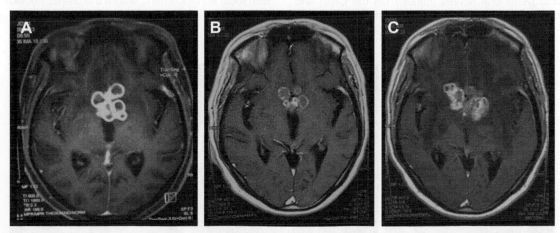

Fig. 22. Paradoxic reaction. Axial T1-weighted postcontrast MR imaging at symptom presentation (A) shows tuberculoma formation at the basal cistern. After treatment with antitubercular therapy, for 8 months the lesion decreased in size (B), but on follow-up after a year, repeat MR imaging shows paradoxic increase in size of the lesion (C).

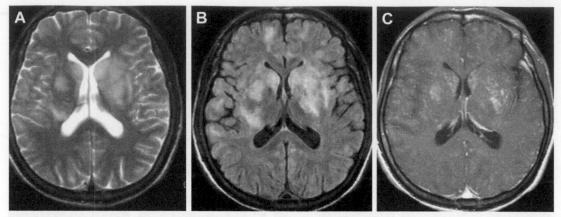

Fig. 23. NTM infection. Axial T2-weighted MR imaging (A) and FLAIR MR imaging (B) show multifocal patchy signal abnormality in the bilateral subcortical white matter and deep gray matter. Axial T1-weighted postcontrast MR imaging (C) shows widespread infiltrative contrast enhancement.

meningitis from other forms of meningitis, including tuberculous meningitis, because NTM infection may also exhibit basal nodular enhancement.[77,80] NTM infection of the CNS has rarely been reported as rhombencephalitis or an abscess that is indistinguishable from other causes of abscess.[78,82] An NTM infection may also manifest as hydrocephalus or brain atrophy, with chronic meningitis.[74,83] Therefore, if an immunocompromised patient has a sign of CNS infection and the pathogen for meningitis is difficult to detect, the clinician should suspect the NTM infection to avoid devastating complications.

LEPROSY

Leprosy is a chronic granulomatous disease caused by M leprae. It primarily affects the skin and peripheral nerves (rather than the CNS) and may cause significant functional impairments and deformities.[84,85] Although the incidence of leprosy has decreased in the past decades, it still remains a global public health issue.[85] A few case reports of CNS leprosy present as leprous ganglionitis and myelitis, mostly at the cervical spine.[86–88] The pathogenesis of spinal cord or brain involvement of leprosy is still unknown and hematogenous spread with direct infection or inflammatory immunologic reactions are suggested.[86]

On imaging, ganglionitis presents as the dorsal root ganglia swelling and contrast enhancement.[87,88] Combined brachial plexus thickening and enhancement may be found.[86] In some cases, there were asymmetrical T2 hyperintense cord signal changes with contrast enhancement at the adjacent cord, suggesting combined myelitis. On brain MR imaging, bilateral symmetric T2/FLAIR hyperintensity is observed in the dorsal brainstem with focal enhancement, where the cranial nucleus is located (Fig. 24).[86]

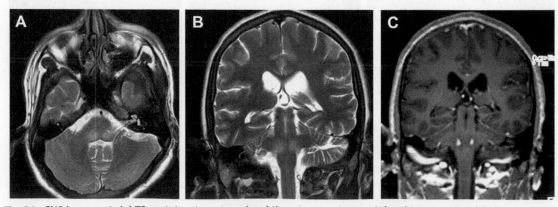

Fig. 24. CNS leprosy. Axial T2-weighted MR imaging (A) and coronal T2-weighted MR imaging (B) show symmetric T2 hyperintensities in the dorsal pons with corresponding contrast enhancement (C).

SUMMARY

TB is a common infectious disease of the CNS in developing countries and developed countries, in association with HIV infection. Cranial and spinal imaging are important in CNS tuberculous infection because understanding typical and atypical imaging findings may help in early diagnosis and disease monitoring in clinical practice. NTM infection is extremely rare in the CNS, and there are no consistent imaging findings. However, a high index of suspicion for CNS-NTM infection in indicative clinical conditions may be helpful.

CLINICS CARE POINTS

- Typical neuroimaging pattern of predominantly basal meningeal enhancement with hydrocephalus, with complications of cerebral infarction, should raise suspicion of tuberculous leptomeningitis, especially in immunocompromised patients and patients living in endemic areas.

- Tuberculomas have different imaging findings according to their clinical staging and radiologists should be aware of their stage-related characteristic imaging findings.

- Destructive, noncontiguous involvement of multiple vertebral bodies sparing intervertebral disks, especially in thoracic spine, is characteristic of tuberculous spondylitis.

DISCLOSURE

The authors have nothing to disclose.

REFERENCES

1. Franco-Paredes C. Infections of the central nervous system caused by nontuberculous mycobacteria. In: Kateryna Kon MR, editor. The Microbiology of central nervous system infections. Academic Press; 2018. p. 141–7.
2. Organization WH. Global tuberculosis report 2020. Geneva: World Health Organization; 2020.
3. Klein NC, Damsker B, Hirschman SZ. Mycobacterial meningitis. Retrospective analysis from 1970 to 1983. Am J Med 1985;79(1):29–34.
4. Ogawa SK, Smith MA, Brennessel DJ, et al. Tuberculous meningitis in an urban medical center. Medicine (Baltimore) 1987;66(4):317–26.
5. Verdon R, Chevret S, Laissy JP, et al. Tuberculous meningitis in adults: review of 48 cases. Clin Infect Dis 1996;22(6):982–8.
6. Yaramis A, Gurkan F, Elevli M, et al. Central nervous system tuberculosis in children: a review of 214 cases. Pediatrics 1998;102(5):E49.
7. Bidstrup C, Andersen PH, Skinhoj P, et al. Tuberculous meningitis in a country with a low incidence of tuberculosis: still a serious disease and a diagnostic challenge. Scand J Infect Dis 2002;34(11):811–4.
8. Banuls AL, Sanou A, Van Anh NT, et al. *Mycobacterium tuberculosis*: ecology and evolution of a human bacterium. J Med Microbiol 2015;64(11):1261–9.
9. Bowen LN, Smith B, Reich D, et al. HIV-associated opportunistic CNS infections: pathophysiology, diagnosis and treatment. Nat Rev Neurol 2016;12(11):662–74.
10. Bernaerts A, Vanhoenacker FM, Parizel PM, et al. Tuberculosis of the central nervous system: overview of neuroradiological findings. Eur Radiol 2003;13(8):1876–90.
11. Solari L, Soto A, Agapito JC, et al. The validity of cerebrospinal fluid parameters for the diagnosis of tuberculous meningitis. Int J Infect Dis 2013;17(12):e1111–5.
12. Chedore P, Jamieson FB. Rapid molecular diagnosis of tuberculous meningitis using the Gen-probe Amplified *Mycobacterium tuberculosis* direct test in a large Canadian public health laboratory. Int J Tuberc Lung Dis 2002;6(10):913–9.
13. Bonington A, Strang JI, Klapper PE, et al. Use of Roche AMPLICOR *Mycobacterium tuberculosis* PCR in early diagnosis of tuberculous meningitis. J Clin Microbiol 1998;36(5):1251–4.
14. Wilkinson RJ, Rohlwink U, Misra UK, et al. Tuberculous meningitis. Nat Rev Neurol 2017;13(10):581–98.
15. Kennedy DH, Fallon RJ. Tuberculous meningitis. JAMA 1979;241(3):264–8.
16. Mezochow A, Thakur K, Vinnard C. Tuberculous meningitis in children and adults: new insights for an ancient foe. Curr Neurol Neurosci Rep 2017;17(11):85.
17. Katrak SM, Shembalkar PK, Bijwe SR, et al. The clinical, radiological and pathological profile of tuberculous meningitis in patients with and without human immunodeficiency virus infection. J Neurol Sci 2000;181(1–2):118–26.
18. Kamran S, Bener AB, Alper D, et al. Role of fluid-attenuated inversion recovery in the diagnosis of meningitis: comparison with contrast-enhanced magnetic resonance imaging. J Comput Assist Tomogr 2004;28(1):68–72.
19. Andronikou S, Smith B, Hatherhill M, et al. Definitive neuroradiological diagnostic features of tuberculous meningitis in children. Pediatr Radiol 2004;34(11):876–85.
20. Bullock MR, Welchman JM. Diagnostic and prognostic features of tuberculous meningitis on CT

scanning. J Neurol Neurosurg Psychiatry 1982; 45(12):1098–101.

21. Mathews VP, Caldemeyer KS, Lowe MJ, et al. Brain: gadolinium-enhanced fast fluid-attenuated inversion-recovery MR imaging. Radiology 1999;211(1): 257–63.

22. Jeevanandham B, Kalyanpur T, Gupta P, et al. Comparison of post-contrast 3D-T1-MPRAGE, 3D-T1-SPACE and 3D-T2-FLAIR MR images in evaluation of meningeal abnormalities at 3-T MRI. Br J Radiol 2017;90(1074):20160834.

23. Berenguer J, Moreno S, Laguna F, et al. Tuberculous meningitis in patients infected with the human immunodeficiency virus. N Engl J Med 1992;326(10): 668–72.

24. Dekker G, Andronikou S, van Toorn R, et al. MRI findings in children with tuberculous meningitis: a comparison of HIV-infected and non-infected patients. Childs Nerv Syst 2011;27(11):1943–9.

25. Raut T, Garg RK, Jain A, et al. Hydrocephalus in tuberculous meningitis: Incidence, its predictive factors and impact on the prognosis. J Infect 2013; 66(4):330–7.

26. Wallace RC, Burton EM, Barrett FF, et al. Intracranial tuberculosis in children: CT appearance and clinical outcome. Pediatr Radiol 1991;21(4):241–6.

27. Patkar D, Narang J, Yanamandala R, et al. Central nervous system tuberculosis: pathophysiology and imaging findings. Neuroimaging Clin N Am 2012; 22(4):677–705.

28. Sanei Taheri M, Karimi MA, Haghighatkhah H, et al. Central nervous system tuberculosis: an imaging-focused review of a reemerging disease. Radiol Res Pract 2015;2015:202806.

29. Gupta RK, Gupta S, Singh D, et al. MR imaging and angiography in tuberculous meningitis. Neuroradiology 1994;36(2):87–92.

30. Misra UK, Kalita J, Srivastava M, et al. Prognosis of tuberculous meningitis: a multivariate analysis. J Neurol Sci 1996;137(1):57–61.

31. Kalita J, Misra UK, Nair PP. Predictors of stroke and its significance in the outcome of tuberculous meningitis. J Stroke Cerebrovasc Dis 2009;18(4): 251–8.

32. McGuinness FE. Intracranial tuberculosis. Clinical imaging in non-pulmonary tuberculosis. Springer; 2000. p. 5–25.

33. Palmer P. Tuberculosis of the central nervous system. The imaging of tuberculosis. Springer; 2002. p. 125–33.

34. Siva A. Vasculitis of the nervous system. J Neurol 2001;248(6):451–68.

35. Rodriguez-Takeuchi SY, Renjifo ME, Medina FJ. Extrapulmonary tuberculosis: pathophysiology and imaging findings. Radiographics 2019;39(7): 2023–37.

36. Essig M, Bock M. Contrast optimization of fluid-attenuated inversion-recovery (FLAIR) MR imaging in patients with high CSF blood or protein content. Magn Reson Med 2000;43(5):764–7.

37. Lehrer H. The angiographic triad in tuberculous meningitis. A radiographic and clinicopathologic correlation. Radiology 1966;87(5):829–35.

38. Kalita J, Singh RK, Misra UK, et al. Evaluation of cerebral arterial and venous system in tuberculous meningitis. J Neuroradiol 2018;45(2):130–5.

39. Kalita J, Prasad S, Maurya PK, et al. MR angiography in tuberculous meningitis. Acta Radiol 2012; 53(3):324–9.

40. Choudhary N, Vyas S, Modi M, et al. MR vessel wall imaging in tubercular meningitis. Neuroradiology 2021;63(10):1627–34.

41. Gupta RK, Kohli A, Gaur V, et al. MRI of the brain in patients with miliary pulmonary tuberculosis without symptoms or signs of central nervous system involvement. Neuroradiology 1997;39(10): 699–704.

42. Khatri GD, Krishnan V, Antil N, et al. Magnetic resonance imaging spectrum of intracranial tubercular lesions: one disease, many faces. Pol J Radiol 2018;83:e524–35.

43. Morgado C, Ruivo N. Imaging meningo-encephalic tuberculosis. Eur J Radiol 2005;55(2):188–92.

44. Jinkins JR, Gupta R, Chang KH, et al. MR imaging of central nervous system tuberculosis. Radiol Clin North Am 1995;33(4):771–86.

45. Pui MH, Ahmad MN. Magnetization transfer imaging diagnosis of intracranial tuberculomas. Neuroradiology 2002;44(3):210–5.

46. Provenzale JM, Jinkins JR. Brain and spine imaging findings in AIDS patients. Radiol Clin North Am 1997;35(5):1127–66.

47. Chakraborti S, Mahadevan A, Govindan A, et al. Clinicopathological study of tuberculous brain abscess. Pathol Res Pract 2009;205(12):815–22.

48. Luthra G, Parihar A, Nath K, et al. Comparative evaluation of fungal, tubercular, and pyogenic brain abscesses with conventional and diffusion MR imaging and proton MR spectroscopy. AJNR Am J Neuroradiol 2007;28(7):1332–8.

49. Krishnan N, Robertson BD, Thwaites G. The mechanisms and consequences of the extra-pulmonary dissemination of *Mycobacterium tuberculosis*. Tuberculosis (Edinb) 2010;90(6):361–6.

50. Trivedi R, Saksena S, Gupta RK. Magnetic resonance imaging in central nervous system tuberculosis. Indian J Radiol Imaging 2009;19(4): 256–65.

51. Lammie GA, Hewlett RH, Schoeman JF, et al. Tuberculous encephalopathy: a reappraisal. Acta Neuropathol 2007;113(3):227–34.

52. Udani PM, Dastur DK. Tuberculous encephalopathy with and without meningitis. Clinical features and pathological correlations. J Neurol Sci 1970;10(6): 541–61.

53. Dastur DK, Manghani DK, Udani PM. Pathology and pathogenetic mechanisms in neurotuberculosis. Radiol Clin North Am 1995;33(4):733–52.

54. Gupta RK, Kumar S. Central nervous system tuberculosis. Neuroimaging Clin N Am 2011;21(4): 795–814. vii-viii.

55. Goyal M, Sharma A, Mishra NK, et al. Imaging appearance of pachymeningeal tuberculosis. AJR Am J Roentgenol 1997;169(5):1421–4.

56. Schaller MA, Wicke F, Foerch C, et al. Central nervous system tuberculosis: etiology, clinical manifestations and neuroradiological features. Clin Neuroradiol 2019;29(1):3–18.

57. Currie S, Galea-Soler S, Barron D, et al. MRI characteristics of tuberculous spondylitis. Clin Radiol 2011; 66(8):778–87.

58. Jung NY, Jee WH, Ha KY, et al. Discrimination of tuberculous spondylitis from pyogenic spondylitis on MRI. AJR Am J Roentgenol 2004;182(6):1405–10.

59. Harada Y, Tokuda O, Matsunaga N. Magnetic resonance imaging characteristics of tuberculous spondylitis vs. pyogenic spondylitis. Clin Imaging 2008; 32(4):303–9.

60. Garg RK, Somvanshi DS. Spinal tuberculosis: a review. J Spinal Cord Med 2011;34(5):440–54.

61. Marais S, Roos I, Mitha A, et al. Spinal tuberculosis: clinicoradiological findings in 274 patients. Clin Infect Dis 2018;67(1):89–98.

62. Gupta RK, Gupta S, Kumar S, et al. MRI in intraspinal tuberculosis. Neuroradiology 1994;36(1):30–40.

63. Sahu SK, Giri S, Gupta N. Longitudinal extensive transverse myelitis due to tuberculosis: a report of four cases. J Postgrad Med 2014;60(4):409–12.

64. Zhang Y, Zhu M, Wang L, et al. Longitudinally extensive transverse myelitis with pulmonary tuberculosis: two case reports. Medicine (Baltimore) 2018;97(3): e9676.

65. Kayaoglu CR, Tuzun Y, Boga Z, et al. Intramedullary spinal tuberculoma: a case report. Spine (Phila Pa 1976) 2000;25(17):2265–8.

66. Compton JS, Dorsch NW. Intradural extramedullary tuberculoma of the cervical spine. Case Report J Neurosurg 1984;60(1):200–3.

67. Sharma MC, Arora R, Deol PS, et al. Intramedullary tuberculoma of the spinal cord: a series of 10 cases. Clin Neurol Neurosurg 2002;104(4):279–84.

68. Garg RK, Malhotra HS, Kumar N. Paradoxical reaction in HIV negative tuberculous meningitis. J Neurol Sci 2014;340(1–2):26–36.

69. Singh AK, Malhotra HS, Garg RK, et al. Paradoxical reaction in tuberculous meningitis: presentation, predictors and impact on prognosis. BMC Infect Dis 2016;16:306.

70. Falkinham JO 3rd. Surrounded by mycobacteria: nontuberculous mycobacteria in the human environment. J Appl Microbiol 2009;107(2):356–67.

71. Gonzalez-Santiago TM, Drage LA. Nontuberculous mycobacteria: skin and soft tissue infections. Dermatol Clin 2015;33(3):563–77.

72. Wu UI, Holland SM. Host susceptibility to nontuberculous mycobacterial infections. Lancet Infect Dis 2015;15(8):968–80.

73. García-Moncó JC, Rodriguez-Sainz A. CNS tuberculosis and other mycobacterial infections. In: García-Moncó JC, editor. CNS infections: a clinical Approach. Cham: Springer International Publishing; 2018. p. 157–79.

74. Jacob CN, Henein SS, Heurich AE, et al. Nontuberculous mycobacterial infection of the central nervous system in patients with AIDS. South Med J 1993;86(6):638–40.

75. Weiss IK, Krogstad PA, Botero C, et al. Fatal Mycobacterium avium meningitis after misidentification of M tuberculosis. Lancet 1995; 345(8955):991–2.

76. Lee MR, Cheng A, Lee YC, et al. CNS infections caused by Mycobacterium abscessus complex: clinical features and antimicrobial susceptibilities of isolates. J Antimicrob Chemother 2012;67(1): 222–5.

77. Talati NJ, Rouphael N, Kuppalli K, et al. Spectrum of CNS disease caused by rapidly growing mycobacteria. Lancet Infect Dis 2008;8(6): 390–8.

78. Karne SS, Sangle SA, Kiyawat DS, et al. Mycobacterium avium-intracellulare brain abscess in HIV-positive patient. Ann Indian Acad Neurol 2012; 15(1):54–5.

79. Cai R, Qi T, Lu H. Central nervous system infection with non-tuberculous mycobacteria: a report of that infection in two patients with AIDS. Drug Discov Ther 2014;8(6):276–9.

80. Kwon LM, Kim ES, Lee K, et al. Nontuberculous mycobacterial meningoencephalitis in a young healthy adult: a case report and literature review. Radiol Infect Dis 2018;5(2):85–90.

81. Gray F, Geny C, Lionnet F, et al. [Neuropathologic study of 135 adult cases of acquired immunodeficiency syndrome (AIDS)]. Ann Pathol 1991;11(4): 236–47.

82. Duong M, Piroth L, Chavanet P, et al. A case of rhombencephalitis with isolation of cytomegalovirus and Mycobacterium avium complex in a woman with AIDS. AIDS 1994;8(9):1356–7.

83. Devi DG, Mallikarjuna H, Chaturvedi A, et al. A case of meningitis caused by Mycobacterium abscessus in a paediatric patient. J Tuberculosis Res 2015; 3(02):54.

84. Lockwood DN, Saunderson PR. Nerve damage in leprosy: a continuing challenge to scientists, clinicians and service providers. Int Health 2012;4(2): 77–85.

85. Rodrigues LC, Lockwood D. Leprosy now: epidemiology, progress, challenges, and research gaps. Lancet Infect Dis 2011;11(6):464–70.

86. Polavarapu K, Preethish-Kumar V, Vengalil S, et al. Brain and spinal cord lesions in leprosy: a magnetic resonance imaging-based study. Am J Trop Med Hyg 2019;100(4):921–31.

87. Rice CM, Oware A, Klepsch S, et al. Leprous ganglionitis and myelitis. Neurol Neuroimmunol Neuroinflamm 2016;3(3):e236.

88. Bafna P, Sahoo RR, Manoj M, et al. Ganglionitis and myelitis: myriad neurological manifestations of Hansen's disease. BMJ Case Rep 2020;13(8).

Imaging of Central Nervous System Parasitic Infections

Thiago Augusto Vasconcelos Miranda, MD[a],*, Kazuhiro Tsuchiya, MD, PhD[b],
Leandro Tavares Lucato, MD, PhD[c,d]

KEYWORDS

- Parasitic neuroinfections • CNS parasitic infections • Neurotoxoplasmosis • Neurocysticercosis
- Cerebral echinococcosis • Neuroschistosomiasis • Neurosparganosis • Toxocariasis

KEY POINTS

- Understanding the epidemiologic relevance of parasitic central nervous system (CNS) infections, still highly prevalent in today's world.
- Radiologists should be familiar with typical imaging presentations of the most common helminthic and protozoan CNS infections, some of which can be diagnostic of the disease, as in neurocysticercosis.
- Clinical and epidemiologic information play a major role in the diagnosis of this group of diseases, particularly as imaging alone can be non-specific in some circumstances.
- Some features, like geographic exposition or eosinophilia, can be of extreme importance to correct clinical suspicion.

INTRODUCTION

Central nervous system (CNS) parasitic infections range from the globally prevalent (such as neurocysticercosis [NCC] and neurotoxoplasmosis) to the exceedingly rare (amebic infection). Table 1 summarizes the main parasites and some epidemiologic information discussed in this review. In the last few decades, worldwide prevalence and annual incidence of new cases have slowly declined, related mainly to improved sanitary policies and better prevention strategies. However, parasites are still endemic in many lower and middle-income countries (LMIC) and are, regrettably, neglected.[1,2] In addition, globalization and the increased movement of people across the globe, either through migration, work, or tourism, have resulted in a vastly interconnected global epidemiologic stage (as recently shown by the coronavirus disease-2019 pandemic), and some of those diseases have been detected a long way from endemic areas.[3,4] One report suggests up to 28% of neuroinfections in a teaching neurology ward in Brazil, were parasitic in etiology.[5] Hence, radiologists should be familiar with typical imaging features, as well as some clinical hallmarks, like eosinophilia. There are two broad categories of parasites: unicellular protozoa and multicellular helminthic worms.

UNICELLULAR PATHOGENS: PROTOZOAN INFECTIONS

Table 2 shows examples of protozoan neuroinfections, diagnostic clues, and imaging findings.

[a] Emergency Radiology Section, Hospital das Clínicas da Faculdade de Medicina da Universidade de São Paulo, Travessa da R. Dr. Ovídio Pires de Campos, 75 - Cerqueira César, São Paulo – SP 05403-010, Brazil; [b] JR Tokyo General Hospital, 2 Chome-1-3 Yoyogi, Shibuya City, Tokyo 151-8528, Japan; [c] Neuroradiology Section, Hospital das Clínicas da Faculdade de Medicina da Universidade de São Paulo, Travessa da R. Dr. Ovídio Pires de Campos, 75 - Cerqueira César, São Paulo – SP 05403-010, Brazil; [d] Grupo Fleury, Av. Gen. Valdomiro de Lima, 508 - Jabaquara, São Paulo - SP, 04344-070, Brazil
* Corresponding author.
E-mail address: thiago.miranda@hc.fm.usp.br

Neuroimag Clin N Am 33 (2023) 125–146
https://doi.org/10.1016/j.nic.2022.07.013
1052-5149/23/© 2022 Elsevier Inc. All rights reserved.

neuroimaging.theclinics.com

Table 1
Summary of common parasitic pathogens with neurologic relevance

Type	Disease	Pathogen	Human Infection Route(s)	Geographic Locations	Population Impact	CNS Involvement
Protozoa (unicellular)	Amebiasis	*Entamoeba histolytica*	Fecal-oral	Worldwide, obligatory parasite	500 million, disease in up to 50 million	Only a few cases reported
		Naegleria fowleri	Nasal mucosa	Worldwide, fresh water sources	<500 cases reported in the literature	
		Acanthamoeba spp. *Balamuthia* spp.	Nasal mucosa	Worldwide, soil and water sources	Only a few cases reported	Only a few cases reported
	Toxoplasmosis	*Toxoplasma gondii*	Contaminated food and water; vertical transmission (congenital)	Worldwide, humans are possible intermediate host	1/3 of the population worldwide. Congenital: 190,000 cases annually worldwide	HIV-AIDS related: up to 30% of reactivation in low lymphocyte CD4+ count. Congenital: 80%–90% of CNS disease
	Trypanosomiasis	*Trypanosoma brucei rhodesiense; Trypanosoma brucei gambiense*	Insect vector bite (tsetse fly)	Africa (mainly sub-Saharan)	<10,000 cases annually	Neurologic symptoms: up to 79%
		Trypanosoma cruzi	Insect vector bite (triatomine). Rarely contaminated food Blood transfusion	Central and South America	6–7 million	Only a few cases reported, usually immunosuppressed patients
	Malaria	*Plasmodium falciparum*	Insect vector bite (*Anopheles* mosquitoes)	Africa, Southeast Asia, Central and South America	241 million worldwide 600,000 deaths annually	1% of malaria patients, mostly children
Metazoa (multicellular)	Schistosomiasis	*Schistosoma japonicum Schistosoma haematobium Schistosoma mansoni*	Larval penetration of skin in contaminated water	Asia Sub-Saharan Africa Central and South America Asia and Africa	240 million worldwide	Cerebral involvement in 4%–28% of brain necropsies Up to 5% of non-traumatic myelopathy in endemic regions
Platyhelminths (flatworms) Trematodes (flukes)	Paragonimiasis				20 million	<1% of cases

		Paragonimus westermani	Contaminated food (crustaceans)			
Cestode (tapeworm)	Cysticercosis	*Taenia solium*	Fecal-oral	Intertropical and subtropical regions	50 million	1st cause of preventable epilepsy worldwide (30% in endemic areas)
	Echinococcosis	*Echinococcus granulosus* *Echinococcus multilocularis*	Contaminated food and water	Middle East, Europe, South America	Up to 7.7/100,000 in endemic areas	<2% of cases
	Sparganosis	*Spirometra mansoni*	Contaminated food and water	Southeast Asia	Uncertain, <2000 cases reported	5%–36% of cases
Nematodes (roundworms)	Toxocariasis	*Toxocara spp.*	Contact with cats and dogs, Contaminated food	Worldwide, especially subtropical and tropical regions	Estimates of up to 30% seropositivity in rural affected areas	<200 cases reported
	Angiostrongyliasis	*Angiostrongylus cantonensis*	Contaminated food (snails)	Southeast Asia and South Pacific	Around 3000 cases reported	
	Trichinellosis	*Trichinella spiralis*	Contaminated food (pork)	Worldwide, cluster-outbreaks	Up to 10,000 cases annually	Up to 10%–15% of all cases
	Gnathostomisasis	*Gnasthostoma spinigerum*	Contaminated food (freshwater fish)	Southeast Asia and Latin America	5000 cases reported	<500 cases reported

There is an important correlation with geographic locations, often affecting the tropical and subtropical regions in different continents. Epidemiologic data can be often imprecise, and there are suggestions of under-reporting in the literature due to low health care access in those regions (See Ref.76), reinforcing the notion of "neglected tropical diseases"

Table 2
Summary of protozoan neuroinfectious, diagnostic clues, and imaging findings

Pathogen	Disease	Clinical Picture and Diagnostic Clues	Imaging Findings
Entamoeba histolytica	Cerebral amebic abscess	CNS symptoms ± extracranial abscess (particularly liver)	Similar to typical brain abscess
Naegleria Fowleri	Primary amebic meningoencephalitis	Fulminant meningoencephalitis History of freshwater exposition Negative tests for other pathogens	Basal meningitis/ meningoencephalitis and cerebral edema
Acanthamoeba spp. *Balamuthia* spp.	Granulomatous amebic encephalitis	Chronic course of meningoencephalitis Specific testing if clinical suspicion	Focal meningitis and meningoencephalitis Cerebral edema, irregular meningeal and brain enhancement
Toxoplasma gondii	Neurotoxoplasmosis	Headaches, seizures, and focal deficit. HIV test (particularly in situations of higher prevalence)	Single/multiple focal nodular enhancing lesions ± central necrosis and edema Eccentric enhancing nodule (eccentric "target" sign) Multiple, bilateral hemorrhagic lesions IRIS-related worsening of lesion after antiretroviral therapy Atypical: pseudotumoral extensive necrotic lesion
	Congenital toxoplasmosis	Routine antenatal monitoring and fetal US fetal growth impairment	Hydrocephalus, periventricular calcifications, and chorioretinitis
Trypanosoma brucei rhodesiense *Trypanosoma brucei gambiense*	African trypanosomiasis (sleeping sickness/tsetse disease)	Early stage: systemic signs of infection. Late stage: sleepiness most frequent; focal neurologic deficits possible	Bilateral, symmetric white matter changes ± enhancement Basal ganglia hemorrhagic foci
Trypanosoma cruzi	American trypanosomiasis (Chagas disease)	Headache, seizures, and focal deficit. Previous diagnosis of the chronic form of the disease in an immunocompromised patient is the most important clue.	Heterogeneous, unspecific, and enhancing lesions Similar to other atypical infections (fungal and tuberculosis) or high-grade tumors
Plasmodium falciparum	Cerebral malaria	Fever, encephalopathy, seizures, and coma (most common in children)	Diffuse brain edema, small cortical infarcts, and microbleeds

Amebiasis

Although some species like *Entamoeba histolytica* are purely parasitic, other amebae are free-living protozoa found almost everywhere in the soil and water; both groups can cause CNS infections via the hematogenous or direct spread.

Cerebral amebic abscess

Entamoeba histolytica is a pure parasitic species and one of the most prevalent intestinal parasitic infections in the world.[6] Feco-oral infection can spread from the digestive system to the CNS in ages but might be more severe in immunocompromised individuals.

Imaging characteristics consist mainly of a cystic abscess with peripheral, irregular enhancement, encasing the necrotic central area with surrounding edema.[7] It can be virtually indistinguishable from bacterial or fungal abscesses. The trophozoite can be shown at the margins of the abscess at biopsy.[8,9] Multiple abscesses can occur in immunocompromised patients.[10] Hemorrhagic foci in the margins of the lesions can also be seen. Because of the embolic nature, liver abscess coexistence with brain abscess is a frequent finding and can be a helpful tip.

Primary amebic meningoencephalitis

Naegleria fowleri is a free-living, freshwater ameba, which can occasionally infect humans through the nasal mucosa to the olfactory nerve, subarachnoid space, and adjacent brain tissue, causing rapid and progressive meningitis and parenchymatous inflammation, with high lethality rates.[11]

Imaging studies can be unremarkable at the beginning of the disease course. Meningeal enhancement, mainly in the basal cisterns, and cerebral edema are most common, sometimes with brain parenchymatous enhancement in the cortico-pial interface (Fig. 1). Brain edema can be severe, with a high risk of herniation.[12–15]

Amebic granulomatous encephalitis

Free-living amebas like *Acanthamoeba* spp., *Balamuthia mandrillaris,* and others can be found widely in lake, rivers, soil, aquatic plants, standing and circulating water circuits, and humidifier tanks.[16] Infection via the nasal mucosa, olfactory apparatus, is common in immunocompromised patients.[16] The infection has a chronic course, with weeks of worsening headache, behavioral changes, with or without focal deficits, and low-grade fever; diagnosis can be challenging.[17]

Imaging findings resemble those of chronic meningitis with extensive focal meningeal enhancement, inflammatory mass, or both, with edema and occasionally enhancement.[14,17,18]

Toxoplasmosis

Toxoplasma gondii is an obligate intracellular parasite of felines; humans are intermediate hosts. Infection occurs by oral ingestion of food or water contaminated by infected cat feces; raw, infected meat, or vertical transmission from mother to child. The parasite will reach the liver of the intermediate host after oral ingestion, commonly affected tissues are muscles, liver, spleen, and CNS.[8,19]

Neurotoxoplasmosis in immunocompromised patients

In patients with HIV-AIDS (human immunodeficiency virus/acquired immunodeficiency syndrome) and extremely low CD4+ lymphocyte count (<50 cells/mm^3), impaired cellular-type immune response becomes insufficient to inhibit parasite reproduction and dissemination, often leading to extensive CNS involvement. Suspicion of toxoplasmosis reactivation should be high in patients with a known history of immunodeficiency.[20]

The most common imaging features include heterogeneous lesions both at computed tomography (CT) and MR, often with alternating attenuation and T2/fluid-attenuated inversion recovery (FLAIR)

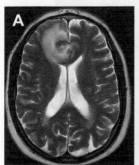 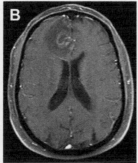 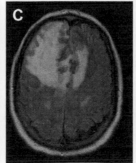 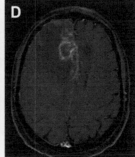

Fig. 1. Primary amebic meningoencephalitis. T2-weighted image (*A*) shows heterogeneous cortical signal with surrounding edema. Postcontrast T1-weighted image (*B*) discloses superficial enhancement. After 11 days, worsening of both perilesional edema on FLAIR (*C*) and postcontrast T1-weighted image (*D*), suggesting an unfavorable prognosis. (*Courtesy of* Maria da Graça Morais Martin, MD, PhD, São Paulo, Brazil.)

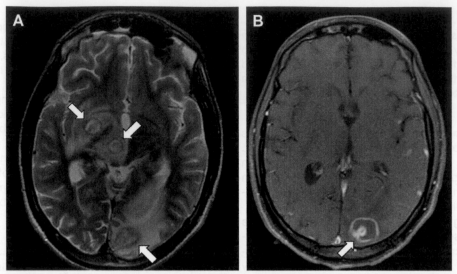

Fig. 2. Neurotoxoplasmosis. T2-weighted image (*A*) show the "target sign" in the right basal ganglia and thalamus (*arrows*), with peripheral edema. Postcontrast T1-weighted images (*B*) show the classic "eccentric target" sign (*arrow*).

signal related to areas of central necrosis, perilesional inflammatory response, and surrounding edema.[21] When the lesion occurs on the brain surface, brain parenchyma and sulcal involvement can give the appearance of an eccentric nodule inside the lesions, which can be highly suggestive of the diagnosis, the so-called eccentric target sign[22] (Fig. 2). Restricted diffusion can sometimes be seen.[23] Worsening of symptoms and imaging after initiation of antiretroviral therapy in HIV-AIDS patients can represent immune reconstitution inflammatory syndrome (IRIS) deterioration. Another uncommon presentation is almost purely hemorrhagic lesions (Fig. 3). In fact, the literature suggests

that most neurotoxoplasmosis lesions can show small intralesional foci of magnetic susceptibility, likely attributable to blood products.[24,25] Single, large, necrotic lesions with extensive adjacent edema (sometimes called acute necrotizing toxoplasmosis) can be almost indistinguishable from lymphoma (Fig. 4). In such tumefactive cases, advanced imaging features such as diffusion, perfusion, and spectroscopy can be sometimes useful to distinguish toxoplasmosis from lymphoma. Slightly higher relative apparent diffusion coefficients values are reported in toxoplasmosis (apparent diffusion coefficient (ADC) $> 1.6 \times 10^{-3}$ mm^2/s suggestive of toxoplasmosis; ADC $< 1.1 \times 10^{-3}$ mm^2/s pointing

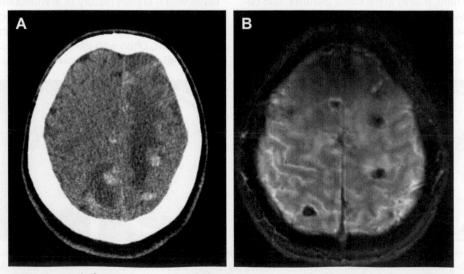

Fig. 3. Neurotoxoplasmosis, hemorrhagic presentation in an HIV-AIDS patient. Multiple hemorrhagic lesions can be appreciated as hyperdensities on CT (*A*), and hypointensities on SWI (*B*).

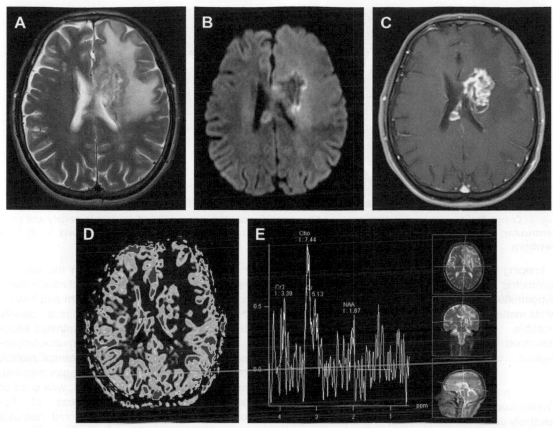

Fig. 4. Neurotoxoplasmosis, pseudotumoral presentation. Irregular periventricular lesion with heterogeneous T2 signal (A), peripheral restricted diffusion (B) and intense contrast enhancement (C). Dynamic susceptibility contrast (DSC) MR perfusion does not show increase in cerebral blood volume (D), and MR spectroscopy shows noisy baseline with slight increase in choline peak, suggesting an increase in cell membrane turnover (E). Although primary CNS lymphoma was suspected, biopsy revealed tachyzoite infiltration and no neoplastic characteristics. Increase in choline peak is likely related to intense inflammatory infiltration (see Ref.[32]).

to lymphoma; intermediate values reported for both), as well as lower relative Cerebral Blood Volume (rCBV) values (rCBV > 1.5 more common in lymphoma).[23,26–28] A markedly increased choline peak at MR spectroscopy could possibly also favor lymphoma over infection, but false positives are possible.[29–31] The coexistence of lymphoma and toxoplasmosis has also been reported.[23,26,27,32] Cerebrospinal fluid (CSF) studies usually confirm the diagnosis; however, particularly in those atypical cases, a trial of therapy and histologic analysis is often needed to establish the diagnosis. After antimicrobial treatment, lesion reduction and edema resolution can be seen; calcifications can arise. Enhancement can persist for weeks to months during treatment.

Congenital toxoplasmosis

Congenital toxoplasmosis occurs when a previously unexposed woman acquires the primary infection during pregnancy. The parasite will reach the placental circulation and the fetus, especially the brain and the eyes. Classical triad is ventriculomegaly, periventricular calcifications, and chorioretinitis.[29,30,33,34] Hydrocephalus and ependymal inflammation can also be seen, often with gross periventricular calcifications. Ocular involvement is characterized by chorioretinitis, with globe wall thickening and later with small, calcified bulbs (Fig. 5).

Trypanosomiasis

African trypanosomiasis

Trypanosoma brucei gambiense and *T brucei rhodesiense* are the two main species causing sleeping sickness, which is endemic in sub-Saharan Africa.[1,2]

Infection occurs by injection of the parasite through the bite of the tsetse fly of *Glossina* genus. Clinically, there are two phases: an acute systemic disease with fever, lymphadenopathy, asthenia, headache, arthralgia; and a late phase, when the parasite reaches other body fluids, like the CSF, leading to a meningoencephalitic stage.[8,35]

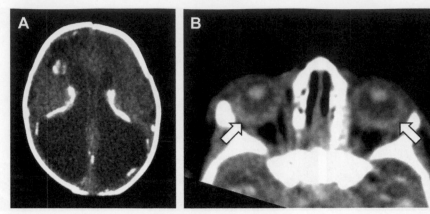

Fig. 5. Congenital toxoplasmosis. Non-contrast CT images disclose the classic triad of ventriculomegaly and periventricular calcification (*A*), and thickened soft-tissue density, signifying chorioretinitis (*arrows* in *B*) in a newborn.

Imaging findings include bilateral extensive and symmetric white matter abnormalities, with hypoattenuation/T2-hyperintensity involving deep white matter and corpus callosum. Enhancement is possible. Hemorrhagic foci have also been described in the basal ganglia and capsular regions.[36,37]

American trypanosomiasis

Trypanosoma cruzi infection (Chagas disease) is relatively common, with estimates of 6 to 7 million individuals affected in Central and South America, where the disease is endemic. Transmission occurs by the insect vector (triatomine bug) bite and inoculation of the parasite in the skin or mouth through vector-infected feces; oral ingestion of contaminated food (palm tree fruit and sugar cane being of particular relevance) and blood transfusion are other possible routes.[38,39]

The presence of an intracellular form in the *T cruzi* life cycle, the amastigote, allows it to develop a chronic, latent disease, in which the parasite "hides" inside cells and can lead to chronic inflammation mainly in the digestive system and heart.

CNS involvement is extremely rare, usually related to an acute, fulminant disseminated infection or reactivating disease in immunocompromised patients (such as heart transplantation patients with a known history of Chagas disease).

Lesions can be single or multiple, with solid or irregular enhancement and areas of T2-hypointensity, sometimes with central necrosis and extensive surrounding edema. These features resemble toxoplasmosis or fungal infections, or high-grade tumors (Fig. 6). Spinal involvement (Fig. 7), is characterized by extensive tumefactive myelitis, heterogeneous T2 signal, and enhancement.[15,40,41]

Cerebral Malaria

Malaria is endemic in Africa, Southeast Asia, and Central and South America.[1,2] *Plasmodium*

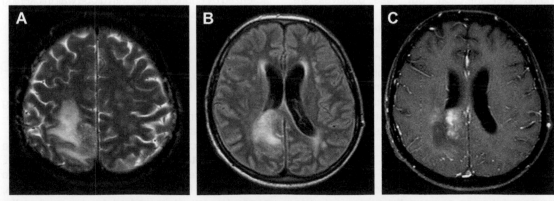

Fig. 6. American trypanosomiasis: Cerebral Chagas disease, status post cardiac transplant. T2-weighted (*A*) and FLAIR (*B*) images show heterogeneous signal, characterized by cortical hypointense areas, perilesional edema, and irregular enhancement (*C*).

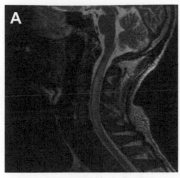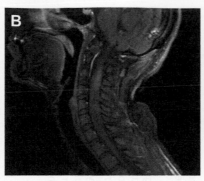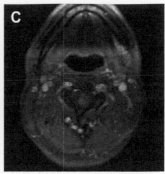

Fig. 7. American trypanosomiasis: Spinal Chagas Disease in an HIV-AIDS patient. Sagittal T2-weighted image shows extensive edema and tumefaction of the cervical cord (*A*), and poorly marginated focal enhancement (*B, C*).

falciparum is by far the most common of the four causative species, accounting for virtually all cases of CNS infection. Mortality rates for cerebral malaria can be as high as 25%.[8] The parasite infects human hosts through the mosquito (*Anopheles*) bite, the sporozoite infects red blood cells (RBCs) and replicates into merozoites that will infect other RBCs or reach other organs, particularly the liver. Sequestration of infected RBCs in the brain capillary circulation can lead to CNS involvement. Obstructed and inflamed small blood vessels can lead to hypoxic and ischemic changes and microbleeds.[8,42]

Imaging changes for CNS involvement are nonspecific and include diffuse brain edema, sulci effacement, small cortical infarcts, and microbleeds. Enhancement is usually absent, but possible. Severe cases can present with multiple lesions with T2-hyperintensity and restricted diffusion in the white matter and basal ganglia, which are thought to be related to hypoxic-ischemic changes and cytotoxic edema.[43–46]

MULTICELLULAR PATHOGENS: METAZOAN (HELMINTHIC) INFECTIONS
Platyhelminths (flatworms)

Trematodes (flukes)
Schistosomiasis Schistosoma species have a complex life cycle, involving freshwater snails as intermediate hosts (Table 3). Human infection occurs through the skin by the larva (cercaria). The clinically relevant species have distinct geographic ranges, including *Schistosoma japonicum* (Asia), *S mansoni* (Americas), and *S haematobium* (Africa). Each year more than 200 million require treatment.[2]

Disease symptoms are related to tissue deposition of the eggs and associated inflammation, usually in the intestines and portal circulation or urogenital tract. Embolization of the eggs through portosystemic or pelvic venous shunts to systemic circulation can gain access to the perivertebral plexus, and thus the CNS. The parasite egg elicits an intense immune reaction, with granuloma formation.[4,8,47,48]

Imaging findings are usually nonspecific and related to granuloma formation and inflammation. Focal lesions showing heterogeneous signal in T2-weighted images and nodular or irregular enhancement, with surrounding vasogenic edema, are the most common findings[47–54] (Fig. 8).

Large lesions with heterogenous signals and multiple irregular nodular and linear enhancement or even "arborized" appearances are also reported in *S japonicum*, which may help differentiate from neoplasm.[55] *Schistosoma mansoni* infection typically affects the *conus* medullaris. Spinal cord T2-hyperintense tumefaction, edema, and abnormal enhancement in a patient with positive epidemiology, can suggest the correct diagnosis[54,55] (Fig. 9).

Paragonimiasis *Paragonimus westermani* is endemic in Asia. Infection occurs through oral ingestion of infected freshwater crustaceans. CNS involvement is uncommon. Extensive inflammation, with hemispheric conglomerates of multiple ring-shaped enhancing lesions ("grape cluster" or "soap bubble") is suggestive. Hemorrhagic lesions and infarction are frequent, related to vascular damage by parasite migration, as well as pseudoaneurysm formation. Calcified lesions have been described.[56–59]

Cestodes (Tapeworm)
Neurocysticercosis *Taenia solium* is one of the most prevalent parasitic diseases in the world, being endemic to most intertropical regions; NCC is the leading cause of acquired epilepsy worldwide. Infection is fecal-oral, and there are two main forms of the disease: (NCC and *taenisasis*). NCC

Table 3
Summary of helminthic neuroinfections, diagnostic clues, and imaging findings

Pathogen	Disease	Clinical Picture and Diagnostic Clues	Imaging Findings
Schistosoma japonicum *Schistosoma mansoni* *Schistosoma haematobium*	Schistosomiasis	Headache, seizures, and focal deficits Cauda equina syndrome Eosinophilia (CSF or blood)	Brain: lesions with heterogeneous T2 signal, nodular, or irregular enhancement, vasogenic edema. "Arborized" enhancement can be suggestive Spine: tumefactive lesion, more frequently in the conus, heterogeneous T2 signal and enhancement
Paragonimus westermani	Paragonimiasis	Seizures, fever Eosinophilia (CSF or blood)	Hemispheric conglomerates of multiple ring-shaped enhancing lesions. Hemorrhagic lesions, infarctions, and pseudoaneurysms (vascular damage).
Taenia solium	Parenchymal Neurocysticercosis (NCC)	Positive epidemiology for NCC Headaches and seizures Meningismus Classic cystic lesion with scolex is the most important clue Eosinophilia is uncommon	Vesicular stage: cystic unilocular CSF-like lesion, and scolex visible—diagnostic Colloidal vesicular stage: cystic lesion with edema (FLAIR) and enhancement. High-protein content. Nodular granular stage: enhancing nodular lesion, residual perilesional inflammation, and edema Nodular calcified stage: small, calcified nodule (SWI or CT), no enhancement, or edema
	Ventricular NCC		Intraventricular lesion (vesicular and vesicular colloidal stages); fourth ventricle most common. CISS and equivalent sequences are helpful.
	Subarachnoid NCC (racemose)		Basal cisterns, sylvian fissure expansion, and meningeal enhancement (scolex usually not identifiable)
	Spinal NCC		Usually subarachnoid disease, in racemose presentation

Echinococcus granulosus	Cystic echinococcosis (hydatid disease)	Positive epidemiology for the disease. Headaches, seizures, and focal deficits. Classic cystic lesion is the most important clue.	CE0/CE1: simple cystic lesion without wall, possible deposited "sand" content inside. CE2: cystic lesion with thin T2-hypointense wall, enhancement and daughter vesicles (diagnostic). CE3: cystic lesion occupied by smaller vesicles and perilesional edema. CE4: degenerated cyst and heterogeneous content. CE5: cystic lesion with peripheral calcifications
Echinococcus multilocularis	Alveolar echinococcosis	Positive epidemiology for the disease. Headaches, seizures and focal deficits. Biopsy often necessary	Heterogeneous multicystic lesions, often with a pseudotumoral appearance.
Spirometra mansoni	Sparganosis	Positive epidemiology for the disease. Headaches, seizures, and focal deficits. Eosinophilia (CSF or blood) is the most important clue	"Tunnel sign": elongated T1-hypointense lesions with a rim of T2-hypointensity and enhancement (granulomatous process, morphology related to the migration of the parasite).
Toxocara spp.	Toxocariasis	Myelitis (most common). Meningoencephalitis. Eosinophilia (CSF or blood) is the most important clue	T2-hyperintense lesions in the spinal cord. Bilateral T2-hyperintense lesions in the white matter, meningeal enhancement. Occasionally ADEM-like appearance (immune-mediated mechanism).
Angiostrongylus cantonensis *Trichinella spiralis* *Gnasthostoma spinigerum*	Eosinophilic meningitis	Headaches and seizures. Meningismus. Eosinophilia (CSF or blood) is the most important clue	Nonspecific: multiple T2-hyperintense lesions in the white matter, and leptomeningeal enhancement. Brain hemorrhagic foci, usually linear. Anterior circulation watershed-infarcts related to severe hypereosinophilia

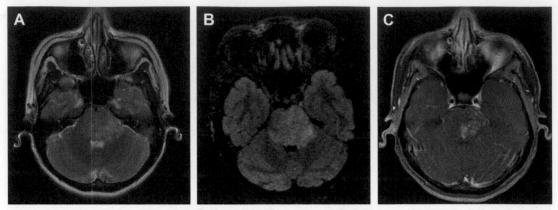

Fig. 8. Cranial neuroschistosomiasis (*Schistosoma mansoni*). T2-weighted (*A*) and FLAIR (*B*) images show tumefaction and hyperintensity of the pons and both middle cerebellar peduncles. There is irregular, patchy enhancement (*C*).

occurs when the eggs are ingested by the intermediate host (swines or humans), and the larva reaches the bloodstream and relocates to the CNS, where it develops into a cystic structure known as *cysticercus*, with the scolex (*T solium* head) inside, avoiding host immune response. *Taeniasis* occurs when the definitive host (usually humans) ingests raw pork meat infected with cysticercus, which will develop into the adult worm in the digestive tract and the production of more eggs, completing the cycle. NCC can be parenchymal, intraventricular, subarachnoid, and spinal; or a combination of these[8,60–63]

Parenchymal   Neurocysticercosis Parenchymal neurocysticercosis has four stages In the *vesicular stage*, the larva develops a well-formed parenchymatous cyst. Imaging features of this stage include visualization of an aqueous cyst and, if big enough, the scolex (parasite) is often distinguishable inside

it, as a small hyperattenuating focus on CT, FLAIR hyperintensity, or restricted diffusion[64] (**Fig. 10**). High-resolution, thin-section constructive interference in steady state (CISS) and equivalent sequences show the parasite and cyst morphology.[65] There is no enhancement or perilesional edema in this phase. The characterization of a cyst with a scolex is diagnostic of the disease.[66,67]

In the *colloidal vesicular stage*, the cyst is degenerating, and this marks the beginning of the active inflammatory phase, characterized by an increase in FLAIR signal intensity inside the cyst related to high protein content, surrounding edema, and peripheral enhancement (**Fig. 11**).[37,43,63] In the *granular nodular stage*, as cyst degeneration progresses, lesion size decreases, and peripheral enhancement is thicker. T2/T2*-hypointensity is more evident, as calcification begins, a process that can be better appreciated by CT. Edema and

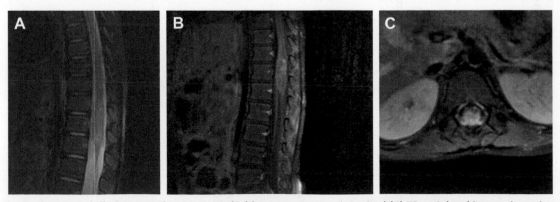

Fig. 9. *Conus medullaris* neuroschistosomiasis (*Schistosoma mansoni*). Sagittal (*A*) T2-weighted image shows heterogeneous hyperintensity and *conus* swelling; there are some foci of internal hypointensity. Sagittal (*B*) and axial (*C*) postcontrast T1-weighted images show heterogeneous nodular enhancement, also involving meninges and cauda equina.

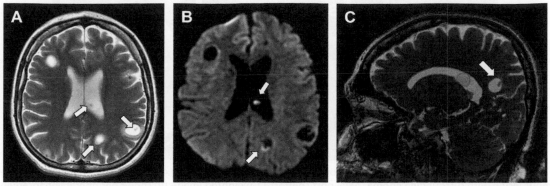

Fig. 10. Vesicular neurocysticercosis. Patient with multiple lesions in different stages. T2-weighted image shows multiple cystic lesions isointense to CSF, (*arrows* in *A*), some with a visible scolex. The scolex is seen on DWI as hyperintense "dots" or "commas" (*arrows* in *B*). 3D-CISS sequences can better depict an intraventricular lesion and the internal structure and scolex within vesicular cyst (*arrow* in *C*).

tumefaction will progressively reduce, leaving an enhancing granulomatous nodule (see Fig. 11).[37,43,63] In the *nodular calcified stage,* the granuloma is characterized by a small, calcified lesion without surrounding edema or enhancement (Fig. 12). A subtle ring enhancement, sometimes associated with residual inflammation, is best seen at MR imaging. Transition between granular nodular and nodular calcified stage should mark the end of the inflammatory phase, although reactivation is possible.[62,63,68,69]

Intraventricular Neurocysticercosis The most common location is the fourth ventricle followed by the third and lateral ventricles. Mass effect of the cyst will often lead to CSF flow disturbances and obstructive hydrocephalus. CISS and equivalent sequences are useful for detection.

Cyst degeneration will lead to a similar FLAIR signal increase as seen in the parenchymatous form. Inflammation inside the ventricular system can lead to ventriculitis and ependymal enhancement, which can by themselves also lead to obstructive hydrocephalus.[37,69,70] (Fig. 13).

Racemose Neurocysticercosis: Subarachnoid and Meningeal Involvement Enlargement and occupation of the basal cisterns and sylvian fissures by multiple cysts are often seen, sometimes arranged in a "grape-like" manner (hence the term

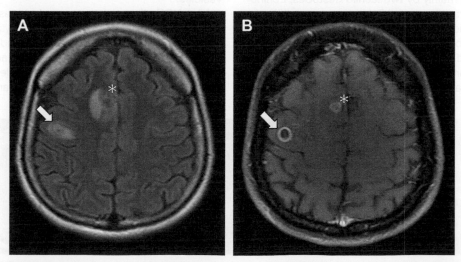

Fig. 11. Colloidal vesicular (*arrow*) and granular nodular (*asterisk*) neurocysticercosis. FLAIR image (*arrow, A*) shows a colloidal vesicular cyst with high signal from protein content, surrounding edema and peripheral enhancement (*arrow, B*) in the frontal lobe. There is a second lesion in the medial frontal region with nodular enhancement typical of granular nodular stage (*asterisks*).

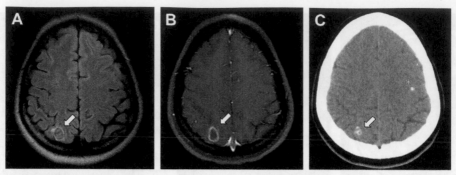

Fig. 12. Granular nodular and calcified neurocysticercosis. Axial FLAIR image (*A*) shows a right parietal heterogeneous lesion with surrounding edema. Axial post contrast T1-weighted image (*B*) shows peripheral enhancement and its cystic nature. After 2 years, CT (*C*) shows lesion shrinkage and partial calcification, as well as edema reduction, showing progression to granular nodular stage (*arrow*). A second, solid calcification in the left frontal region with no edema depicts the typical calcified stage (*asterisk*).

racemose). Frequently no scolex is seen. Imaging findings include localized sulci enlargement and meningeal enhancement (Fig. 14). CISS sequences help to identify the cyst wall within the subarachnoid space. Other findings include hydrocephalus from meningitis and obstruction of ventricular openings. Prognosis is often worse compared with other forms.[69,71–73]

Spinal Neurocysticercosis Spinal NCC is rare, usually represented by racemose cysts in the subarachnoid space, leading to cord compression and meningitis (see Fig. 14). Intramedullary disease is even rarer, when present it is similar to brain parenchymal NCC.[43,74,75]

Echinococcosis (Hydatid Disease) Echinococcosis is caused mainly by two taeniid cestodes, *Echinococcus granulosus* and *Echinococcus multilocularis*, which causes cystic and alveolar echinococcosis, respectively. Definitive hosts are dogs, and humans are intermediate hosts. Infection occurs by ingestion of the parasite eggs in contaminated food or water. *Echinococcus*

granulosus is found in Oceania, the Middle East, and South America, and *E multilocularis* is prevalent in the northern hemisphere.[2,76]

CNS disease is rare, and the following forms can be found: cystic cerebral, cystic subarachnoid/ventricular, and spinal forms, related to *E granulosus;* and cerebral alveolar echinococcosis, related to *E multilocularis*.

Parenchymal Cystic Echinococcosis The most common presentation is a large unilocular cyst surrounded by brain parenchyma. The cystic lesion comprises an outer layer, the pericyst (a host-derived fibrous and inflammatory tissue); the ectocyst (a middle acellular layer, derived from the parasite); and an inner layer, the endocyst, a germinal layer that can produce the typical daughter vesicles.

Like NCC, there are proposed stages to help guide therapy. Initially, there is a simple cystic lesion without wall, and possible deposited "sand" content inside (classified as CE0/CE1, indicating active disease). Then one can appreciate a cystic lesion with a thin T2-hypointense wall, possible enhancement,

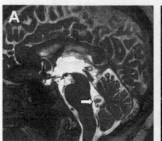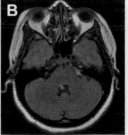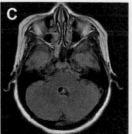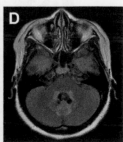

Fig. 13. Intraventricular cysticercosis. MR 3D-CISS image (*A*) depicts a typical IV ventricle cyst, with scolex (*arrow*). Sequential axial FLAIR images over 4 years show progression: from typical aqueous cyst with scolex (*B*); cyst degeneration and heterogeneously increased signal content (*C*); IV ventricle dilation and edema of the surrounding cerebellum from inflammatory synechia and adhesions obstructing the CSF flow (*D*).

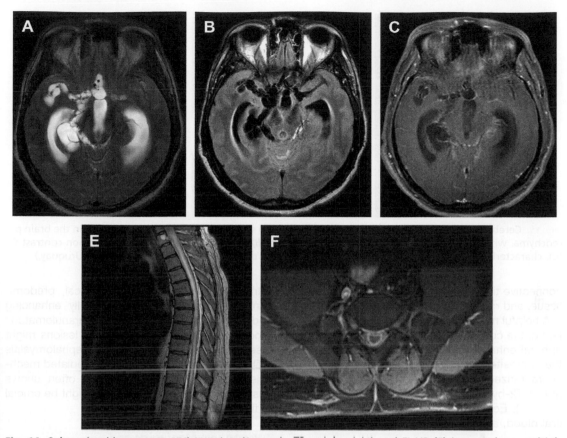

Fig. 14. Subarachnoid racemose and spinal cysticercosis. T2-weighted (A) and FLAIR (B) images show multiple cisternal cysts and hydrocephalus with interstitial edema, corresponding postcontrast T1-weighted image (C) shows enhancement of cyst walls and leptomeninges. No scolex is seen, a common finding in racemose cysticercosis. On sagittal T2-weighted spinal image, there is extensive intramedullary increased signal (D) and peripheral enhancement on axial postcontrast T1-weighted image (E).

smaller peripheral daughter vesicles (also related to active disease, CE2, which is the most typical for the diagnosis of echinococcosis). The following stage is represented by a cystic lesion occupied by smaller vesicles and perilesional edema (transitional form, CE3). The latter two stages represent inactive disease, CE4 (degenerated cyst, heterogeneous content) and CE5 (cystic lesion with peripheral calcifications)[43,77–79] (Fig. 15).

MR spectroscopy shows peaks from lactate, succinate, and acetate, similarly to spectra from pyogenic bacteria; however, a pyruvate peak can suggest cestode parasite infection.[80–82]

Subarachnoid and Ventricular Echinococcosis It is an unusual form of the disease. Only one unilocular or multilocular subarachnoid cyst is present, with variable dimensions. Meningitis and leptomeningeal enhancement are possible.[37,78,83]

Spinal Echinococcosis Rarely, the disease can affect the spinal cord, and slow growth can lead to vertebral bony remodeling, compressive myelopathy, and extension to adjacent structures[79,84] (Fig. 16).

Alveolar cerebral echinococcosis Echinococcus multilocularis forms heterogeneous lesions that can be mistaken for malignancies rather than simple cysts.[85]

Imaging characteristics include collections of small cysts, often forming an irregular mass of inflammatory tissue. There can be a peripheral enhancement, with a T2-hypointense irregular rim. Partially calcified walls are possible. Often, extensive surrounding edema leads to mass effect.[78,79,85,86]

Sparganosis The cestode *Spirometra mansoni* affects small carnivores and causes a migrating larval disease in Asia. Infection occurs mainly by oral ingestion, with humans acting as the intermediate hosts. Migration of the larva through

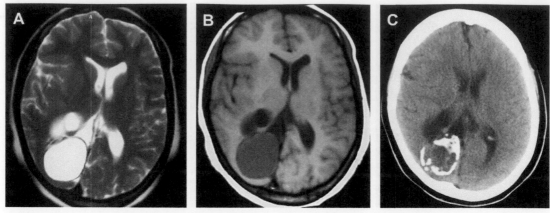

Fig. 15. Cerebral cystic echinococcosis. T2-weighted image (*A*) shows large, complex cystic lesions in the brain parenchyma, with intermediate signal intensity (T1-weighted, *B*) and peripheral calcifications on non-contrast CT (*C*), characterizing an inactive form of the disease. (*Courtesy of* Jorge Boschi, MD, Montevideo, Uruguay.)

connective tissue affects the eyes, subcutaneous tissue, and rarely, the CNS.[8,53,87]

A helpful neuroimaging feature is the visualization of the curvilinear T1-hypointensities with peripheral enhancement ("tunnel sign"), formed as the parasite migrates. Granuloma formation characterized by T1-hypointense lesions with a rim of T2-hypointensity has also been reported (Fig. 17). Eosinophilia, both at CSF and peripheral blood, are clues to the diagnosis.[88–94]

Nematodes (Roundworms)

Toxocariasis
Toxocariasis is caused by the *Toxocara* spp., common ascarid roundworms found in domesticated animals worldwide. Humans are accidental hosts, after ingestion of the eggs or larvae in contaminated meat or water, visceral (liver, lungs, musculoskeletal system), and ocular toxocariasis is commoner than myelitis or meningoencephalitis.[8,95,96]

Imaging findings include multifocal, predominantly T2-hyperintense, occasionally enhancing nodular lesions likely related to the granulomatous process.[76–81,95–102] Sometimes the lesions might resemble acute disseminated encephalomyelitis (ADEM), with a possible immune-mediated mechanism[101] (Fig. 18). CSF analysis often shows eosinophilia, and this information might be crucial to the correct diagnosis.[102]

Eosinophilic Meningitis and Meningoencephalitis

Eosinophilic meningitis is defined by the presence of 10 or more eosinophils/μL in the CSF or a CSF eosinophilia of at least 10%. This is a very helpful feature for narrowing the differential diagnosis since the commonest cause is a helminthic invasion. Although reported in correlation with most of the other helminths discussed before, it should be noted that *Angiostrongylus*

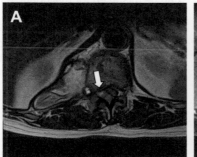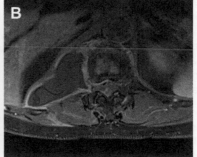

Fig. 16. Spinal echinococcosis (same patient as Fig. 15). T2-weighted images (*A*) show a small, partially collapsed epidural spinal cyst (*arrow*) and larger paraspinal complex soft tissue cyst with internal linear hypointensities. Postcontrast T1-weighted image (*B*) shows extensive perilesional enhancement. (*Courtesy of* Jorge Boschi, MD, Montevideo, Uruguay.)

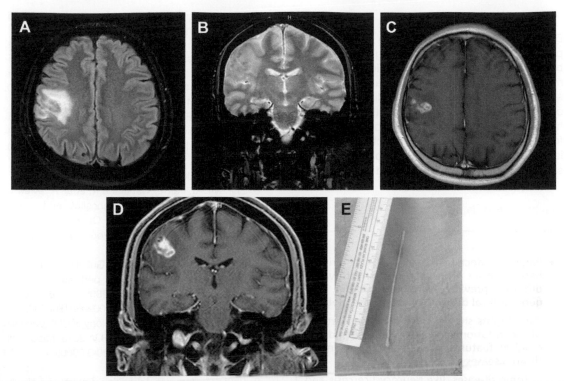

Fig. 17. Sparganosis. Axial FLAIR (*A*) and coronal T2-weighted (*B*) images show heterogeneous abnormal cortical signal with surrounding vasogenic edema. Corresponding postcontrast T1-weighted images (*C*, *D*) show curvilinear non-enhancing areas with intense peripheral enhancement. This could represent the migrating tracks of the parasite in the parenchyma ("tunnel sign"). At surgery, the parasite was removed (*E*). (*Courtesy of* A Boongird, MD, Mahidol University, Bangkok, Thailand.)

cantonensis is reported as the most frequent cause.[53,103–107] Other causes of eosinophilic meningitis include the helminths *Trichinella spiralis* and *Gnasthostoma spinigerum*, fungi such as *Coccidioides immitis*, bacteria, rickettsia, malignancies, and drugs.[107]

Imaging findings are nonspecific and can include multiple bilateral T2-hyperintense lesions in the white matter, extensive meningitis (with or without leptomeningeal enhancement).[108] Anterior circulation watershed infarcts, likely related to severe hypereosinophilia, have been reported in trichinellosis.[109] Brain hemorrhagic foci, sometimes linear, have been reported in association with angiostrongyliasis, and could represent parasite migration "tracks."[108,110]

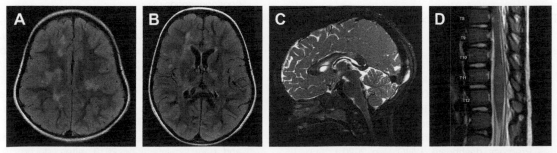

Fig. 18. Toxocariasis. FLAIR images (*A*, *B*) show multiple irregular areas of hyperintensity in the cerebral white matter and basal ganglia bilaterally. Sagittal reformatted 3D-T2-weighted image (*C*) shows a lesion in the body of the corpus callosum. There were no enhancing lesions. Sagittal T2-weighted image (*D*) depicts a tumefactive lesion in the *conus medullaris* consistent with ADEM-like pattern, a reported feature in toxocara infection (see Ref.[101]). CSF eosinophilia was fundamental to reach the correct diagnosis.

SUMMARY

Despite recent reductions in the prevalence of parasitic diseases worldwide, the global morbidity burden of protozoan and helminthic infections remains high not only in endemic areas. Although some parasitic diseases have distinct imaging characteristics that are diagnostic, others are highly dependent on clinical and epidemiologic information: eosinophilia (either peripheral or in CSF) is especially important to alert radiologists to parasitic diseases in today's globalized world.

CLINICS CARE POINTS

- Parasitic infections of the CNS comprise a heterogenous group of diseases, with vastly different prevalences, clinical pictures, and geographical distribution across the globe.

- Radiologists should know common patterns of presentation and key clinical and epidemiological features of the most prevalent of those diseases.

- In some diseases, like Neurocysticercosis and Cerebral Echinococcosis, some imaging patterns can be diagnostic of the disease, or even very suggestive, as in congenital or AIDS-related Neurotoxoplasmosis.

- In most other CNS parasitic infections, imaging alone is usually not sufficient for diagnosis. In those cases, the radiologist should always work along with clinicians to review relevant clinical, epidemiological and laboratory studies, in order to correctly identify these conditions.

- In the context of a suspected CNS pathology, the presence of eosinophilia should raise suspicion for parasitic etiology.

DISCLOSURE

The authors declare no conflict of interest.

REFERENCES

1. WHO. Integrating Neglected Tropical Diseases into Global Health and Development: Fourth WHO Report on Neglected Tropical Diseases; 2017.
2. World Health Organization. Accelerating work to overcome the global impact of NTDs: 2011–2020. Progress dashboard. WHO Rep 2020;1. https://www.who.int/teams/control-of-neglected-tropical-diseases/progress-dashboard-2011-2020.
3. Norman FF, Monge-Maillo B, Á Martínez-Pérez, et al. Parasitic infections in travelers and immigrants: Part i protozoa. Future Microbiol 2015;10(1):69–86. https://doi.org/10.2217/fmb.14.105.
4. Norman FF, Monge-Maillo B, Á Martínez-Pérez, et al. Parasitic infections in travelers and immigrants: Part II helminths and ectoparasites. Future Microbiol 2015;10(1):87–99. https://doi.org/10.2217/fmb.14.106.
5. Marchiori PE, Lino AM, Machado LR, et al. Neuroinfection survey at a neurological ward in a Brazilian tertiary teaching hospital. Clinics 2011;66(6):1021–5. https://doi.org/10.1590/S1807-59322011000600017.
6. Shirley DAT, Farr L, Watanabe K, et al. A review of the global burden, new diagnostics, and current Therapeutics for amebiasis. Open Forum Infect Dis 2018;5(7):1–9. https://doi.org/10.1093/ofid/ofy161.
7. Celik H, Karaosmanoglu DA, Gultekin S, et al. Cerebral amebiasis: MRI, DWI, perfusion and MRS features. Riv di Neuroradiol 2005;18(5–6):559–63. https://doi.org/10.1177/197140090501800506.
8. Pittella JEH. 1st edition. Pathology of CNS parasitic infections, vol. 114. Elsevier B.V; 2013. https://doi.org/10.1016/B978-0-444-53490-3.00005-4. All rights reserved.
9. Petri WA, Haque R. 1st edition. *Entamoeba histolytica* brain abscess, vol. 114. Elsevier B.V; 2013. https://doi.org/10.1016/B978-0-444-53490-3.00009-1. All rights reserved.
10. Tamer GS, Öncel S, Gökbulut S, et al. A rare case of multilocus brain abscess due to Entamoeba histolytica infection in a child. Saudi Med J 2015;36(3):356–8. https://doi.org/10.15537/smj.2015.3.10178.
11. Cooper AM, Aouthmany S, Shah K, et al. Killer amoebas: Primary amoebic meningoencephalitis in a changing climate. J Am Acad Physician Assist 2019;32(6):30–5. https://doi.org/10.1097/01.JAA.0000558238.99250.4a.
12. Yoder JS, Eddy BA, Visvesvara GS, et al. The epidemiology of primary amoebic meningoencephalitis in the USA, 1962-2008. Epidemiol Infect 2010;138(7):968–75. https://doi.org/10.1017/S0950268809991014.
13. Jahangeer M, Mahmood Z, Munir N, et al. Naegleria fowleri: Sources of infection, pathophysiology, diagnosis, and management; a review. Clin Exp Pharmacol Physiol 2020;47(2):199–212. https://doi.org/10.1111/1440-1681.13192.
14. Singh P, Kochhar R, Vashishta RK, et al. Amebic meningoencephalitis: Spectrum of imaging findings. Am J Neuroradiol 2006;27(6):1217–21.
15. Freddi T, de Godoy LL, Goncalves FG, et al. Fungal and parasitic infections 2019. https://doi.org/10.1007/978-3-319-61423-6_47-2.
16. Healy JF. Balamuthia amebic encephalitis: Radiographic and pathologic findings. Am J Neuroradiol 2002;23(3):486–9.

17. Sarica FB, Tufan K, Cekinmez M, et al. A Rare But Fatal Case of Granulomatous Amebic Encephalitis with Brain Abscess : The First Case Reported from Turkey Nadir Gözlenen Ölümcül Seyirli Beyin Absesinin Efllik Etti ᴑ i Olgusu : Türkiye ' den Bildirilen ilk. Turk Neurosurg 2009;19(3):256–9.

18. Schimmel M, Mehta I. Granulomatous Amebic Encephalitis. N Engl J Med 2020;383(13):1262. https://doi.org/10.1056/nejmicm2002401.

19. McKeever PE. Pathologic Basis of Central Nervous System Infections. Neuroimaging Clin N Am 2012; 22(4):773–90. https://doi.org/10.1016/j.nic.2012.06.001.

20. Vidal JE. HIV-Related Cerebral Toxoplasmosis Revisited: Current Concepts and Controversies of an Old Disease. J Int Assoc Provid AIDS Care 2019;18: 1–20. https://doi.org/10.1177/2325958219867315.

21. Mahadevan A, Ramalingaiah AH, Parthasarathy S, et al. Neuropathological correlate of the "concentric target sign" in MRI of HIV-associated cerebral toxoplasmosis. J Magn Reson Imaging 2013; 38(2):488–95. https://doi.org/10.1002/jmri.24036.

22. Kumar GGS, Mahadevan A, Guruprasad AS, et al. Eccentric target sign in cerebral toxoplasmosis: Neuropathological correlate to the imaging feature. J Magn Reson Imaging 2010;31(6):1469–72. https://doi.org/10.1002/jmri.22192.

23. Schroeder PC, Post MJD, Oschatz E, et al. Analysis of the utility of diffusion-weighted MRI and apparent diffusion coefficient values in distinguishing central nervous system toxoplasmosis from lymphoma. Neuroradiology 2006;48(10):715–20. https://doi.org/10.1007/s00234-006-0123-y.

24. Benson JC, Cervantes G, Baron TR, et al. Imaging features of neurotoxoplasmosis: A multiparametric approach, with emphasis on susceptibility-weighted imaging. Eur J Radiol Open 2018; 5(September 2017):45–51. https://doi.org/10.1016/j.ejro.2018.03.004.

25. Smith AB, Smirniotopoulos JG, Rushing EJ. Central nervous system infections associated with human immunodeficiency virus infection: Radiologicpathologic correlation. Radiographics 2008;28(7): 2033–58. https://doi.org/10.1148/rg.287085135.

26. Camacho DLA, Smith JK, Castillo M. Differentiation of toxoplasmosis and lymphoma in AIDS patients by using apparent diffusion coefficients. Am J Neuroradiol 2003;24(4):633–7.

27. da Rocha AJ, Sobreira Guedes BV, da Silveira da Rocha TMB, et al. Modern techniques of magnetic resonance in the evaluation of primary central nervous system lymphoma: Contributions to the diagnosis and differential diagnosis. Rev Bras Hematol Hemoter 2016;38(1):44–54. https://doi.org/10.1016/j.bjhh.2015.12.001.

28. Dibble EH, Boxerman JL, Baird GL, et al. Toxoplasmosis versus lymphoma: Cerebral lesion characterization using DSC-MRI revisited. Clin Neurol Neurosurg 2017;152:84–9. https://doi.org/10.1016/j.clineuro.2016.11.023.

29. Raizer JJ, Koutcher JA, Abrey LE, et al. Proton magnetic resonance spectroscopy in immunocompetent patients with primary central nervous system lymphoma. J Neurooncol 2005;71(2): 173–80. https://doi.org/10.1007/s11060-004-1360-8.

30. Zacharia TT, Law M, Naidich TP, et al. Central nervous system lymphoma characterization by diffusion-weighted imaging and MR spectroscopy. J Neuroimaging 2008;18(4):411–7. https://doi.org/10.1111/j.1552-6569.2007.00231.x.

31. Arpit Nagar V, Ye J, Xu M, et al. 309 MR Spectroscopy in Tumours-Veena Arpit Nagar et Al Multivoxel MR Spectroscopic Imaging-Distinguishing Intracranial Tumours from Non-Neoplastic Disease. Vol 36.; 2007.

32. Chaudhari VV, Yim CM, Hathout H, et al. Atypical imaging appearance of toxoplasmosis in an HIV patient as a butterfly lesion. J Magn Reson Imaging 2009;30(4):873–5. https://doi.org/10.1002/jmri.21924.

33. Surendrababu NRS, Kuruvilla KA, Jana AK. Unusual pattern of calcification in congenital toxoplasmosis: The tram-track sign. Pediatr Radiol 2006; 36(6):569. https://doi.org/10.1007/s00247-005-0098-6.

34. Norton ME, Fox NS, Monteagudo A, et al. Fetal Ventriculomegaly. Am J Obstet Gynecol 2020; 223(6):B30–3. https://doi.org/10.1016/j.ajog.2020.08.182.

35. Kennedy PGE. Clinical features, diagnosis, and treatment of human African trypanosomiasis (sleeping sickness). Lancet Neurol 2013;12(2): 186–94. https://doi.org/10.1016/S1474-4422(12)70296-X.

36. MacLean L, Myburgh E, Rodgers J, et al. Imaging African trypanosomes. Parasite Immunol 2013; 35(9–10):283–94. https://doi.org/10.1111/pim.12046.

37. Abdel Razek AAK, Watcharakorn A, Castillo M. Parasitic diseases of the central nervous system. Neuroimaging Clin N Am 2011;21(4):815–41. https://doi.org/10.1016/j.nic.2011.07.005.

38. Nóbrega AA, Garcia MH, Tatto E, et al. Oral transmission of chagas disease by consumption of Açaí palm fruit, Brazil. Emerg Infect Dis 2009;15(4): 653–5. https://doi.org/10.3201/eid1504.081450.

39. dos Santos VRC, de Meis J, Savino W, et al. Acute chagas disease in the state of Pará, amazon region: Is it increasing? Mem Inst Oswaldo Cruz 2018;113(5):2–7. https://doi.org/10.1590/0074-02760170298.

40. Lury KM, Castillo M. Chagas' disease involving the brain and spinal cord: MRI findings. Am J

Roentgenol 2005;185(2):550–2. https://doi.org/10.2214/ajr.185.2.01850550.

41. Do Carmo RL, Simão AKA, Do Amaral LLF, et al. Neuroimaging of emergent and reemergent infections. Radiographics 2019;39(6):1649–71. https://doi.org/10.1148/rg.2019190020.

42. Sierro F, Grau GER. The ins and outs of cerebral malaria pathogenesis: Immunopathology, extracellular vesicles, immunometabolism, and trained immunity. Front Immunol 2019;10(MAR):1–11. https://doi.org/10.3389/fimmu.2019.00830.

43. Shih R, Koeller KK. Bacterial, fungal, and parasitic infections of the central nervous system: Radiologic-pathologic correlation and historical perspectives. Radiographics 2015;35(4):1141–69. https://doi.org/10.1148/rg.2015140317.

44. Sahu PK, Hoffmann A, Majhi M, et al. Brain Magnetic Resonance Imaging Reveals Different Courses of Disease in Pediatric and Adult Cerebral Malaria. Clin Infect Dis 2020;(Xx Xxxx):1–10. https://doi.org/10.1093/cid/ciaa1647. c.

45. Gamanagatti S, Kandpal H. MR imaging of cerebral malaria in a child. Eur J Radiol 2006;60(1):46–7. https://doi.org/10.1016/j.ejrad.2006.05.014.

46. Nickerson JP, Tong KA, Raghavan R. Imaging cerebral malaria with a susceptibility-weighted MR sequence. Am J Neuroradiol 2009;30(6):85–6. https://doi.org/10.3174/ajnr.A1568.

47. Vale TC, De Sousa-Pereira SR, Ribas JGR, et al. Neuroschistosomiasis mansoni: Literature Reviewand Guidelines. Neurologist 2012;18(6):333–42. https://doi.org/10.1097/NRL.0b013e3182704d1e.

48. Suthiphosuwan S, Lin A, Gao AF, et al. Delayed presentation of cerebral schistosomiasis presenting as a tumor-like brain lesion. Neuroradiol J 2018;31(4):395–8. https://doi.org/10.1177/1971400917703991.

49. Shen J, Yuan L, Sun Y, et al. Case report: Multiple schistosomiasis japonica cerebral granulomas without gastrointestinal system involvement: Report of two cases and review of literature. Am J Trop Med Hyg 2020;102(6):1376–81. https://doi.org/10.4269/ajtmh.19-0797.

50. Bennett GM, Provenzale J. Schistosomal myelitis: Findings at MR imaging. Eur J Radiol 1998;27(3):268–70. https://doi.org/10.1016/S0720-048X(98)00006-0.

51. Sanelli PC, Lev MH, Gonzalez RG, et al. Unique linear and nodular MR enhancement pattern in schistosomiasis of the central nervous system: Report of three patients. Am J Roentgenol 2001;177(6):1471–4. https://doi.org/10.2214/ajr.177.6.1771471.

52. Huang J, Luo J, Peng J, et al. Cerebral schistosomiasis: Diffusion-weighted imaging helps to differentiate from brain glioma and metastasis. Acta Radiol 2017;58(11):1371–7. https://doi.org/10.1177/0284185116687173.

53. Lv S, Zhang Y, Steinmann P, et al. Helminth Infections of the Central Nervous System Occurring in Southeast Asia and the Far East. Adv Parasitol 2010;72(C):351–408. https://doi.org/10.1016/S0065-308X(10)72012-1.

54. Saleem S, Belal AI, El-Ghandour NM. Spinal cord schistosomiasis: MR imaging appearance with surgical and pathologic correlation. Am J Neuroradiol 2005;26(7):1646–54.

55. Liu H, Tchoyoson Lim CC, Feng X, et al. MRI in cerebral schistosomiasis: Characteristic nodular enhancement in 33 patients. Am J Roentgenol 2008;191(2):582–8. https://doi.org/10.2214/AJR.07.3139.

56. Chen J, Chen Z, Lin J, et al. Cerebral paragonimiasis: A retrospective analysis of 89 cases. Clin Neurol Neurosurg 2013;115(5):546–51. https://doi.org/10.1016/j.clineuro.2012.06.025.

57. Li L, Zhang Y, Zhu J, et al. Intracranial Pseudoaneurysm Caused by Cerebral Paragonimiasis in Pediatric Patients. Pediatr Neurol 2020;109:47–51. https://doi.org/10.1016/j.pediatrneurol.2020.03.018.

58. Zhang JS, Huan Y, Sun LJ, et al. MRI features of pediatric cerebral paragonimiasis in the active stage. J Magn Reson Imaging 2006;23(4):569–73. https://doi.org/10.1002/jmri.20546.

59. Wang Q, Hou L, Liu L. Diagnosis and treatment of hemorrhagic cerebral paragonimiasis: Three case reports and literature review. Turk Neurosurg 2020;30(4):624–8. https://doi.org/10.5137/1019-5149.JTN.22666-18.3.

60. Rahalkar MD, Shetty DD, Kelkar AB, et al. The many faces of cysticercosis. Clin Radiol 2000;55(9):668–74. https://doi.org/10.1053/crad.2000.0494.

61. Del Brutto OH, García HH. Taenia solium Cysticercosis - The lessons of history. J Neurol Sci 2015;359(1–2):392–5. https://doi.org/10.1016/j.jns.2015.08.011.

62. Garcia HH, Gonzalez AE, Gilman RH. Taenia solium cysticercosis and its impact in neurological disease. Clin Microbiol Rev 2020;33(3). https://doi.org/10.1128/CMR.00085-19.

63. de Souza A, Nalini A, Kovoor JME, et al. Natural history of solitary cerebral cysticercosis on serial magnetic resonance imaging and the effect of albendazole therapy on its evolution. J Neurol Sci 2010;288(1–2):135–41. https://doi.org/10.1016/j.jns.2009.09.018.

64. Santos GT, Leite CC, Machado LR, et al. Reduced diffusion in neurocysticercosis: Circumstances of appearance and possible natural history implications. Am J Neuroradiol 2013;34(2):310–6. https://doi.org/10.3174/ajnr.A3198.

65. Govindappa SS, Narayanan JP, Krishnamoorthy VM, et al. Improved detection of

intraventricular cysticercal cysts with the use of three-dimensional constructive interference in steady state MR sequences. Am J Neuroradiol 2000;21(4):679–84.

66. Del Brutto OH, Nash TE, White AC, et al. Revised diagnostic criteria for neurocysticercosis. J Neurol Sci 2017;372:202–10. https://doi.org/10.1016/j.jns.2016.11.045.

67. Garcia HH, Del Brutto OH. Neurocysticercosis: updated concepts about an old disease. Lancet Neurol 2005;4(10):653–61. https://doi.org/10.1016/S1474-4422(05)70194-0.

68. Wagner RG, Newton CR. Do helminths cause epilepsy? Parasite Immunol 2009;31(11):697–705. https://doi.org/10.1111/j.1365-3024.2009.01128.x.

69. Raibagkar P, Berkowitz AL. The Many Faces of Neurocysticercosis. J Neurol Sci 2018;390:75–6. https://doi.org/10.1016/j.jns.2018.04.018.

70. De Araujo ALE, Rodrigues RS, Marchiori E, et al. Migrating intraventricular cysticercosis: Magnetic resonance imaging findings. Arq Neuropsiquiatr 2008;66(1):111–3. https://doi.org/10.1590/S0004-282X2008000100031.

71. Do Amaral LLF, Ferreira RM, Da Rocha AJ, et al. Neurocysticercosis: Evaluation with advanced magnetic resonance techniques and atypical forms. Top Magn Reson Imaging 2005;16(2):127–44. https://doi.org/10.1097/01.rmr.0000189106.78146.98.

72. Vieira E, Faquini IV, Silva JL, et al. Subarachnoid neurocysticercosis and an intracranial infectious aneurysm: Case report. Neurosurg Focus 2019;47(2):1–5. https://doi.org/10.3171/2019.5.FOCUS19280.

73. Foerster BR, Thurnher MM, Malani PN, et al. Intracranial infections: Clinical and imaging characteristics. Acta Radiol 2007;48(8):875–93. https://doi.org/10.1080/02841850701477728.

74. Shin DA, Shin HC. A case of extensive spinal cysticercosis involving the whole spinal canal in a patient with a history of cerebral cysticercosis. Yonsei Med J 2009;50(4):582–4. https://doi.org/10.3349/ymj.2009.50.4.582.

75. Amaral L, Maschietto M, Maschietto R, et al. Unusual manifestations of neurocysticercosis in MR imaging: Analysis of 172 cases. Arq Neuropsiquiatr 2003;61(3 A):533–41. https://doi.org/10.1590/s0004-282x2003000400002.

76. Tamarozzi F, Legnardi M, Fittipaldo A, et al. Epidemiological distribution of echinococcus granulosus s.L. infection in human and domestic animal hosts in european mediterranean and balkan countries: A systematic review. Plos Negl Trop Dis 2020;14(8):1–23. https://doi.org/10.1371/journal.pntd.0008519.

77. Razek AAKA, El-Shamam O, Wahab NA. Magnetic resonance appearance of cerebral cystic echinococcosis: World Health Organization (WHO) classification. Acta Radiol 2009;50(5):549–54. https://doi.org/10.1080/02841850902878161.

78. Bükte Y, Kemanoğlu S, Nazaroğlu H, et al. Cerebral hydatid disease: CT and MR imaging findings. Swiss Med Wkly 2004;134(31–32):459–67. https://doi.org/10.14260/jemds/2014/3737.

79. Cemil B, Tun K, Gurcay AG, et al. Cranial epidural hydatid cysts: Clinical report and review of the literature. Acta Neurochir (Wien) 2009;151(6):659–62. https://doi.org/10.1007/s00701-009-0276-7.

80. Jayakumar PN, Chandrashekar HS, Ellika S. Imaging of parasitic infections of the central nervous system. Handbook Clin Neurol 2013;114:37–64. https://doi.org/10.1016/B978-0-444-53490-3.00004-2. Elsevier B.V.

81. Jayakumar PN, Chandrashekar HS, Srikanth SG, et al. MRI and in vivo proton MR spectroscopy in a racemose cysticercal cyst of the brain. Neuroradiology 2004;46(1):72–4. https://doi.org/10.1007/s00234-003-1108-8.

82. Jayakumar PN, Srikanth SG, Chandrashekar HS, et al. Pyruvate: An in Vivo Marker of Cestodal Infestation of the Human Brain on Proton MR Spectroscopy. J Magn Reson Imaging 2003;18(6):675–80 https://doi.org/10.1002/jmri.10409.

83. Pandey S, Pandey D, Shende N, et al. Cerebral intraventricular echinococcosis in an adult. Surg Neurol Int 2015;6(1). https://doi.org/10.4103/2152-7806.163177.

84. Lotfinia I, Sayyahmolli S, Mahdkhah A, et al. Intradural extramedullary primary hydatid cyst of the spine: A case report and review of literature. Eur Spine J 2013;22(SUPPL.3):329–36. https://doi.org/10.1007/s00586-012-2373-1.

85. Senturk S, Oguz KK, Soylemezoglu F, et al. Cerebral alveolar echinoccosis mimicking primary brain tumor. Am J Neuroradiol 2006;27(2):420–2. https://doi.org/10.1016/s0098-1672(08)70486-7.

86. Al Zain TJ, Al-Witry SH, Khalili HM, et al. Multiple intracranial hydatidosis. Acta Neurochir (Wien) 2002;144(11):1179–85. https://doi.org/10.1007/s00701-002-0987-5.

87. Sundaram C, Prasad VSSV, Reddy JJM. Cerebral sparganosis. J Assoc Physicians India 2003;51(NOV):1107–9. https://doi.org/10.3171/jns.1990.73.1.0147.

88. Bo G, Xuejian W. Neuroimaging and pathological findings in a child with cerebral sparganosis: Case report. J Neurosurg 2006;105 PEDIAT(-SUPPL. 6):470–2. https://doi.org/10.3171/ped.2006.105.6.470.

89. Moon WK, Chang KH, Cho SY, et al. Cerebral sparganosis: MR imaging versus CT features. Radiology 1993;188(3):751–7. https://doi.org/10.1148/radiology.188.3.8351344.

90. Migration : A Notable Feature of Cerebral Sparganosis on. Ajnr Published Online 2013;327–33.

91. Li H-X, Luan S-H, Guo W, et al. Sparganosis of the brain: a case report and brief review. Neuroimmunol Neuroinflammation 2017;4(11):238. https://doi.org/10.20517/2347-8659.2017.16.

92. Song T, Wang WS, Zhou BR, et al. CT and MR characteristics of cerebral sparganosis. Am J Neuroradiol 2007;28(9):1700–5. https://doi.org/10.3174/ajnr.A0659.

93. Tran QR, Tran MC, Mehanna D. Sparganosis: An under-recognised zoonosis in Australia? BMJ Case Rep 2019;12(5):10–3. https://doi.org/10.1136/bcr-2018-228396.

94. Peh WM, Hean GG, Clement YHR. The tunnel sign revisited: A novel observation of cerebral melioidosis mimicking sparganosis. J Radiol Case Rep 2018;12(8):1–11. https://doi.org/10.3941/jrcr.v12i8.3441.

95. Nicoletti A. Toxocariasis. Handb Clin Neurol 2013;114:217–28. https://doi.org/10.1016/B978-0-444-53490-3.00016-9.

96. Meliou M, Mavridis IN, Pyrgelis ES, et al. Toxocariasis of the Nervous System. Acta Parasitol 2020;65(2):291–9. https://doi.org/10.2478/s11686-019-00166-1.

97. Nicoletti A. Neurotoxocariasis Adv Parasitol 2020;109(5):219–31. https://doi.org/10.1016/bs.apar.2020.01.007.

98. FINSTERER J, KALLAB V, AUER H. Neurotoxocariasis associated with lower motor neuron disease: Report of one case TT - Neurotoxocariasis asociada a enfermedad de motoneurona inferior: Presentación de un caso. Rev Med Chil 2010;138(4):483–6. Available at: http://www.scielo.cl/scielo.php?script=sci_arttext&pid=S0034-98872010000400014&lang=pt%0Ahttp://www.scielo.cl/pdf/rmc/v138n4/art14.pdf.

99. Bossi G, Bruno R, Novati S, et al. Cerebral Toxocariasis as a Cause of Epilepsy: A Pediatric Case. Neuropediatrics 2021;52(02):142–5.

100. Abir B, Malek M, Ridha M. Toxocariasis of the central nervous system: With report of two cases. Clin Neurol Neurosurg 2017;154(2):94–7. https://doi.org/10.1016/j.clineuro.2017.01.016.

101. Marx C, Lin J, Masruha MR. Toxocariasis of the CNS simulating Acute Disseminated Encephalomyelitis. Neurology 2007;69:806–7. https://doi.org/10.1212/01.wnl.0000267664.53595.75.

102. Duprez TPJ, Bigaignon G, Delgrange E, et al. MRI of cervical cord lesions and their resolution in Toxocara canis myelopathy. Neuroradiology 1996;38(8):792–5. https://doi.org/10.1007/s002340050350.

103. Starr MC, Montgomery SP. Soil-transmitted helminthiasis in the United States: A systematic review - 1940-2010. Am J Trop Med Hyg 2011;85(4):680–4. https://doi.org/10.4269/ajtmh.2011.11-0214.

104. Dzikowiec M, Góralska K, Błaszkowska J. Neuroinvasions caused by parasites. Ann Parasitol 2017;63(4):243–53. https://doi.org/10.17420/ap6304.111.

105. Eamsobhana P. Eosinophilic meningitis caused by Angiostrongylus cantonensis–a neglected disease with escalating importance. Trop Biomed 2014;31(4):569–78.

106. Schmutzhard E, Helbok R. 1st edition. Rickettsiae, Protozoa, and Opisthokonta/Metazoa, 121. Elsevier B.V.; 2014. https://doi.org/10.1016/B978-0-7020-4088-7.00096-1.

107. Graeff-Teixeira C, Da Silva ACA, Yoshimura K. Update on eosinophilic meningoencephalitis and its clinical relevance. Clin Microbiol Rev 2009;22(2):322–48. https://doi.org/10.1128/CMR.00044-08.

108. Kanpittaya J, Jitpimolmard S, Tiamkao S, et al. MR findings of eosinophilic meningoencephalitis attributed to Angiostrongylus cantonensis. Am J Neuroradiol 2000;21(6):1090–4.

109. Rosca EC, Simu M. Border zone brain lesions due to neurotrichinosis. Int J Infect Dis 2018;67:43–5. https://doi.org/10.1016/j.ijid.2017.12.011.

110. Senthong V, Chindaprasirt J, Sawanyawisuth K. Differential diagnosis of CNS angiostrongyliasis: a short review. Hawaii J Med Public Health 2013;72(6 Suppl 2):52–4.

Human Immunodeficiency Virus

Opportunistic Infections and Beyond

Rekha Siripurapu, MBBS, MRCP, FRCR[a],*, Yoshiaki Ota, MD[b]

KEYWORDS

- Human immunodeficiency virus (HIV) • Opportunistic infections
- HIV-associated neurocognitive disorder (HAND)
- Immune reconstitution inflammatory syndrome (IRIS) • Lymphoma • JC Virus • Tuberculosis
- Progressive multifocal leukoencephalopathy (PML)

KEY POINTS

- Central nervous system (CNS) involvement in human immunodeficiency virus (HIV) can be due to primary HIV infection, secondary to opportunistic infections (OIs), or due to immune reconstitution associated with antiretroviral therapy (ART).
- In this era of ART and increased survival, OIs are decreasing, but prevalent, with increasing recognition of inflammatory syndromes and treatment complications.
- OIs in HIV have unique imaging features that can help in early diagnosis and management.
- Immune reconstitution may significantly alter the imaging appearances of OIs.
- Interpretation of imaging in correlation with the HIV status (viral load and CD4 count) and treatment is important to avoid potential pit falls.

Abbreviations	
JC Virus	John Cunningham virus

INTRODUCTION

Human immunodeficiency virus (HIV) is a retrovirus that infects cells of the immune system and destroys or disrupts their function.[1] Infection by HIV-1 accounts for most of the global HIV cases, with only 1 to 2 million of the 33 million HIV infections being caused by the less common HIV-2 virus.[2] Since its first description in the 1980s, the epidemiology and imaging patterns of HIV infection have changed due to increased access to combination antiretroviral therapy (ART).[3]

Central nervous system (CNS) diseases in HIV-infected patients result directly from HIV itself or from a variety of opportunistic infections (OI), depending on the extent of immunosuppression. Others include malignancy such as lymphoma, cerebral infarction,[4] and immune reconstitution inflammatory syndrome (IRIS).

Although radiological findings of HIV-associated diseases are diverse, typical features of atypical presentations have been recognized, which help in differential diagnosis.

In this article, we reviewed imaging findings of primary HIV infection, opportunistic CNS infections, malignancy, and inflammatory syndromes in the setting of HIV and ART.

[a] Department of Neuroradiology, Manchester Centre for Clinical Neurosciences, Salford Royal Hospital, Northern Care Alliance NHS Foundation Trust, Stott Lane, Salford, M6 8HD, UK; [b] Division of Neuroradiology, Department of Radiology, University of Michigan, 1500 East Medical Center Drive, UH B2, Ann Arbor, MI 48109, USA
* Corresponding author.
E-mail address: rekha.siripurapu@nca.nhs.uk
Twitter: @rekhasiripurapu (R.S.); @GattsukiRadiol (Y.O.)

Neuroimag Clin N Am 33 (2023) 147–165
https://doi.org/10.1016/j.nic.2022.07.014
1052-5149/23/Crown Copyright © 2022 Published by Elsevier Inc. All rights reserved.

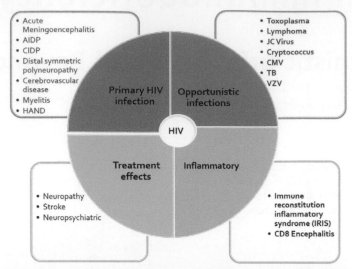

Fig. 1. The range of neurologic manifestations associated with HIV infection. AIDP, acute inflammatory demye-linating polyneuropathy; CIDP, chronic inflammatory demyelinating polyneuropathy; CMV, cytomegalovirus; HAND, HIV-associated neurocognitive disorder; TB, tuberculosis; VZV, varicella-zoster virus.

Fig. 1 shows the wide spectrum of neurologic manifestations beyond OIs. It is important to note the changing epidemiology in the ART era with increasing number of people living with HIV, decreasing OIs, and increasing awareness of inflammatory and dysimmune conditions.[3]

Human Immunodeficiency Virus Biomarkers and Terminology

Understanding the common terminology used in clinical management of HIV is essential for avoiding potential pitfalls and appropriate assessment of imaging features.[5]

Acquired immunodeficiency syndrome: Acquired immunodeficiency syndrome (AIDS) is the most advanced stage of HIV infection. To be diagnosed with AIDS, a person with HIV must have an AIDS-defining condition *or* have a CD4 count less than 200 cells/mm³ (regardless of whether the person has an AIDS-defining condition).

ART or highly active antiretroviral therapy (previous terminology) refers to the combination of medicines to treat HIV infection.

Two surrogate markers are used to monitor the health of people living with HIV: viral load and CD4 count.

Viral load (VL) is the amount of HIV in a sample of blood, reported as the number of HIV RNA copies per milliliter. It is a marker of response to ART, used to monitor the effectiveness of therapy. An important goal of ART is to suppress the VL to undetectable levels.

CD4 count is the most important laboratory indicator of the strength of immune function in HIV patients and the strongest predictor of subsequent

disease progression and survival. Most OIs occur in patients when CD4 counts reduce to less than 200 cells/mm³. It is used to assess a patient's immunologic response to ART.

CNS viral escape: The presence of HIV in the CSF at a concentration greater than that in plasma is called CSF HIV RNA escape.[6]

PRIMARY HUMAN IMMUNODEFICIENCY VIRUS INFECTION

HIV invades the CNS early in infection, crossing the blood–brain (BBB) barrier through infected monocytes described as a "Trojan Horse" mechanism[7] with evidence of virus in CSF as early as 1 to 2 weeks and changes in brain structure within 3 months of primary infection. Most of these are mild neurologic manifestations. More severe neurologic manifestations may occur during seroconversion, including acute meningoencephalitis and AIDP,[3] with usually nonspecific or no imaging findings.

Human Immunodeficiency Virus-Associated Neurocognitive Disorder

HIV-associated neurocognitive disorder (HAND) is one of the most common neurologic complications of primary HIV infection that occurs due to the direct effect of HIV infection. The clinical spectrum includes asymptomatic neurocognitive impairment (ANI), mild neurocognitive disorder (MND), and HIV-associated dementia (HAD).[8] What was previously called "AIDS dementia complex" in the pre-ART era is now referred to as HAD. Although overall prevalence of HAND is similar to

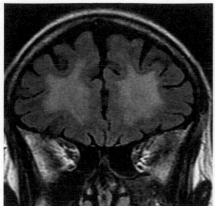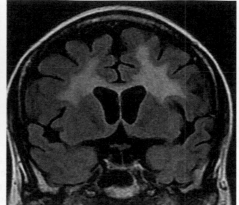

Fig. 2. HIV-associated dementia (HAD). Coronal FLAIR images in a 30-year-old patient with cognitive changes show bilateral symmetric confluent white matter hyperintensity with generalized volume loss.

pre-ART era, severe dementia (HAD) rarely develops in patients on effective ART.[3]

ANI and MND usually show no abnormality on conventional imaging. Imaging features of HAD include generalized volume loss with (or without) abnormal bilateral, usually symmetric, nonenhancing signal change within the white matter[9] (Fig. 2). Predominant periventricular and deep white matter involvement, symmetric nature, and the absence of low signal on T1-weighted images help distinguish this from progressive multifocal leukoencephalopathy (PML).

Volumetric imaging has shown changes in both cortical volumes and subcortical white matter, which accrue early after seroconversion and may continue to persist even after ART.[10]

Advanced neuroimaging techniques, which may help in early detection of HAND, include diffusion tensor imaging, blood oxygen level-dependent functional MR imaging, and ASL. A decrease in blood flow was seen soon after seroconversion with HIV-positive patients including those without neuropsychological impairment.[11] Functional MR imaging has shown compromised function of the caudate and connected prefrontal regions in HIV.[12]

Human Immunodeficiency Virus-Associated Cerebrovascular Complications

Several studies in the ART era have shown higher rates of ischemic[13–15] and hemorrhagic[16] stroke in HIV-affected individuals compared with HIV-uninfected controls, after adjustment for established stroke risk factors. In a study of a large virtual cohort of veterans, those with CD4 count of less than 200 cells/mm^3 or HIV RNA 500 or greater copies/mL were shown to be at highest risk of incident ischemic stroke.[15] Several

mechanisms proposed for HIV-associated stroke include premature atherosclerosis, OIs, hypercoagulable states, cardio embolism, and HIV vasculopathy.[3]

HIV vasculopathy is primarily an aneurysmal arteriopathy characterized by fusiform aneurysmal dilatation[17–20] (Fig. 3). Pathologic studies on HIV vasculopathy have shown large and medium vessel involvement with leukocytoclastic vasculitis of vasa vasora and periadventitial vessels, significant arteria media layer disruption and fragmentation of internal elastic lamina[21,22] with thinning of the arterial media layer postulated as a possible preclinical stage.[18] The diagnosis of HIV vasculopathy can be made only after the exclusion of other causes of stroke in HIV such as OIs such as tuberculosis (TB),[23] syphilis,[24] and varicella-zoster virus.[20,25]

Due to the changing epidemiology of HIV infection after introduction of ART, increasing proportion of individuals aged older than 65 years, the spectrum of cerebrovascular disease in HIV-infected individuals is changing with increase in atherosclerotic disease.[26]

OPPORTUNISTIC CENTRAL NERVOUS SYSTEM INFECTIONS

Although the overall incidence of CNS OIs has decreased in the last 30 years,[27] it continues to be a major cause of mortality and morbidity in HIV, and radiologists should be familiar with the typical imaging features.

OIs typically result from reactivation of latent viral, fungal, or parasitic infection, and they most commonly occur when the CD4 cell count is 200 cells/mm^3 or less, and, in up to 15% of HIV-infected patients, more than one OI can be present.[2] Patients with severe immune suppression

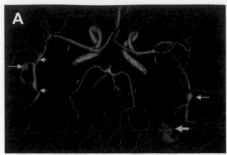
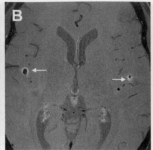
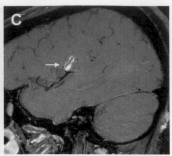

Fig. 3. HIV vasculopathy. Volume-rendered MR angiogram (*A*) in a 44-year-old woman, newly diagnosed HIV with CSF anti-VZV IgG antibodies shows multiple fusiform aneurysms (*arrows*) of both MCA along with a partially thrombosed large aneurysm (*bold arrow*) and fusiform dilatation of a long segment of M3 (short *arrows*). High-resolution intracranial vessel wall images using postcontrast T1-weighted black blood sequences (*B, C*) show avid concentric enhancement of the vessel wall (*white arrows*) at the sites of aneurysmal dilatation. This patient was treated for both HIV and VZV.

(CD4-cell count lower than 200 cells/mm^3) are at risk of toxoplasma encephalitis, cryptococcal meningitis, cytomegalovirus (CMV) infection, primary CNS lymphoma, and PML, whereas patients with moderate immune suppression (CD4-cell counts of 200–500 cells/mm^3) are at risk of tuberculous meningitis and PML.[2]

The incidence of OIs varies based on loco regional and socioeconomic differences and the relative availability of ART[28]; for example, in the United Kingdom, common OIs include toxoplasmosis, TB, PML, cryptococcal meningitis, CMV, and varicella zoster.

Toxoplasmosis

Toxoplasmosis is caused by *Toxoplasma gondii*, an intracellular protozoan that is found worldwide, and is transmitted to humans primarily by ingestion of cysts in undercooked meat, contaminated vegetables, or through direct contact with cat feces.[29] Cerebral toxoplasmosis is more commonly seen in immunocompromised patients; nearly 25% to 50% of patients with HIV infection who have latent toxoplasma infection have reactivation of the disease and develop cerebral toxoplasmosis in the absence of antimicrobial prophylaxis.[30,31] Pathologically, acute toxoplasmosis usually manifests as necrotizing abscess formation in the basal ganglia, thalami, and the gray–white matter junctions. Necrotizing abscesses are usually characterized by 3 zones: central zone consisting of coagulative necrosis, intermediate zone consisting of numerous neutrophils and mononuclear cells as well as numerous reactive astrocytes and microglia, and peripheral zone composed primarily of astrogliosis.[31] It is important to note that the pathologic findings depend on the degree of immune impairment

with less inflammation and fibrosis seen in severely immunocompromised patients.

On computed tomography (CT), lesions are hypodense to isodense with surrounding vasogenic edema and mass effect. On MR imaging, these lesions are usually seen as T1 hypointense, T2 and FLAIR hyperintense, or isointense areas with peripheral T1 hyperintensity (a feature that helps distinguish toxoplasmosis from lymphoma; Fig. 4).[29] After contrast injection, rim-like enhancement with an "eccentric target sign" is well described.[32]

DWI of a toxoplasma lesion has been reported to usually show no diffusion restriction in the core of the lesion, which is helpful in differentiating from bacterial abscesses and possibly lymphoma.[33]

Tuberculosis

CNS tuberculosis (TB) remains a leading cause of morbidity and mortality and occurs in up to 10% of HIV-infected patients with a predilection for younger patients.[34] No differences in neuroimaging have been reported between HIV-infected and non-HIV-infected patients.

Basal meningitis with ring-enhancing lesions in the basal cisterns and adjacent parenchyma is the classic feature of TB meningitis. The spectrum includes opticochiasmatic, cranial nerve, and leptomeningeal enhancement. Hydrocephalus is a frequent complication. Infarction due to vasculitis complicating basal exudative meningitis is considered a poor prognostic factor.[23]

The prognosis is better when treatment is started before the development of focal neurologic signs and altered state of consciousness. Therefore, anti-TB therapy should be promptly initiated based on strong clinical suspicion without waiting

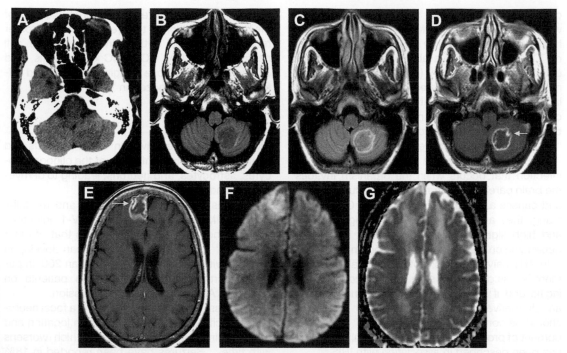

Fig. 4. Toxoplasmosis. A 62-year-old HIV-positive woman with fatigue, cognitive difficulties, and headache. CT (*A*) shows a hypodense left cerebellar mass. T1-weighted (*B*) and FLAIR images (*C*) show a centrally hypointense mass with slight peripheral linear hyperintensity. Contrast-enhanced images (*D*, *E*) show rim enhancement with an eccentric nodule (*arrow*). DWI (*F*) shows hyperintensity without restricted diffusion on ADC (*G*).

for laboratory confirmation, in combination with HIV treatment in order to enhance the antibacterial effect, cover the possibly resistant infection, and reduce the likelihood of emerging therapy resistance.[35]

Cryptococcosis

CNS infection caused by *Cryptococcus neoformans*, the most common form of fungal infection in HIV patients[36] occurs due to hematogenous spread from lungs and usually when CD4 count

is less than 100 cells/mm^3. *Cryptococcus gattii* has been reported to cause infection in immunocompetent as well as immunocompromised.

Imaging findings include dilated perivascular spaces (VR spaces), pseudocysts, cryptococcomas, miliary disease, basal meningitis, and hydrocephalus with dilated perivascular spaces (Fig. 5) being the most commonly reported, particularly in the profoundly immunecompromised.[37,38]

Perivascular spaces that become dilated and filled with fungus are commonly seen as decreased

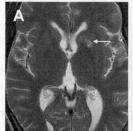
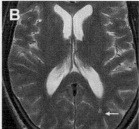
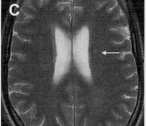
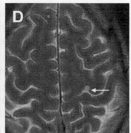

Fig. 5. Cryptococcal infection. A 30-year-old man with new diagnosis of HIV, headaches, and decreased vision. Axial T2-weighted images show mild hydrocephalus with dilated perivascular spaces in the left basal ganglia (*A*, *arrow*) and in left peritrigonal white matter (*B*, *arrow*). Focal parenchymal lesions in left corona radiata (*C*, *arrow*) and left motor strip (*D*, *arrow*) are in keeping with cryptococcoma, which did not enhance after contrast injection (images not shown).

density in basal ganglia, thalami, midbrain, and white matter on CT. On MR imaging, they show high signal on T2, slightly higher than CSF signal on T1(mucin), can be variable signal on fluid attenuated inversion recovery (FLAIR), and usually do not enhance. When dilated VR spaces coalesce into larger lesions or when they enlarge due to large quantities of capsular mucoid material, they become gelatinous pseudocysts, which have a "soap-bubble" appearance.[38]

Cryptococcoma is the parenchymal form of infection that occurs when the organism invades the brain parenchyma from the perivascular spaces and causes a granulomatous reaction. On MR imaging, they are intermediate to low signal on T1 and high signal on T2. Enhancement is variable depending on the degree of immunocompromise.[38]

In ART naïve patients, leptomeningeal enhancement is less commonly seen in cryptococcal meningitis and if prominent meningeal enhancement, an alternative diagnosis such as TB meningitis should be considered.[36] Following ART, the development of prominent leptomeningeal enhancement has been described in association with IRIS.[39]

Cytomegalovirus

Cytomegalovirus (CMV) infection occurs due to the reactivation of a latent virus and has been described to cause 5 distinct neurologic syndromes in the immunocompromised: retinitis, myelitis, ventriculoencephalitis, micronodular encephalitis, and mononeuritis multiplex.[36] With increased ART availability, CMV incidence has decreased[3] because this is a late-stage manifestation of HIV infection usually occurring at CD4 count less than 50 cells/mm.[3] The most common imaging findings in patients who have CMV encephalitis are cortical atrophy, periventricular enhancement, and diffuse white matter abnormalities.[36,40] In ventriculoencephalitis, the features include hydrocephalus with diffuse ependymal enhancement (Fig. 6).

John Cunningham Virus (JC Virus) Infection

Named after its first victim, John Cunningham (JC) virus is a polyomavirus that destroys oligodendrocytes and their myelin processes.

Although HIV is the most common predisposing factor for JC virus reactivation, increasing incidence is also reported in non-HIV settings such as monoclonal antibody therapy, transplant recipients, primary immune deficiency syndromes, and in patients with minimal or occult immunosuppression.[41]

During the last 3 decades, and particularly since the advent of ART, there have been significant changes in epidemiology, pathogenesis, clinical and radiological features of JC virus infection of the brain. In addition to the well-known PML, other recently described entities include granule cell neuronopathy (JCV GCN), JC encephalitis, and JC meningitis,[42] whose imaging findings and differentials are summarized in Table 1.

Progressive Multifocal Leukoencephalopathy

PML, caused by reactivation of the JC virus and characterized by lytic infection of the oligodendrocytes, astrocytes, and neurons, leading to demyelination and neuronal damage.[43]

ART has reduced the incidence and mortality due to PML in patients with HIV-1 infection, although not to the same extent as that of other CNS OIs.[44] Unlike other OIs, PML can develop in patients with CD4 counts greater than 200, in patients starting ART and rarely, in patients on long-term ART with full viral suppression.[45]

The classic presentation of PML is a focal neurologic deficit depending on the lesion location and often begins as a partial deficit, which worsens with time.[44] Seizures have been reported in 18% of patients.[46]

MR imaging has been incorporated into PML diagnostic criteria and is the recommended screening tool in the surveillance of immunocompromised patients.[47] Definitive diagnosis of PML requires neuropathological demonstration of the typical triad of demyelination, bizarre astrocytes, and enlarged oligodendroglia nuclei. The presence of clinical and imaging manifestations consistent with the diagnosis and not better explained by other disorders coupled with the demonstration of JC virus by PCR in CSF is also considered diagnostic according to the American association of Neurology consensus statement.[47]

Typically, PML is a confluent supratentorial white matter disease with bilateral asymmetric involvement of frontal or/and parietooccipital lobe subcortical white matter especially the U fibers[48] (Figs. 7 and 8). With disease progression, it may also extend to deep and rarely into periventricular white matter including the corpus callosum. Posterior fossa is next commonly involved with lesions in the middle cerebellar peduncles, adjacent pons, and peri-dentate region. Isolated posterior fossa involvement is rare,[49] and spinal cord involvement is exceedingly rare.[50,51]

Two patterns of imaging abnormalities have been described: classic PML and inflammatory PML. On CT, these are typically hypodense lesions with scalloped borders.[48] On MR, classic PML (see Fig. 7) lesions are characteristically decreased in signal intensity on T1 compared with normal white matter,[42,43] which is a useful

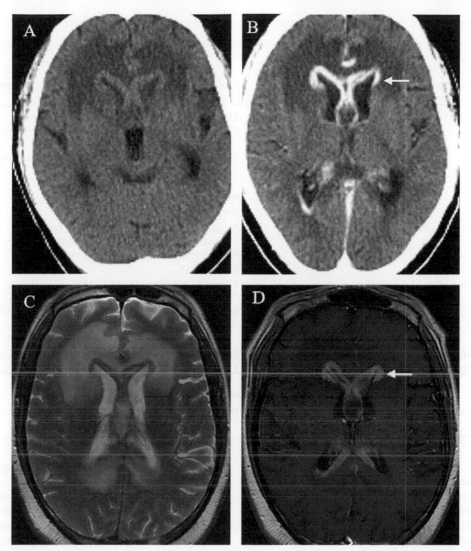

Fig. 6. CMV ventriculitis (case courtesy of Dr A Herwadkar). Precontrast (A) and postcontrast CT (B) show florid bilateral ventricular ependymal thickening and enhancement. Axial T2-weighted (C) and postcontrast T1-weighted images (D) show extensive edema in the subjacent brain parenchyma with prominent ependymal enhancement (arrow).

differentiating feature from leukoencephalopathy in HAD. Less commonly they may be isointense or show an incomplete rim of high signal at the advancing edge.[42] On T2 and FLAIR, PML is hyperintense to white matter with some cases showing microcysts at the center of an active lesion[42] (see Fig. 7). Lack of enhancement and mass effect are typical in classic PML.

Inflammatory PML is less common than classic PML and is characterized radiologically by peripheral contrast enhancement and/or mass effect with vasogenic edema. This can be encountered in 2 different scenarios: in the setting of IRIS in HIV-positive patients following treatment with ART (see "Immune Reconstitution inflammatory Syndrome" section on IRIS), and very rarely,

inflammatory PML may be the presenting phenotype in HIV patients without ART[42] (see Fig. 8).

DWI appearances of PML vary according to the stage of the disease. Restricted diffusivity in newer lesions and advancing edge of large lesions has been reported to signify active infection.[52] Ill-defined rim of high signal at the advancing edge and a hypointense core within a large lesion is better visualized on high b-value DWI[53] and may help differentiate PML from other demyelinating diseases.[54]

A recent study[55] reported that a thin, uniformly linear, gyriform SWI hypointense rim in the paralesional U fibers may represent an end point stage of the neuroinflammatory process in long-term survivors of PML.[55]

Table 1
Imaging features and differential diagnosis of varied manifestations of John Cunningham virus infection

JC Virus CNS Manifestations	Typical Location	Typical Imaging Features	Important Differential Diagnosis
Classic PML	Frontal, parietal, and occipital subcortical white matter Posterior fossa—middle cerebellar peduncle, pons, and cerebellum	T1 hypointense T2 and Flair hyperintense Restricted diffusivity of the peripheral margins No enhancement No mass effect	HIV-associated leukoencephalopathy (HAD/HIV encephalopathy
Inflammatory PML	Same as classic PML	Peripheral enhancement Perilesional edema Mass effect	Tumefactive demyelination Lymphoma
JC encephalitis	Diffuse cortical involvement Subcortical white matter involvement later in disease	T2 and FLAIR high signal intensity Mass effect No enhancement	HIV encephalitis CD8 encephalitis
JC granule cell neuronopathy	Cerebellar cortex, middle cerebellar peduncle, and pontine white matter	Cerebellar atrophy T2/Flair high signal in white matter Pontine "hot cross bun"	Multiple system atrophy Spinocerebellar ataxia SCA 2 and 3
JC meningitis	Meninges	No specific imaging findings	Other causes of viral meningitis

Proton MR Spectroscopy shows reduced levels of N-acetyl aspartate, elevated levels of choline, and normal or elevated levels of myoinositol depending on stage of disease. Myoinositol/creatine ratio has been described as a prognostic marker of the disease.[56]

Granule Cell Neuronopathy

JCV GCN is a rare JC virus-related disease in immunocompromised patients caused by lytic infection of the cerebellar granule cell layer, first described in 2003.[57] Initially, thought to be confined to the cerebellum,[42] it is now understood to involve cerebellar cortex as well as adjacent infratentorial white matter.[58]

Imaging in the early stages may be normal, and the common imaging feature in the later stages include cerebellar atrophy, followed by increased T2 signal intensity.[42] Additional features include T2 and FLAIR high-signal intensity in the brainstem and middle cerebellar peduncles[58] (Fig. 9).

John Cunningham Encephalitis

JC encephalitis is a recently described encephalopathic form of JC virus infection with preferential infection of cortical pyramidal neurons and astrocytes with necrosis.[59]

MR imaging typically shows multiple cortical lesions without enhancement initially restricted to the gray matter and subsequently, with disease progression, involving the subcortical white matter.[59]

MALIGNANCY
Primary Central Nervous System Lymphoma

Primary central nervous system lymphoma (PCNSL) can arise from the brain, spinal cord, and leptomeninges without systemic lymphoma and is the most common CNS neoplasm in AIDS. HIV-related PCNSL is a B-cell non-Hodgkin lymphoma that is almost always positive for Epstein-Barr virus.[60]

PCNSLs have varied imaging findings depending on the patient's immune status (Table 2).

On CT, these seem as heterogeneously enhancing multifocal, necrotic, or hemorrhagic lesions, most frequently involving the basal ganglia, followed by the frontal lobes.[61,62] On MR imaging, the lesions are T1 hypointense and T2 isointense to hyperintense with varying degrees of enhancement (Fig. 10).[61,62] It can be difficult to differentiate these lesions from

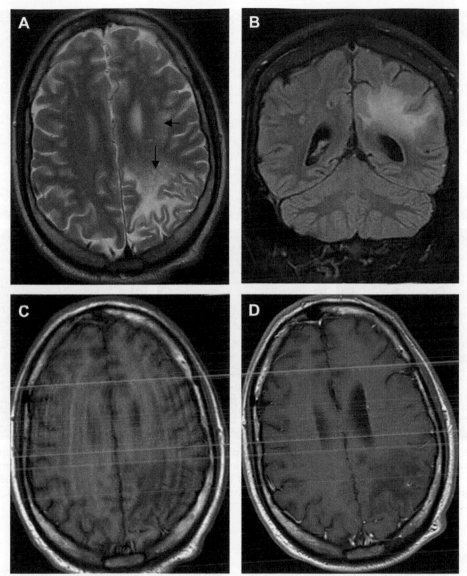

Fig. 7. Classic PML. A 32-year-old man with a new diagnosis of HIV and right-sided weakness. Axial T2-weighted image (A) shows a large confluent left parietal subcortical white matter lesion with microcysts (arrows). Note the absence of mass effect and cortical sparing on T2-weighted and FLAIR images (B), typical low signal intensity on T1-weighted image (C) without contrast enhancement (D).

cerebral toxoplasmosis, which also manifests as multifocal ring-enhancing lesions but increased rCBV in MR perfusion and FDG PET uptake in PCNSL can be helpful.[63,64]

INFLAMMATORY SYNDROMES
Immune Reconstitution Inflammatory Syndrome

IRIS is a complex phenomenon seen most commonly in HIV-infected patients after the initiation of ART and is characterized by an intense inflammatory reaction to dead or latent organisms, or to self-antigens due to a heightened but probably dysregulated immune response.[39,45,65,66,67,68,69] Although usually self-limiting, it can rarely be fulminating, leading to death in a short interval.[65]

IRIS is typically diagnosed when there is worsening of neurologic status after the initiation of ART in the setting of immune reconstitution (increasing CD4 counts and decreasing VL), with new or worsening radiological findings that cannot be explained by OI, drug toxicity, or treatment noncompliance.[65,68]

Incidence of IRIS, severity and mortality rates vary with the specific type of patient population,

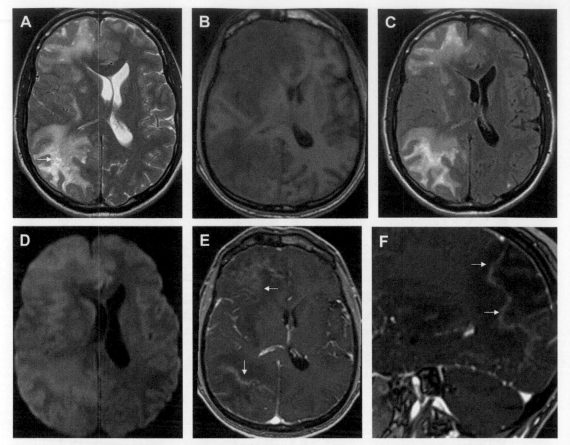

Fig. 8. Inflammatory PML. A 38-year-old man with new diagnosis of HIV, not on ART. Extensive right hemispheric, predominantly white matter abnormality, high signal intensity on T2-weighted (*A*) and FLAIR (*C*) images, low signal on T1-weighted image (*B*) and significant mass effect shows peripheral high signal on b1000 DWI (*D*) with florid enhancement of the advancing edge (*arrows*) on postcontrast T1-weighted images (*E, F*). Extensive demyelination was detected subsequently on biopsy.

type of AIDS-defining illness and the geographic location.[68] It usually develops within weeks or months, are rarely years, after initiation of ART.[39]

In a systematic review and meta-analysis, the proportion of patients developing IRIS was highest in those with CMV retinitis, cryptococcal meningitis, PML, or TB.[67]

Reported risk factors for IRIS include ART Naïve,[65] severely immunocompromised with CD4 counts less than 50 at ART initiation,[66,67] high pre-ART HIV VL, rapid decrease in HIV VL following ART[66] and OI.[66]

Two forms of IRIS have been described: delayed IRIS (previously called paradoxic IRIS) and simultaneous IRIS (previously called unmasking IRIS).[65]

Simultaneous IRIS (s IRIS; **Fig. 11**): Patients develop IRIS and a newly diagnosed OI at the same time due to inflammatory response to a viable pathogen related to a latent infection.

Delayed IRIS (d IRIS; **Fig. 12**): Patients develop IRIS sometime after being treated for an OI and occurs due to delayed inflammatory response to previously identified and treated antigen.

A significant change in the imaging features compared with classic appearances can be seen in PML and Cryptococcus in the setting of IRIS, whereas not much change occurs in Toxoplasma or TBM-related IRIS.[39,68] Increasing parenchymal high signal on FLAIR, increasing size of existing lesions or development of new lesions, enhancement of parenchymal lesions or leptomeninges, and restricted diffusion are features that predominate in CNS IRIS.[39,68]

The varied spectrum of IRIS across different OIs and comparison to classic features without IRIS is described in **Table 3**.

Depending on the severity, CNS-IRIS can be classified as (1) asymptomatic, where only

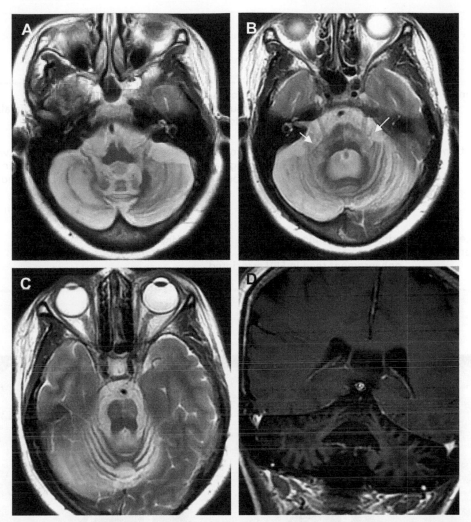

Fig. 9. Granule cell neuronopathy. A 49-year-old woman with ataxia had a normal MR imaging scan (not shown) at presentation. Follow-up MR imaging a few months later shows severe, bilaterally symmetric atrophy of the cerebellum with increased signal intensity on axial T2-weighted images (*A–C*). Abnormal high signal also seen involving the pons and middle cerebellar peduncles bilaterally (*arrows, B*) with volume loss. Coronal T1 postcontrast (*D*) shows corresponding nonenhancing low signal with severe atrophy, in contrast, to the normal supratentorial brain.

radiological changes such as increased enhancement may be present; (2) symptomatic, where clinical deterioration in neurologic function accompanies new changes on MR imaging; or (3) catastrophic, where severe neurologic deficits occur such as coma and imminent signs of cerebral herniation.[65]

Radiologists play an important role in early recognition of this condition, and it is important to consider IRIS in a HIV patient recently started on ART, whose neurologic condition worsens in the face of rising CD4 counts and reducing VLs, as appropriate containment of the inflammatory response can improve long-term outcome.

CD8 Encephalitis

CD8 encephalitis is a steroid-responsive severe inflammatory cerebral disease dominated by infiltration of brain by CD8 + T lymphocytes. Most of the reported cases occurred in long-standing HIV patients with well-controlled HIV and systemic viral suppression.[70,71] It is an emerging clinical entity whose exact pathophysiology is yet to be determined but is histopathologically characterized by diffuse white matter parenchymal infiltration by CD8+ T cells but little or no CD4+ T cell or B cell involvement and with microglial activation.[71]

Clinical presentation is usually with symptoms and signs of diffuse brain swelling such as

Table 2
Primary central nervous system lymphoma—differences in imaging between immunocompetent adults and human immunodeficiency virus

	PCNSL in Immunocompetent Patients	HIV-Related PCNSL
Location	Periventricular regions, often in contact with ventricular or meningeal surfaces Frontal lobes and basal ganglia also often affected	May be cortical or subcortical Frontal lobes and basal ganglia also often affected
Conventional MR	Usually isointense to gray matter on all spin echo sequences (hemorrhage and necrosis can be seen in EBV-associated lymphoma)	The lesions are often associated with central T2WI and FLAIR hyperintense areas due to *necrosis and hemorrhage*
DWI	Marked restricted diffusion	Restricted diffusion sparing the necrotic areas
Enhancement pattern	Predominantly homogeneous enhancement (Heterogenous enhancement seen in EBV associated lymphoma)	Highly variable; predominantly *heterogenous enhancement*

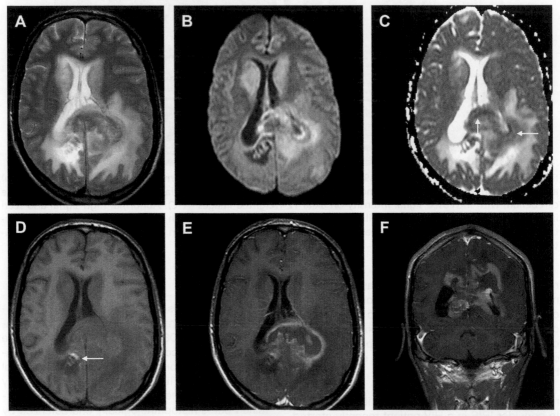

Fig. 10. PCNSL. A 23-year-old man with seizures and CD4 count of 100. Axial T2-weighted image (*A*) shows a large mass involving the corpus callosal splenium and the bilateral peritrigonal regions, with heterogenous high signal centrally and extensive perilesional edema. Note the nonenhancing increased signal involving caudate nuclei bilaterally. DWI (*B*) shows high signal and low ADC (*arrows, C*) of the periphery and focal high signal blood products on corresponding T1-weighted image (*D, arrow*). There is heterogenous peripheral enhancement on post-contrast images (*E, F*).

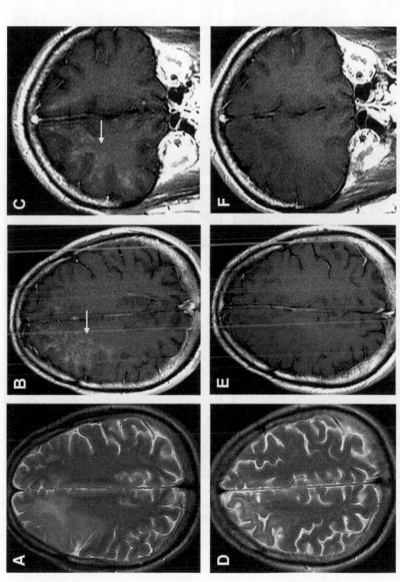

Fig. 11. PML and simultaneous IRIS. A 54-year-old male patient developing IRIS and PML simultaneously after the initiation of ART. On axial T2-weighted images (A), right frontal subcortical white matter hyperintensity with local swelling and mass effect shows speckled enhancement postcontrast (B, C). Lower panel (D–F) shows decrease in mass effect on Axial T2 (D) and resolution of enhancement on postcontrast sequences (E, F) following steroid therapy. Mass effect and enhancement are features typical of IRIS in PML; these are not seen in classic PML.

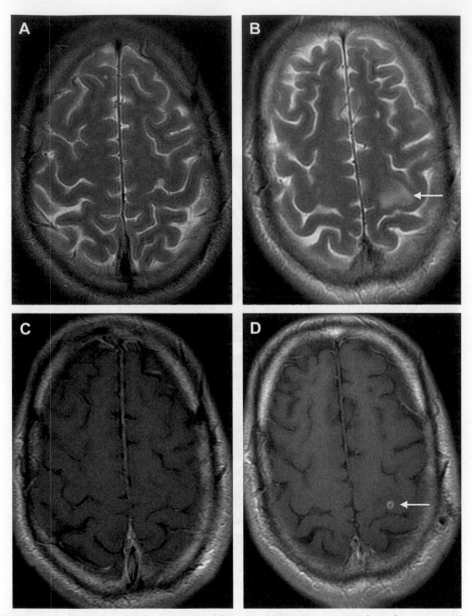

Fig. 12. Cryptococcus and delayed IRIS. A 33-year-old known HIV patient on ART for a few years and previously treated for cryptococcal meningitis presented with a seizure. Axial T2-weighted (*A, B*) and postcontrast T1-weighted (*C, D*) images show previously nonenhancing left motor strip cryptococcoma (*A, C*) develops new enhancement (*arrow, D*) and perilesional edema (*arrow, B*). CSF evaluation was unremarkable except for mild elevation of protein and CSF cryptococcal antigen negative in this case of delayed IRIS.

headache, confusion, and seizures.[70] In the largest case series of HIV-associated CD8 encephalitis[71] so far, the risk factors suggested were Black African ethnicity, interruption of ART, IRIS after commencement of ART, intercurrent infection, and drug resistance, with CNS viral escape probably being the immunologic phenomenon responsible.

Imaging shows diffuse brain swelling with bilateral, fairly symmetric, confluent white matter high signal change on T2 and FLAIR sequences involving both supratentorial and infratentorial compartments[71] (Fig. 13) with severe mass effect. Diffuse perivascular enhancement on postcontrast T1 spin echo sequence with magnetization transfer has been

Table 3
Differences in the imaging appearances of opportunistic infections in the setting of immune reconstitution inflammatory syndrome

Entity	Classic Imaging Features	Imaging Features in IRIS
CMV	Ventriculitis Retinitis	*Vasculitis with infarcts* Vitreitis
Cryptococcus	Hydrocephalus Leptomeningeal enhancement—less common Nonenhancing distended VR spaces/gelatinous pseudocysts	Hydrocephalus *Florid leptomeningeal enhancement* *Enhancement of VR spaces with secondary involvement of brain parenchyma*
PML	Confluent lesion in the subcortical white matter, low signal on T1 No mass effect No enhancement DWI peripheral incomplete restricted diffusivity of large/new lesions	Confluent lesion in the subcortical white matter, low signal on T1 *Mass effect* *Peripheral enhancement* *Edema*
TB[a]	Basal meningitis Hydrocephalus Granulomata Infarcts	Basal meningitis Hydrocephalus Granulomata Infarcts *New lesions or worsening of preexisting lesions with increasing edema*
Toxoplasma[a]	Ring-enhancing lesion with edema	Ring-enhancing lesion *Worsening edema*
VZV	Vasculopathy with beading, infarcts	Vascular beading and infarcts *Leptomeningeal, brain parenchymal and cord enhancement*

These have been listed in decreasing order of the proportion of patients with a specific OI developing IRIS, the highest proportion being reported in CMV retinitis.[67]

[a] Denotes OIs where the imaging can be very similar between IRIS and non-IRIS state.

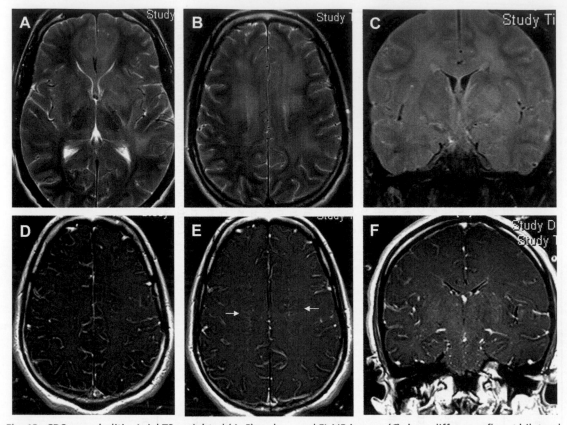

Fig. 13. CD8 encephalitis. Axial T2-weighted (*A*, *B*) and coronal FLAIR images (*C*) show diffuse confluent bilateral, symmetric white matter high signal with significant mass effect and complete effacement of CSF cisterns. Postcontrast axial (*D*, *E*) and coronal T1-weighted images (*F*) show prominent perivascular (*arrows*) and leptomeningeal enhancement.

reported,[70] as has relapsing and remitting course.[72]

CSF analysis may be difficult to obtain due to the contraindication for lumbar puncture in patients with severe brain swelling but there is typically mild protein elevation with a predominant CD8 pleocytosis (>90%).[70] CSF flow cytometry studies show definitive reversed CD4:CD8 ratio.[70,73]

It is important for the radiologist to be aware and consider this entity in the context of a long-standing, well-controlled, HIV patient who presents with a sudden and rapid neurologic deterioration, where the imaging shows a diffuse leukoencephalopathy with mass effect ± perivascular enhancement, as prompt treatment with steroids has been shown to save lives.[70,71]

SUMMARY

Radiologists should be familiar with imaging features of primary HIV infection, OI, malignancy, and inflammatory syndromes. ART has led to a changing spectrum with decreasing incidence of OIs and greater recognition of inflammatory

conditions, including IRIS. Being familiar with varied spectrum of imaging findings, the impact of ART and interpretation of imaging in the context of clinical and laboratory findings is important for radiologists as well as clinicians in the management of HIV-infected patients.

CLINICS CARE POINTS

- Patients with severe immune suppression (CD4 count <200 cells/mm^3) are at risk of toxoplasma encephalitis, cryptococcal meningitis, cytomegalovirus infection, primary CNS lymphoma, and PML, and patients with moderate immune suppression (CD4 counts of 200–500 cells/mm^3) are at risk of tuberculous meningitis and PML.

- T1 hyperintensity on precontrast images and postcontrast eccentric nodule of enhancement in ring-enhancing lesions can be useful distinguishing features of toxoplasmosis.

- PML is a confluent supratentorial white matter disease with asymmetric involvement of subcortical white matter and U fibers with characteristic low signal on T1 and absence of mass effect or enhancement.

- HIV-related PCNSL is a B-cell non-Hodgkin lymphoma that is almost always positive for Epstein-Barr virus and has a heterogenous appearance.

- IRIS is a complex phenomenon seen after initiation of cART, characterized by an intense inflammatory reaction to dead or latent organisms and can significantly alter the imaging appearances of opportunistic infections.

DISCLOSURE

The authors have nothing to disclose.

REFERENCES

1. Smith AB, Smirniotopoulos JG, Rushing EJ. Central nervous system infections associated with human immunodeficiency virus infection: Radiologicpathologic correlation. Radiographics 2008;28(7): 2033–58.
2. Tan IL, Smith BR, von Geldern G, et al. HIV-associated opportunistic infections of the CNS. Lancet Neurol 2012;11(7):605–17.
3. Thakur KT, Boubour A, Saylor D, et al. Global HIV neurology: A comprehensive review. AIDS 2019; 33(2):163–84.
4. Connor MD, Lammie GA, Bell JE, et al. Cerebral infarction in adult AIDS patients: Observations from the Edinburgh HIV Autopsy Cohort. Stroke 2000; 31(9):2117–26.
5. Dube MP, Stein JH, AJ. Panel on Antiretroviral Guidelines for Adults and Adolescents. Guidelines for the Use of Antiretroviral Agents in Adults and Adolescents with HIV. Dep Heal Hum Serv 2018; 40(Build 29393). Available at: https://aidsinfo.nih. gov/contentfiles/lvguidelines/adultandadolescentgl. pdf.
6. Winston A, Antinori A, Cinque P, et al. Defining cerebrospinal fluid HIV RNA escape: Editorial review AIDS. Aids 2019;33(January):S107–11.
7. Liu NQ, Lossinsky AS, Popik W, et al. Human Immunodeficiency Virus Type 1 Enters Brain Microvascular Endothelia by Macropinocytosis Dependent on Lipid Rafts and the Mitogen-Activated Protein Kinase Signaling Pathway. J Virol 2002;76(13): 6689–700.
8. Antinori A, Arendt G, Becker JT, et al. HHS Public Access 2015;69(18):1789–99.
9. Clifford DB, Ances BM. HIV-associated neurocognitive disorder. Lancet Infect Dis 2013;13(11):976–86.
10. Fennema-Notestine C, Ellis RJ, Archibald SL, et al. Increases in brain white matter abnormalities and subcortical gray matter are linked to CD4 recovery in HIV infection. J Neurovirol 2013;19(4):393–401.
11. Ances BM, Sisti D, Vaida F, et al. Resting cerebral blood flow. Neurology 2009;73(9):702–8.
12. Melrose RJ, Tinaz S, Castelo JMB, et al. Compromised fronto-striatal functioning in HIV: An fMRI investigation of semantic event sequencing. Behav Brain Res 2008;188(2):337–47.
13. Marcus JL, Leyden WA, Chao CR, et al. HIV infection and incidence of ischemic stroke. Aids 2014;28(13): 1911–9.
14. Chow FC, Regan S, Zanni MV, et al. Elevated ischemic stroke risk among women living with HIV infection. Aids 2018;32(1):59–67.
15. Sico JJ, Chang CCH, So-Armah K, et al. HIV status and the risk of ischemic stroke among men. Neurology 2015;84(19):1933–40.
16. Chow FC, He W, Bacchetti P, et al. Elevated rates of intracerebral hemorrhage in individuals from a US clinical care HIV cohort. Neurology 2014;83(19): 1705–11.
17. Goldstein DA, Timpone J, Cupps TR. HIV-associated intracranial aneurysmal vasculopathy in adults. J Rheumatol 2010;37(2):226–33.
18. Gutierrez J, Glenn M, Isaacson RS, et al. Thinning of the arterial media layer as a possible preclinical stage in HIV vasculopathy: A pilot study. Stroke 2012;43(4):1156–8.
19. Robbs JV, Paruk N. Management of HIV Vasculopathy - A South African Experience. Eur J Vasc Endovasc Surg 2010;39(SUPPL. 1). https://doi.org/10. 1016/j.ejvs.2009.12.028.
20. Gutierrez J, Ortiz G. HIV/AIDS patients with HIV vasculopathy and VZV vasculitis: A case series. Clin Neuroradiol 2011;21(3):145–51.
21. Chetty R, Batitang S, Nair R. Large artery vasculopathy in HIV-positive patients: Another vasculitic enigma. Hum Pathol 2000;31(3):374–9.
22. Brent Tipping MBChB, Linda de Villiers MBChB, Candy Sally, et al. Stroke caused by human immunodeficiency virus-associated vasculopathy. Arch Neurol 2006;63:1640–2.
23. Lammie GA, Hewlett RH, Schoeman JF, et al. Tuberculous cerebrovascular disease: A review. J Infect 2009;59(3):156–66.
24. Zetola NM, Klausner JD. Syphilis and HIV infection: An update. Clin Infect Dis 2007;44(9):1222–8.
25. Nagel M, Cohrs R, Mahalingam R, et al. The varicella zoster virus vasculopathies: Clinical, CSF, imaging, and virologic features. Neurology 2008;70(11):853–60.
26. Cruse B, Cysique LA, Markus R, et al. Cerebrovascular disease in HIV-infected individuals in the era of highly active antiretroviral therapy. J Neurovirol 2012;18(4):264–76.

27. Bowen LN, Smith B, Reich D, et al. HIV-associated opportunistic CNS infections: Pathophysiology, diagnosis and treatment. Nat Rev Neurol 2016; 12(11):662–74.
28. C C Tchoyoson Lim. HIV and related conditions. In: Magnetic Resonance Imaging of Neurological Diseases in Tropics. ; 2014:198-205. doi:DOI: 10.5005/jp/books/12139_13.
29. Lee GT, Antelo F, Mlikotic AA. Best cases from the AFIP: Cerebral toxoplasmosis. Radiographics 2009;29(4):1200–5.
30. Grant IH, Gold JWM, Rosenblum M, et al. Toxoplasma gondii serology in HIV-infected patients: The development of central nervous system toxoplasmosis in AIDS. Aids 1990;4(6):519–21.
31. Chacko G. Parasitic diseases of the central nervous system. Semin Diagn Pathol 2010;27(3):167–85.
32. Kumar GGS, Mahadevan A, Guruprasad AS, et al. Eccentric target sign in cerebral toxoplasmosis: Neuropathological correlate to the imaging feature. J Magn Reson Imaging 2010;31(6):1469–72.
33. Moritani Toshio, Ota Yoshiaki, Patricia A, et al. Infectious diseases. In: diffusion-weighted MR imaging of the brain, Head and Neck, and spine. Switzerland AG: Springer Nature; 2021. p. 429–86.
34. Schaller MA, Wicke F, Foerch C, et al. Central Nervous System Tuberculosis: Etiology, Clinical Manifestations and Neuroradiological Features. Clin Neuroradiol 2019;29(1):3–18.
35. leonard John M. Central nervous system tuberculosis. Microbiol Spectr 2017;5(2). https://doi.org/10.1128/microbiolspec.TNMI7-0044-2017.
36. Thurnher MM, Donovan Post MJ. Neuroimaging in the Brain in HIV-1-Infected Patients. Neuroimaging Clin N Am 2008;18(1):93–117.
37. Loyse A, Moodley A, Rich P, et al. Neurological, visual, and MRI brain scan findings in 87 South African patients with HIV-associated cryptococcal meningoencephalitis. J Infect 2015;70(6):668–75.
38. Offiah CE, Naseer A. Spectrum of imaging appearances of intracranial cryptococcal infection in HIV/AIDS patients in the anti-retroviral therapy era. Clin Radiol 2016;71(1):9–17.
39. Post MJD, Thurnher MM, Clifford DB, et al. CNS-immune reconstitution inflammatory syndrome in the setting of HIV infection, Part 1: Overview and discussion of progressive multifocal leukoencephalopathy-immune reconstitution inflammatory syndrome and cryptococcal- Immune reconstitution inflammatory syndrome. Am J Neuroradiol 2013;34(7):1297–307.
40. Post MJD, Hensley G, Moskowitz LB, et al. Cytomegalic inclusion virus encephalitis in patients with AIDS: CT, clinical, and pathological correlation. Am J Roentgenol 1986;146(6):1229–34.
41. Gheuens S, Pierone G, Peeters P, et al. Progressive multifocal leukoencephalopathy in individuals with minimal or occult immunosuppression. J Neurol Neurosurg Psychiatry 2010;81(3):247–54.
42. Bag AK, Curé JK, Chapman PR, et al. JC virus infection of the brain. Am J Neuroradiol 2010;31(9):1564–76.
43. Wüthrich C, Cheng YM, Joseph JT, et al. Frequent infection of cerebellar granule cell neurons by polyomavirus JC in progressive multifocal leukoencephalopathy. J Neuropathol Exp Neurol 2009;68(1):15–25.
44. Cinque P, Koralnik IJ, Gerevini S, et al. Progressive multifocal leukoencephalopathy in HIV-1 infection. Lancet Infect Dis 2009;9(10):625–36.
45. Falcó V, Olmo M, Del Saz SV, et al. Influence of HAART on the Clinical Course of HIV-1-infected patients with progressive multifocal leukoencephalopathy: Results of an observational multicenter study. J Acquir Immune Defic Syndr 2008;49(1):26–31.
46. Lima MA, Drislane FW, Koralnik IJ. Seizures and their outcome in progressive multifocal leukoencephalopathy. Neurology 2006;66(2):262–4.
47. Berger JR, Aksamit AJ, Clifford DB, et al. PML diagnostic criteria: Consensus statement from the AAN neuroinfectious disease section. Neurology 2013;80(15):1430–8.
48. Whiteman MLH, Post MJD, Berger JR, et al. Progressive multifocal leukoencephalopathy in 47 HIV-seropositive patients: Neuroimaging with clinical and pathologic correlation. Radiology 1993;187(1):233–40.
49. Mudau A, Suleman FE, Schutte CM, et al. Isolated posterior fossa involvement of progressive multifocal leucoencephalopathy in HIV: A case series with review of the literature. South Afr J Radiol 2017;21(2):1–6.
50. Bernal-Cano F, Joseph JT, Koralnik IJ. Spinal cord lesions of progressive multifocal leukoencephalopathy in an acquired immunodeficiency syndrome patient. J Neurovirol 2007;13(5):474–6.
51. Murayi R, Schmitt J, Woo JH, et al. Spinal cord progressive multifocal leukoencephalopathy detected premortem by MRI. J Neurovirol 2015;21(6):688–90.
52. Bergui M, Bradac GB, Oguz KK, et al. Progressive multifocal leukoencephalopathy: Diffusion-weighted imaging and pathological correlations. Neuroradiology 2004;46(1):22–5.
53. Godi C, De Vita E, Tombetti E, et al. High b-value diffusion-weighted imaging in progressive multifocal leukoencephalopathy in HIV patients. Eur Radiol 2017;27(9):3593–9.
54. Finelli PF, Foxman EB. The etiology of ring lesions on diffusion-weighted imaging. Neuroradiol J 2014;27(3):280–7.
55. Thurnher MM, Boban J, Rieger A, et al. Susceptibility-weighted MR imaging hypointense rim in progressive multifocal leukoencephalopathy: The end

point of neuroinflammation and a potential outcome predictor. Am J Neuroradiol 2019;40(6):994–1000.

56. Katz-Brull R, Lenkinski RE, Du Pasquier RA, et al. Elevation of myoinositol is associated with disease containment in progressive multifocal leukoence-phalopathy. Neurology 2004;63(5):897–900.

57. Du Pasquier RA, Corey S, Margolin DH, et al. Productive infection of cerebellar granule cell neurons by JC virus in an HIV+ individual. Neurology 2003; 61(6):775–82.

58. Wijburg MT, Van Oosten BW, Murk JL, et al. Hetero-geneous imaging characteristics of JC virus granule cell neuronopathy (GCN): A case series and review of the literature. J Neurol 2015;262(1):65–73.

59. Wüthrich C, Dang X, Westmoreland S, et al. Fulmi-nant JC virus encephalopathy with productive infec-tion of cortical pyramidal neurons. Ann Neurol 2009; 65(6):742–8.

60. Brandsma D, Bromberg JFC. 1st ed. Primary CNS lymphoma in HIV infection, 152. Elsevier B.V.; 2018. https://doi.org/10.1016/B978-0-444-63849-6. 00014-1.

61. Javadi S, Menias CO, Karbasian N, et al. HIV-related malignancies and mimics: Imaging findings and management. Radiographics 2018;38(7):2051–68.

62. Bathla G, Hegde A. Lymphomatous involvement of the central nervous system. Clin Radiol 2016;71(6): 602 9.

63. Dibble EH, Boxerman JL, Baird GL, et al. Toxoplas-mosis versus lymphoma: Cerebral lesion character-ization using DSC-MRI revisited. Clin Neurol Neurosurg 2017;152:84–9.

64. Hoffman John M, Waskin Hetty A, Tobias Schifter, et al. FDG-PET in differentiating lymphoma from nonmalignant central nervous system lesions in pa-tients with AIDS. J Nucl Med 1993;34:567–75.

65. Johnson T, Nath A. Neurological complications of immune reconstitution in HIV-infected populations. Ann N Y Acad Sci 2010;1184:106–20.

66. Shelburne SA, Visnegarwala F, Darcourt J, et al. Inci-dence and risk factors for immune reconstitution in-flammatory syndrome during highly active antiretroviral therapy. Aids 2005;19(4):399–406.

67. Müller M, Wandel S, Colebunders R, et al. Immune reconstitution inflammatory syndrome in patients starting antiretroviral therapy for HIV infection: a sys-tematic review and meta-analysis. Lancet Infect Dis 2010;10(4):251–61.

68. Post MJD, Thurnher MM, Clifford DB, et al. CNS-im-mune reconstitution inflammatory syndrome in the setting of HIV infection, part 2: Discussion of neuro-immune reconstitution inflammatory syn-drome with and without other pathogens. Am J Neu-roradiol 2013;34(7):1308–18.

69. Bahr N, Boulware DR, Marais S, et al. Central ner-vous system immune reconstitution inflammatory syndrome. Curr Infect Dis Rep 2013;15(6):583–93.

70. Lescure FX, Moulignier A, Savatovsky J, et al. CD8 encephalitis in HIV-infected patients receiving ART: A treatable entity. Clin Infect Dis 2013;57(1):101–8.

71. Lucas SB, Wong KT, Nightingale S, et al. HIV-Asso-ciated CD8 Encephalitis: A UK Case Series and Re-view of Histopathologically Confirmed Cases. Front Neurol 2021;1–20. https://doi.org/10.3389/fneur. 2021.628296.

72. Salam S, Mihalova T, Ustianowski A, et al. Relapsing CD8+ encephalitis-looking for a solution. BMJ Case Rep 2016. https://doi.org/10.1136/bcr-2016.

73. Kerr C, Adle-Biassette H, Moloney PB, et al. CD8 en-cephalitis with CSF EBV viraemia and HIV drug resistance, a case series. Brain Behav Immun - Heal 2020;100164. https://doi.org/10.1016/j.bbih. 2020.100164.

Spinal Infections

Hajime Yokota, MD, PhD[a],*, E. Turgut Tali, MD[b]

KEYWORDS

- Spinal infection • Myelitis • Meningitis • Arachnoiditis • Spondylitis

KEY POINTS

- Spinal infections should always be considered as differential diagnoses because they present with a wide variety of imaging findings.
- In infectious myelitis, differential diagnoses can be refined by focusing on the distribution of the lesions.
- For arachnoiditis, care should be taken to differentiate it from neoplasms.
- Infectious spondylitis has many mimickers and requires careful interpretations of images, clinical findings, and follow-up information.

INTRODUCTION

The spine consists of organs of both the nervous system and skeletal systems in close proximity, and a variety of pathologic conditions can occur. Infectious diseases may affect either or both systems, and it is often difficult to determine the specific diagnosis based on imaging alone. It is extremely important to differentiate between infectious and noninfectious diseases because it has a significant impact on treatment strategies. The prevalence and range of pathogens of spinal infections varies significantly according to the geographic region. Clinical and/or laboratory findings can show wide variations, and if tests for specific markers are not promptly performed, the diagnosis may be delayed. Imaging assessment is required for confirmation and localization. Radiologists need to list proper differential diagnoses.

When interpreting images, it is essential to review the patient's medical history.[1] Then, the location of the lesion must be considered. If neurologic symptoms, such as paresthesia and paralysis are the main presentations, spinal cord lesions should be suspected. In some cases, the spinal cord is directly affected by myelitis, whereas in other cases, neurologic symptoms may be caused by external compression of the spinal cord and/or nerve roots. Rarely, there may be peripheral neuropathy. In contrast, if pain is the main symptom, a spinal bone lesion should be suspected. Although myelopathy can rarely present with pain, neurologic deficit is the main symptom.

Infections generally follow an acute course, and serum inflammatory biomarkers are often elevated. Nevertheless, it is important not to forget infections in the differential diagnosis because some infections have a chronic progressive course, in which inflammatory biomarkers are often difficult to detect. Conversely, fever and leukocytosis can sometimes be present in noninfectious causes.[2,3] Imaging findings of spinal infections are often atypical and other diseases can mimic them. This article highlights both typical and atypical imaging findings of spinal infections.

SPINAL CORD INFECTIONS

Infections that affect the spinal cord are typically viral in origin, and often preferentially affect the gray matter.[4–6] Table 1 shows the typical imaging features and the differential diagnosis of spinal cord infection by anatomic location. Diseases that mainly affect the anterior horn include poliovirus infection and poliomyelitis-like syndromes. Varicella-zoster virus (VZV) tends to form lesions

[a] Department of Diagnostic Radiology and Radiation Oncology, Graduate School of Medicine, Chiba University, 1-8-1 Inohana, Chuo-ku, Chiba 2608670, Japan; [b] Section of Neuroradiology, Lokman Hekim University School of Medicine, Sogutozu, Ankara 06510 Turkey
* Corresponding author.
E-mail address: hjmykt@chiba-u.jp

Neuroimag Clin N Am 33 (2023) 167–183
https://doi.org/10.1016/j.nic.2022.07.015
1052-5149/23/© 2022 Elsevier Inc. All rights reserved.

Table 1
Differential diseases by site of myelitis/myelopathy

	Infection	Noninfectious
Anterior horn	Poliomyelitis Poliomyelitis-like syndrome	Spinal cord infarction Compressive myelopathy Hopkins syndrome
Posterior horn	Herpes zoster myelitis	
Posterior column	HIV myelopathy	Subacute combined degeneration of the spinal cord
	Syphilis	Folate deficiency
	Herpes zoster myelitis	Atopic myelopathy Wallerian degeneration due to peripheral neuropathy Myelopathy after intrathecal chemotherapy Cerebrotendinous xanthomatosis
Lateral column	Human T-cell leukemia virus type 1 associated myelopathy	Amyotrophic lateral sclerosis
	HIV myelopathy	Adrenomyeloneuropathy Paraneoplastic syndrome Krabbe disease Wallerian degeneration Subacute combined degeneration of the spinal cord

in and around the posterior horn. Human immuno-deficiency virus (HIV) and syphilis are known to form lesions in the posterior horn, and human T-lymphotropic virus type 1 (HTLV-1) can form lesions in the lateral and posterior columns.

Myelitis, whether infectious or noninfectious, does not always have specific biomarkers, and therefore, imaging plays a significant role. MR imaging is the imaging modality of choice.[7] Contrast enhancement can be useful in detecting active myelitis. However, the absence of contrast does not indicate the absence of active myelitis. Once the extent of the lesion is known, it is important to direct appropriate imaging to that area.

For bone lesions, fat-suppressed T2-weighted imaging (FS-T2WI), short-tau inversion recovery (STIR) imaging is essential. Gradient sequences providing T2* images are also useful to detect bleeding, calcifications and diffusion-weighted image (DWI) is useful to evaluate lesions suspected of restricting diffusions, such as abscesses, infarction, and tumors. Postcontrast imaging with or without fat saturation is helpful for detecting acute lesions and the distribution of diseases.

Poliomyelitis and Poliomyelitis-like Syndrome

With widespread vaccination, the number of new cases of polio virus infection has decreased dramatically worldwide. In the past, due to the use of live polio vaccines, cases of vaccine-associated poliomyelitis were reported.[8] Viruses

other than poliovirus can also cause anterior horn myelitis. The condition is referred to as poliomyelitis-like syndrome.[9,10] As with poliomyelitis, it is more common in children and presents with signs and symptoms of acute or progressive flaccid paralysis. On MR imaging, the anterior horn of the spinal cord shows abnormal signals bilaterally or unilaterally, with an extension to the surrounding structures (**Fig. 1**). This may be associated with mild swelling. Enhancement of the anterior roots can also be seen.

Postpolio Syndrome

New muscle weakness, atrophy, myalgia, arthralgia, fatigue, sleep disturbance, respiratory dysfunction, and dysphagia may be seen in 20% to 85% of patients with a distant past history of poliomyelitis.[11]

In these patients, MR imaging is often performed to rule out other diseases and can show high signal localized to the anterior horn on T2WI but not accompanied by swelling (**Fig. 2**).

Herpes Zoster or Varicella-Zoster Virus myelitis

VZV affecting the spinal cord is often associated with herpes zoster skin lesions but myelitis without skin lesions has also been reported. Because myelitis spreads from the virus latent in the dorsal root ganglia, posterior horn and posterior columns

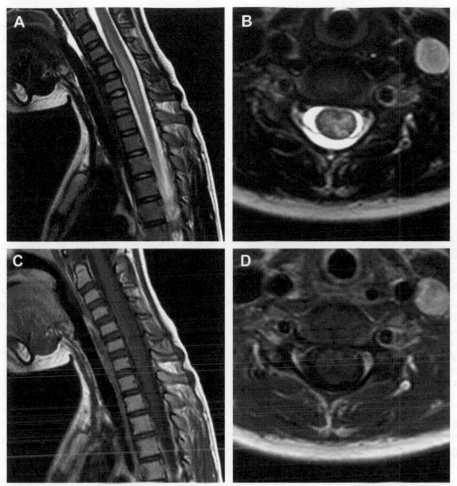

Fig. 1. Poliomyelitis-like syndrome. An 8-year-old girl presented with fever, sore throat for 4 days, and difficulty in using the left upper extremity, with right upper limb weakness, chest pain, and respiratory distress the next day. T2-weighted (*A, B*) and precontrast T1-weighted images (*C, D*) in the sagittal and axial planes showed both the anterior horns and the right posterior horn are involved, and there is a mild swelling. Contrast enhancement was unclear.

are typically affected[12,13] (**Fig. 3**). However, there are cases in which the lesions are more extensive, resembling transverse myelitis. In these cases, the dorsal root may also be enhanced.

Human Immunodeficiency Virus myelopathy

Patients with HIV-AIDS are susceptible to 2 types of myelopathy namely, HIV-associated myelopathy and myelitis associated with opportunistic infections. Vacuolar myelopathy associated with HIV presents with slowly progressive spastic paraplegia, bladder and rectal disturbance, and ataxia. Pathologic condition shows demyelination in the posterior and lateral columns (**Fig. 4**), which is similar to that of subacute combined spinal cord degeneration.[14,15] However, because patients with HIV may also suffer vitamin B12 deficiency

due to low nutrition,[16] care should be taken to differentiate between HIV myelopathy and subacute combined spinal cord degeneration because the latter can be treated.

Human T-lymphotropic Virus Type I-Associated myelopathy

HTLV-1 virus may cause HTLV-1 associated myelopathy (HAM) or tropical spastic paraparesis more common in Japan, the Caribbean, South America, Melanesian islands, Papua New Guinea, and Africa.[17] HAM typically presents with slowly progressive spastic paraparesis and urinary disturbance. MR imaging show abnormal signal areas in the lateral column and central gray matter with enlargement during the early stage[18,19] (**Fig. 5**). Later, spinal cord atrophy develops,

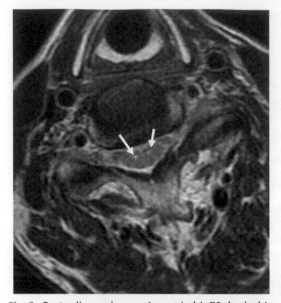

Fig. 2. Postpolio syndrome. A man in his 70s had a history of poliomyelitis at 8 months of age and subsequent disuse of the right upper extremity. Muscle weakness in the left upper extremity began in his 20s and progressed gradually. T2-weighted image shows hyperintense spots in the anterior horns bilaterally, sparing the rest of the cord (arrows).

especially in the thoracic spinal cord (Fig. 6).[20] During the period of atrophy, abnormal intramedullary signals become less distinct.

Intramedullary Spinal Cord Abscess

Intramedullary spinal cord abscess is rare, and differentiation from tumors or transverse myelitis may be challenging. Imaging appearance varies according to the stage of infection. Patchy

hyperintensity of inflammation due to pyogenic and/or hypointensity caused by granulomatous infections may be seen on T2WI with no or mild enhancement during the myelitis stage. Progression to abscess form shows decrease of the patchy hyperintensity and ring-like capsule formation seen as iso-hypointense on T2WI, hyperintense on T1WI, with ring-like enhancement on postcontrast T1WI (Fig. 7).[21,22] The signal intensity of central necrosis into the capsule varies according to the causative agent. Pyogenic abscess shows high signal on both T2WI and T1WI. DWI usually shows diffusion restriction in pyogenic abscesses while granulomatous abscesses may not demonstrate diffusion restriction.[23] Widespread edema is usually seen during the acute stage but during subacute and chronic stage, surrounding edema and contrast enhancement both decrease. The enhancing capsule becomes irregular and disappears during the chronic stage together with the normalization of DWI and apparent diffusion coefficient (ADC) signal changes.

DIFFERENTIAL DIAGNOSIS OF INFECTIOUS MYELITIS

Distribution of the involved site is important to differentiate among myelitis. The list of differential diagnoses by the involved site is shown in Table 1.

Diseases Involving the Anterior Horn

Occlusion of the anterior spinal artery can result in spinal cord infarction, typically depicted as abnormal signal in the anterior horns bilaterally. Spinal cord infarction has an acute onset,[24] and neurologic deficits are typically complete at time of presentation.[10] In contrast, viral myelitis

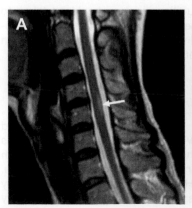
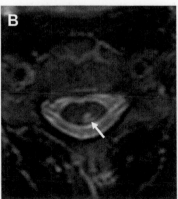
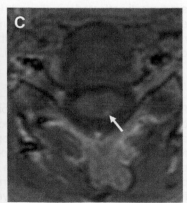

Fig. 3. Herpes zoster myelitis. A woman in her 40s developed herpes zoster on the left side of her abdomen a week ago, with subsequent lower limb muscle weakness, dysuria, plantar numbness, and sensory disturbances. T2-weighted sagittal and axial images show hyperintensity involving the left posterior horn and posterior column (A, B: arrows). The postcontrast T1-weighted image shows spot enhancement (C: arrow).

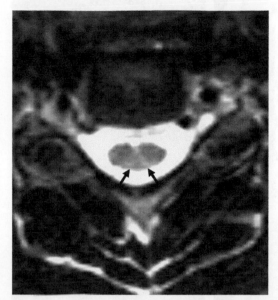

Fig. 4. HIV vacuolar myelopathy. A man in his 20s complained of gait disturbance for 1 year, frequent urination for 3 months, and difficulty in carrying heavy objects for 2 months. T2-weighted images show increased signal intensity mainly in the posterior column (*arrows*). No cord enlargement was observed.

typically presents with an acute to subacute course that is completed in days to weeks. Myelopathy caused by cervical spondylosis may also cause abnormal signals of the anterior horn.[25] Hopkins syndrome is a rare condition of acute flaccid paralysis after an asthma attack, in which high T2WI signals are confined to the anterior horn.[26]

Neuromyelitis optica spectrum disorders and myelin oligodendrocyte glycoprotein antibody-associated disorders typically demonstrate longitudinally extensive lesions predominantly in the central part of the spinal cord, with a transverse myelitis pattern.[27,28] Atypically, abnormal signal can be smaller and limited to the anterior horn.

Diseases Involving the Posterior Horn

Diseases that affect the dorsal horn and posterior column include subacute combined spinal cord degeneration from vitamin B12 deficiency, and iatrogenic posterior column injury after intrathecal injections, particularly of chemotherapeutic agents.[29–31] Vitamin B12 levels and history are the most important factors in the differentiation of these diseases. Copper and folic acid deficiencies can also show similar findings. In VZV myelitis, asymmetrical involvement of the posterior column is typical. HIV myelopathy may be diagnosed by exclusion when the symptoms do not improve with vitamin B12 treatment, especially in patients who are both HIV-positive and have low vitamin B12 levels.

Diseases Involving the Lateral Column

Diseases that systematically affect the lateral columns include degenerative diseases, such as amyotrophic lateral sclerosis, adrenomyeloneuropathy, and drug-induced diseases.[32,33] The motor nerves in adjacent spinal segments above and below are often affected simultaneously, and the history and neurologic findings differ from those of viral myelitis. Paraneoplastic syndromes may also involve the lateral columns.[34] Although subacute combined degeneration of the spinal cord typically involves the posterior columns, sometimes the lateral columns can also be affected in isolation.[35]

Disease Presenting as a Mass-like Lesion

Intramedullary abscesses are challenging to differentiate from tumors and transverse myelitis.[36] Typically, the history of tumors tends to follow a subacute progressive course during a few weeks. In contrast, abscesses tend to follow an acute course. Moreover, inflammatory markers are often elevated in abscesses but not tumors.

SUBARACHNOID SPACE INFECTIONS

Painful inflammation of the subarachnoid space and spinal nerves is called arachnoiditis. It often spreads from intracranial meningitis because there is no anatomic barrier to cerebrospinal fluid (CSF) flow. Abnormalities of the subarachnoid space are difficult to detect on conventional T1WI and T2WI, and abnormal contrast enhancement may be the only imaging finding observed along the spinal cord surface and nerve roots during the acute stage.

Infectious Meningitis/Arachnoiditis

The clinical manifestations of meningitis are headache, meningeal irritation, and increased inflammatory markers. MR imaging detects abnormal thickening and enhancement along the surface of the spinal cord and nerve roots or cauda equina (Figs. 8 and 9).[37,38] This may be accompanied by abnormal signal, suggestive of inflammation spreading into the spinal cord parenchyma. Later in the course of infection, adhesive arachnoiditis may also be seen as irregular meningeal thickening, adhesions, and loculations of CSF or pus.[39] These can obliterate the subarachnoid space and may cause blockage of the CSF circulation. Cranial imaging is usually necessary to assess the upward extent of spread.

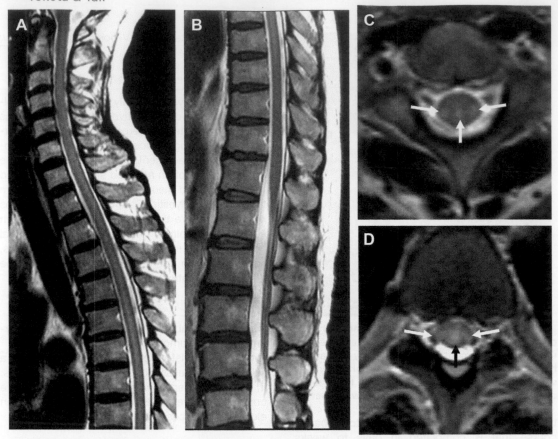

Fig. 5. HAM (early stage). A woman in her 50s without known past medical history presented with slowly progressive spastic paraplegia, paresthesia, and dysuria for 1.5 years. T2-weighted sagittal images show multifocal hyperintense areas in the spinal cord (A, B). T2-weighted axial images show these hyperintense areas are located in the central gray matter and the lateral column (C, D: arrows).

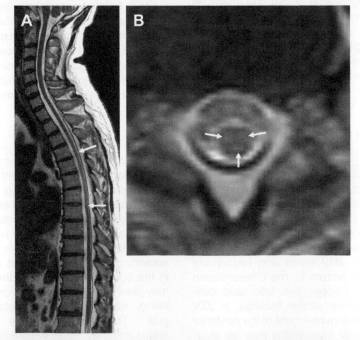

Fig. 6. HAM (late stage). A man in his 50s with known HTLV-1 infection presented with gradually progressive spastic paraplegia and dysuria for the past 10 years. T2-weighted sagittal images show atrophic thinning of the thoracic spine (A; arrows). T2-weighted axial image shows spotty hyperintensities in the anterior horn, lateral, and posterior columns (B: arrows).

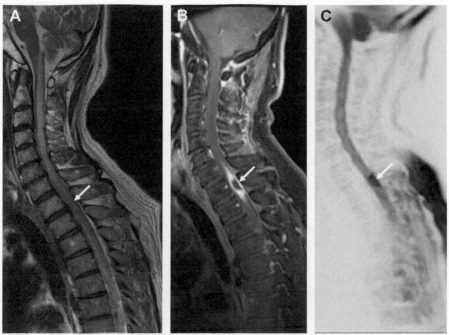

Fig. 7. Intramedullary spinal cord abscess. A man in his 60s developed difficulty walking and bladder and rectal disturbance 4 days earlier. His symptoms rapidly worsened despite steroid treatment, and he developed respiratory depression. T2-weighted sagittal image showing a long segment spinal cord swelling and hyperintensity (*A: arrow*). A fat-suppressed T1-weighted image showing contrast-enhancing lesion with a nonenhancing center (*B: arrow*). DWI shows hyperintensity corresponding to the poorly enhanced area, consistent with pyogenic abscess (*C: arrow*). (*Courtesy of* C Bamba, MD, Kyoto, Japan.)

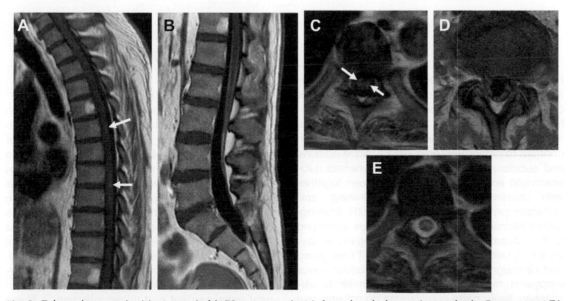

Fig. 8. Tuberculous meningitis. A man in his 50s presented with fever, headache, and tetraplegia. Postcontrast T1-weighted images show contrast enhancement on the surface of the spinal cord and cauda equina (*A–D: arrows*). On T2-weighted images, intramedullary hyperintensity is suggestive of myelitis or meningitis-related myelopathy (*E*).

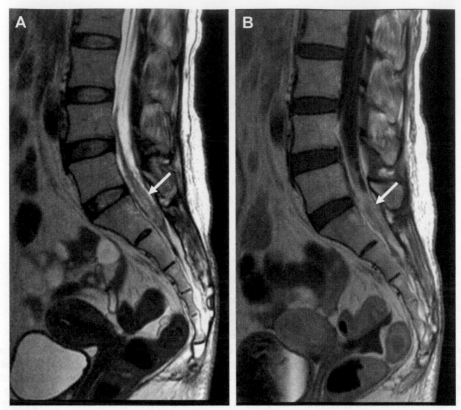

Fig. 9. Postoperative infectious arachnoiditis. A woman in her 40s underwent surgical resection of an ependymoma of the fourth ventricle 2 months ago. Follow-up MR imaging performed to search for tumor dissemination revealed an abnormality within the subarachnoid space at the caudal end of the dural sac, inseparable from the cauda equina (*A: arrow*). The lesion is slightly hyperintense to normal cauda and strongly enhanced (*B: arrow*). The patient had a fever and neck stiffness for several days after surgery but was improving at the time of MR imaging. The CSF analysis confirmed infection by *Klebsiella* species bacteria.

Empyema

Focal collection of purulent material results in subarachnoid, subdural, or epidural empyema and is often seen with the spread from neighboring infections, mainly meningitis.[40] Long segment lesions can be seen into all the spaces of the spine in contrast to intracranial empyema. Unique epidural and subdural empyema are rare, whereas subarachnoid empyema is frequently seen together with meningitis. Meningeal thickening and enhancement is usually seen on MR imaging. Signal intensity of the empyema varies according to the causative agent. Usually, pyogenic empyema is hyperintense to CSF on both T1-weighted and T2-weighted images, whereas granulomatous empyema may be hypointense. Similar to abscesses, liquid parts in empyema do not enhance while neighboring meninges enhance on postcontrast images; loculations can be seen due to adhesions.[41,42]

DIFFERENTIAL DIAGNOSIS OF MENINGITIS/ ARACHNOIDITIS

Contrast enhancement along the spinal cord surface and nerve roots may also be observed in neoplastic, depositional, and noninfectious granulomatous diseases (Box 1). After brain tumor surgery, drop metastases may be detected in the spinal canal. However, in the first few months after surgery or following interventions such as lumbar puncture, contrast enhancement due to subarachnoid hemorrhage or meningitis may be observed, so it is important not to simply assume that all MR imaging abnormalities are the result of drop metastases.[43] Many other causes, including certain administered drugs, hyperoxygenation, and anesthesia may also cause meningeal enhancement and mimic infection.[44] These may be difficult to differentiate on imaging and require additional clinical information and CSF analysis.

Box 1
Differential diagnosis of arachnoiditis

Neoplasm
    Leptomeningeal dissemination/drop metastasis, lymphoma
Infection
    Infectious meningitis
Others
    Sarcoidosis
    Amyloidosis

SPONDYLITIS/SPONDYLODISCITIS

Spondylitis is a general term for vertebral osteomyelitis and disc infection caused by bacteria, fungi, and parasites. In a patient with neurologic deficits localized to the spinal level, if pain is a prominent symptom, a spinal bone lesion is suspected, rather than a spinal cord lesion. Back pain is a common chief complaint, and imaging studies are of limited benefit in cases of nonspecific back pain in the general population, unless "red flags" (Box 2) justify MR imaging evaluation for clinically critical lesions like malignancy or infection.[45,46] The sensitivity of MR imaging for spondylitis has been reported as 96%, with 92% specificity, and 94% accuracy.[47]

Pyogenic spondylitis

In pyogenic spondylitis, fever and white blood cell elevation is present in less than 50% but elevated C-reactive protein is present in more than 80% of cases.[48,49] Risk factors include injection drug use, infective endocarditis, degenerative spine disease, prior spinal surgery, diabetes mellitus, and corticosteroid therapy.

Box 2
Red flags of lumber pain

Age less than 20 or greater than 55 years
Back pain not related to time or activity
Chest pain
History of cancer, diabetes mellitus, HIV steroids, drug usage
Malnutrition
Weight loss
Widespread neurologic symptoms
Spinal deformity
Fever

Typical pyogenic spondylitis occurs in the lower lumbar vertebrae but it can also occur at any level.[50–52] The typical progression of pyogenic spondylitis is as follows (Figs. 10 and 11). (1) Infection frequently begins in the anterior corners, which is rich in blood flow and corresponds to the end of the artery. (2) The infection spreads through the endplate to the intervertebral discs, and the intervertebral space initially widens, followed by narrowing. (3) The infection spreads to the adjacent vertebral bodies. (4) Infection extends underneath the anterior and posterior longitudinal ligaments, to the epidural space and neighboring paraspinal soft tissues, paraspinal muscles, and even to the retroperitoneum. In rare cases, an abscess forms immediately around the vertebral body (Fig. 12). In children, the infection begins near the growth plate and quickly spreads to the intervertebral discs, which may present as discitis. If the lesion is confined to one vertebral body in the early stages of infection, it may be difficult to differentiate it from other diseases, such as compression fractures.

On MR imaging, infection of the perivertebral soft tissues (98%), nonanatomic high signal in the intervertebral disc on T2WI in pyogenic infections (93%; and low signal for the granulomatous infections), contrast enhancement of the intervertebral disc (95%), and narrowing of the intervertebral space (84%) are common findings.[47,50,53] However, imaging features are not specific and should be considered in combination with clinical and laboratory findings. On FS-T2WI, the high-intensity signal region of the vertebral body can be difficult to distinguish in patients with red marrow reconversion or gelatinous transformation.[54] Fractures or degeneration of the spine can also mask the early stage infection.[55] Treatment strategies are different; hence, imaging findings may help identify the causative pathogen (Table 2).

Septic arthritis of the facet joint is easily overlooked, so care must be taken because this can easily develop into an epidural abscess (Fig. 13).[50] It is important to detect fluid accumulation in the facet joint and contrast enhancement. An abnormal signal can also be seen around the joint. Other locations of infection including the spinous process, vertebral arch, and dental process have been reported.

Spondylitis may be caused by infection spreading from the adjacent structures; hence, patients undergoing complex neck, mediastinal, and retroperitoneal surgery, tracheal, esophageal and aortic stenting, transrectal prostate biopsy, and BCG intravesical infusion (Fig. 14) should be closely monitored.

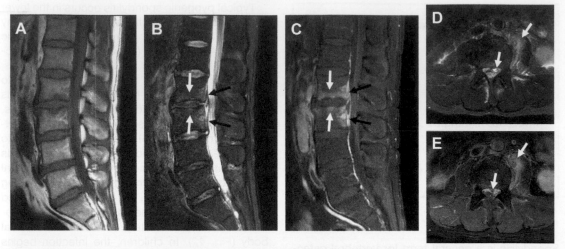

Fig. 10. Appearance of pyogenic spondylitis using different imaging techniques. T1-weighted image (*A*). Fat-suppressed T2-weighted image (*B, D*). Contrast-enhanced fat-suppressed T1-weighted image (*C, E*). The extent of the lesion can be determined on the fat-suppressed T2-weighted images. However, the contrast-enhanced fat-suppressed T1-weighted images are more revealing (*B–E: arrows*).

Tuberculous spondylitis

Compared with pyogenic spondylitis, tuberculous spondylitis has a longer course and less inflammatory response. Thoracolumbar spine is the most common site. The intervertebral discs tend to be preserved, whereas the vertebral bodies are destroyed. It tends to involve multiple vertebral bodies with skip lesions and often spreads to the posterior component. Abscesses may be formed that are larger than the extent of bone destruction (**Fig. 15**).[42] Calcification may also occur.

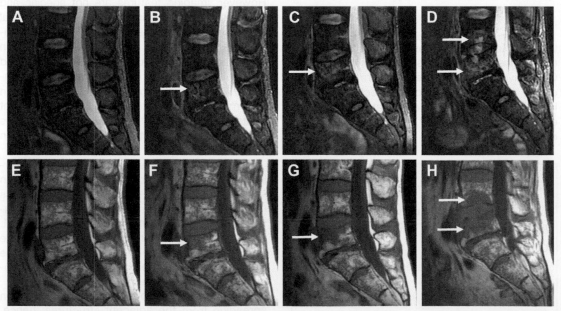

Fig. 11. The typical course of pyogenic spondylitis. The upper panel shows fat-suppressed T2-weighted sagittal images (*A–D*), and the lower panel shows T1-weighted sagittal images (*E–H*). There was no obvious abnormal signal on MR imaging 1 week before symptoms (*A, E*). At the onset of fever and back pain, there was an abnormal signal area limited to the anterior endplate of the L5 vertebra (*B, F: arrows*). Two weeks after onset, the abnormal signal area is enlarged (*C, G: arrows*). Five weeks after the onset, the abnormal signal area in the L5 vertebral body extended to the intervertebral disc and L4 vertebral body (*D, H: arrows*).

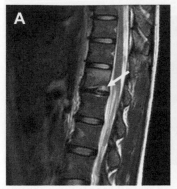 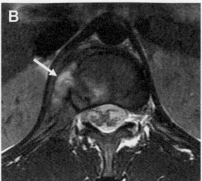 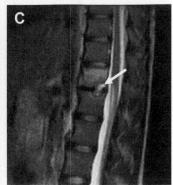

Fig. 12. Early formation of a paravertebral abscess following pyogenic spondylitis. On T2-weighted sagittal image, there is abnormal increased signal in the caudal endplate of the vertebral body, also involving the intervertebral disc (*A: arrow*). The adjacent vertebrae are normal but T2-weighted axial image shows abscess formation in the paravertebral body (*B, arrow*). Four weeks later, the lesion has spread to the adjacent vertebral body (*C: arrow*).

The anterior meningovertebral ligament anchors the posterior longitudinal ligament to the posterior surface of the vertebral body. When an epidural abscess forms, this ligament tends to be destroyed in pyogenic spondylitis but is preserved in tuberculous spondylitis.[56] Moreover, pyogenic spondylitis tends to exhibit osteoporotic changes.[57] In contrast, vertebral body destruction in tuberculous spondylitis is characterized by concave destruction of the vertebral body with clear boundaries (Fig. 16).

Brucella spondylitis

Brucella spondylitis is caused by oral ingestion of infected dairy products. Similar to tuberculosis, it can affect multiple vertebrae.[58,59,60] It differs from tuberculosis in that the lower lumbar vertebrae are the primary sites of involvement. The vertebral body height is typically maintained but the intervertebral discs tend to be destroyed (Fig. 17). Perivertebral abscesses are relatively rare.

Disseminated Nontuberculous Mycobacterium infection

Disseminated nontuberculous mycobacterium (NTM) presents with pulmonary, lymph node, bone, and soft tissue lesions, most often from acquired immunodeficiency due to anti-interferon-gamma (INFγ) antibodies (80%). Bone lesions may be seen as nonspecific abnormal bone signals and may not be accompanied by disc destruction or abscess formation.[61] In such cases, the differentiation of NTM from tumors or spondyloarthropathy becomes difficult.[62,63] Disseminated NTM in HIV rarely presents with bone and soft tissue involvement, which suggests a different pathogenesis of immunodeficiency. The sensitivity of biopsy for mycobacteriosis is limited, and a negative biopsy does not rule out mycobacteriosis.[64]

DIFFERENTIAL DIAGNOSIS OF SPONDYLITIS

Differential diagnoses of spondylitis are noted in Box 3.

Table 2
Differential diagnosis of pyogenic, tuberculous and brucella spondylitis

	Pyogenic	Tuberculous	Brucella
Clinical progression	Acute	Relatively slow	Relatively slow
Frequent location	Lower lumber	Lower thoracic	Lower lumber
Bone destruction	Relatively mild	Severe	Relatively maintained
Intervertebral space narrowing	Relatively severe	Relatively mild	Relatively severe
Posterior involvement	Relatively rare	Relatively common	Relatively rare
Multiple lesion	Relatively rare	Relatively common	Relatively common
Paraspinal abscess	Relatively common	Common	Rare

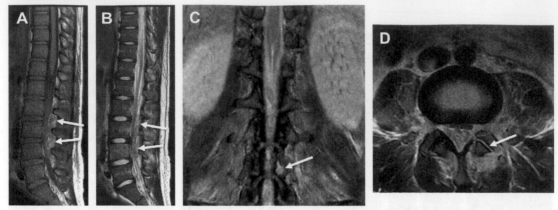

Fig. 13. Septic arthritis of the lumber facet joint. T1-weighted and T2-weighted sagittal images show abnormal dorsal extradural high signal compressing the filum terminale (*A, B*: *arrows*). T2-weighted coronal and axial images show abnormal high signal fluid accumulation in the left facet joint and abnormal signal in the surrounding muscle and epidural soft tissue (*C, D*: *arrows*).

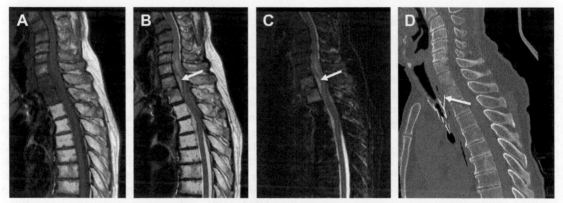

Fig. 14. Spondylitis after tracheal stent placement for lung cancer. T1-weighted, T2-weighted, and fat-suppressed T2-weighted sagittal images show abnormal signals in 2 of the vertebral bodies and an extensive epidural abscess (*A–C*). Computed tomography (CT) shows a partially disrupted tracheal stent impinging on the anterior vertebral body (*D*: *arrow*).

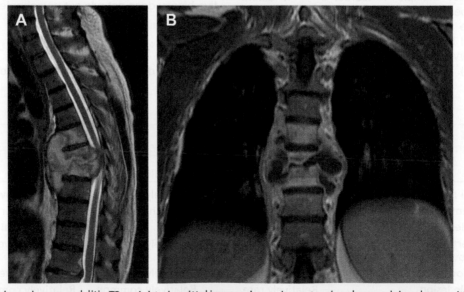

Fig. 15. Tuberculous spondylitis. T2-weighted sagittal images showed an extensive abnormal signal area with subligamentous extension over 3 vertebral bodies and wedge-shaped bone destruction (*A*). An abscess was formed in the intervertebral space to the epidural space and the anterior surface of the vertebral body. A contrast-enhanced T1-weighted image shows contrast enhancement in the vertebral body and abscess wall with nonenhancing cavity (*B*).

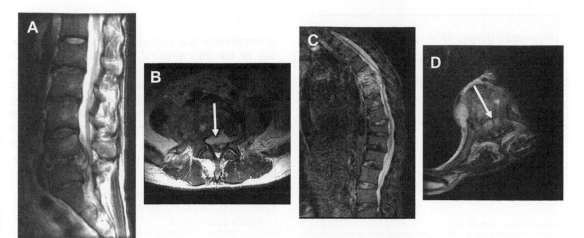

Fig. 16. Differentiating the diagnosis of pyogenic versus tuberculous spondylitis, based on the anterior meningo-vertebral ligament finding. Pyogenic spondylitis with epidural abscess (*A, B*). The anterior meningovertebral ligament is not detected (*B: arrow*). Tuberculous spondylitis with epidural abscess (*C, D*). The anterior meningovertebral ligament is preserved in tuberculous spondylitis (*D: arrow*).

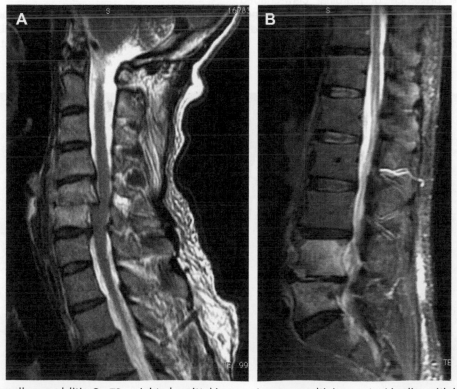

Fig. 17. Brucella spondylitis. On T2-weighted sagittal image, there are multiple vertebral bodies with high signal in the cervical and lumbar spine (*A, B*). The intervertebral discs are narrowed and destroyed but the vertebral bodies are relatively intact.

Box 3
Differential diagnosis of spondylitis

Modic type1 degeneration

Acute cartilage nodule (Schmorl nodule)

Ankylosing spondylitis

SAPHO syndrome

Neuropathic spine

Limbus vertebra

Metastases

Compression Fracture

Contrast enhancement of the vertebral body and perivertebral regions is not specific and can also be caused by compression fracture; hence, it should not be immediately taken for a sign of spondylitis.[65]

Modic Type 1 Endplate Change

Modic type I endplate change, an acute form of vertebral degeneration, can be difficult to differentiate from early stage of pyogenic spondylitis because of the overlapping preferred site and pain. The presence of marginal claw-shaped high-intensity signal on DWI in Modic type I endplate helps distinguish it from pyogenic spondylitis, in which the claw sign is absent (**Figs. 18** and **19**).[66,67]

Schmorl Node

Schmorl node is a herniation of the nucleus pulposus of the intervertebral disc into the vertebral body.[68] A weak signal on the T2-weighted image corresponding to sclerosis is often seen around the protruding nucleus pulposus, with surrounding bone marrow edema in the acute stage.[42] Corner dissection is a condition in which the anterior margin of the endplate is absent but it is thought to be caused by Schmorl node or a cleavage fracture in the same region.

Synovitis, Acne, Pustulosis, Hyperostosis Osteitis Syndrome

Synovitis, acne, pustulosis, hyperostosis osteitis (SAPHO) syndrome may present with multiple vertebral lesions.[69,70] Hyperostosis of the sternoclavicular joint is typical and should be sought. Palmoplantar pustulosis is a characteristic clinical manifestation of SAPHO syndrome. However, skin lesions, such as generalized pustulosis, have been reported in anti-INFγ autoantibody-positive disseminated nontuberculous mycobacteriosis and may require differentiation.[62]

Metastases

Metastases may mimic early stage of the spondylitis. Multiple vertebral involvement, absence of soft tissue extension or disc involvement, is typical for metastases.

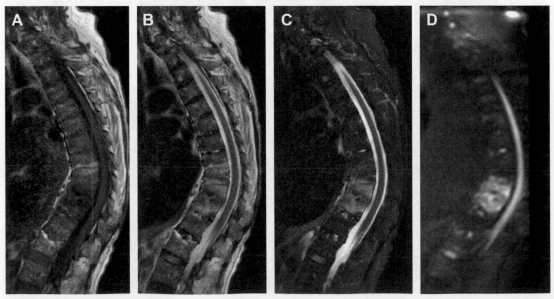

Fig. 18. DWIs to differentiate pyogenic spondylitis. T1, T2, and fat-suppressed T2-weighted sagittal images show abnormal signals over 2 adjacent vertebrae (*A–C*). DWI shows corresponding hyperintense signals over the vertebral body and the intervertebral disc in the middle, suggestive of pyogenic spondylitis (*D*).

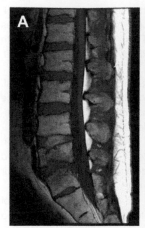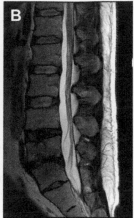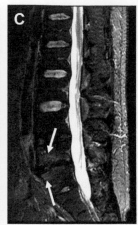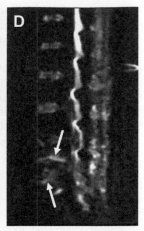

Fig. 19. DWIs to differentiate Modic type 1. T1, T2, and fat-suppressed T2-weighted sagittal image shows abnormal signal in 2 vertebral bodies from possible infection or Modic change (*A–C: arrows*). DWI shows a linear high-signal area in a distant region with inconspicuous signals near the endplate, positive for claw sign and suggestive of Modic type 1 (*D: arrows*).

SUMMARY

Spinal infections can affect the spinal cord, meninges and meningeal spaces, bony vertebrae, and neighboring soft tissue. Spinal infections are of critical importance, and early detection and diagnosis are paramount because infection is an emergency and often can be treated. Imaging is essential to optimize treatment and ultimately improve patient care and prevent mortality.

This article describes spinal infections and lists differential diagnoses according to anatomic structures from the cord to the bone. There are many atypical presentations and mimics for infection. It is necessary to identify the site where the abnormal findings are present and to list the differential diagnoses. To arrive at a correct diagnosis, radiologists must unify clinical and anatomic imaging features and prepare proper differential diagnoses, and be familiar with variations in clinical and imaging findings.

CLINICS CARE POINTS

- Radiologists must aggregate clinical, laboratory, and follow-up information in order to interpret images in patients suspected of spinal infections.

- It is necessary to customize the MR imaging sequences and acquisition direction according to the site of abnormal findings.

- Where the lesions are located and the site of greatest destruction are key to differentiating spinal infections from mimics.

DISCLOSURE

The authors have nothing to disclose.

REFERENCES

1. Duarte Rui M, Vaccaro Alexander R. Spinal infection: state of the art and management algorithm. Eur Spine J 2013;22(12):2787 99.
2. DeWitt Sarah, Chavez Summer A, Perkins Jack, et al. Evaluation of fever in the emergency department. Am J Emerg Med 2017;35(11):1755–8.
3. Long Brit, Liang Stephen Y. Koyfman Alex, et al. Tuberculosis: a focused review for the emergency medicine clinician. Am J Emerg Med 2020;38(5):1014–22.
4. Yokota Hajime, Yamada Kei. Viral infection of the spinal cord and roots. Neuroimaging Clin N Am 2015;25(2):247–58.
5. Irani David N. Aseptic meningitis and viral myelitis. Neurol Clin 2008;26(3):635–55, vii–viii.
6. Archana Asundi, Cervantes-Arslanian Anna M, Lin Nina H, et al. Infect Myelitis. Semin Neurol 2019;39(4):472–81.
7. Balériaux Danielle L, Carine N. Spinal and spinal cord infection. Eur Radiol 2004;14(Suppl 3):E72–83.
8. DeVries Aaron S, Harper Jane, Murray Andrew, et al. Vaccine-derived poliomyelitis 12 years after infection in Minnesota. N Engl J Med 2011;364(24):2316–23.
9. Shen WC, Chiu HH, Chow KC, et al. MR imaging findings of enteroviral encephalomyelitis: an outbreak in Taiwan. AJNR Am J Neuroradiol 1999;20(10):1889–95.
10. Murphy Olwen C, Kevin Messacar, Leslie Benson, et al. Acute flaccid myelitis: cause, diagnosis, and management. Lancet 2021;397(10271):334–46.

11. Boyer F-C, Tiffreau V, Rapin A, et al. Post-polio syndrome: Pathophysiological hypotheses, diagnosis criteria, drug therapy. Ann Phys Rehabil Med 2010; 53(1):34–41.

12. Devinsky O, Cho ES, Petito CK, et al. Herpes zoster myelitis. Brain 1991;114(Pt 3):1181–96.

13. Friedman DP. Herpes zoster myelitis: MR appearance. AJNR Am J Neuroradiol 1992;13(5):1404–6.

14. Thurnher MM, Post MJ, Jinkins JR. MRI of infections and neoplasms of the spine and spinal cord in 55 patients with AIDS. Neuroradiology 2000;42(8): 551–63.

15. Yoshio Shimojima, Masahide Yazaki, Kaneko Kazuma, et al. Characteristic spinal MRI findings of HIV-associated myelopathy in an AIDS patient. Intern Med 2005;44(7):763–4.

16. Remacha AF, Cadafalch J. Cobalamin deficiency in patients infected with the human immunodeficiency virus. Semin Hematol 1999;36(1):75–87.

17. Araujo Abelardo QC, Silva Marcus Tulius T. The HTLV-1 neurological complex. Lancet Neurol 2006; 5(12):1068–76.

18. Shakudo M, Inoue Y, Tsutada T. HTLV-I-associated myelopathy: acute progression and atypical MR findings. AJNR Am J Neuroradiol 1999;20(8):1417–21.

19. Fujio Umehara, Hirohisa Nose, Saito Mineki, et al. Abnormalities of spinal magnetic resonance images implicate clinical variability in human T-cell lymphotropic virus type I-associated myelopathy. J Neurovirol 2007;13(3):260–7.

20. Shila A, Govind N, Enose-Akahata Y, et al. Imaging spinal cord atrophy in progressive myelopathies: HTLV-I-associated neurological disease (HAM/TSP) and multiple sclerosis (MS). Ann Neurol 2017; 82(5):719–28.

21. Murphy KJ, Brunberg JA, Quint DJ, et al. Spinal cord infection: myelitis and abscess formation. AJNR Am J Neuroradiol 1998;19(2):341–8.

22. Simon Jakub K, Lazareff Jorge A, Diament Michael J, et al. Intramedullary abscess of the spinal cord in children: a case report and review of the literature. Pediatr Infect Dis J 2003;22(2):186–92.

23. Eun RJ, Seung Young L, Sang-Hoon C, et al. Sequential magnetic resonance imaging finding of intramedullary spinal cord abscess including diffusion weighted image: a case report. Korean J Radiol 2011;12(2):241–6.

24. Asaf Honig, Gomori John M, Ronen Schneider, et al. Spinal ischemic stroke following dialysis: clinical and radiologic findings. Neurology 2013;80(9):865–6.

25. Mizuno Junichi, Nakagawa Hiroshi, Inoue Tatsushi, et al. Clinicopathological study of "snake-eye appearance" in compressive myelopathy of the cervical spinal cord. J Neurosurg 2003;99(2 Suppl):162–8.

26. Liedholm LJ. Eeg-Olofsson O., Ekenberg B. E., et al. Acute postasthmatic amyotrophy (Hopkins' syndrome). Muscle Nerve 1994;17(7):769–72.

27. Dubey Divyanshu, Pittock Sean J, Krecke Karl N, et al. Clinical, radiologic, and prognostic features of myelitis associated with myelin oligodendrocyte glycoprotein autoantibody. JAMA Neurol 2019; 76(3):301–9.

28. Tadahiro Yonezu, Ito Shoichi, Mori Masahiro, et al. Bright spotty lesions" on spinal magnetic resonance imaging differentiate neuromyelitis optica from multiple sclerosis. Mult Scler 2014;20(3):331–7.

29. Ilniczky S, Jelencsik I, Kenéz J, et al. MR findings in subacute combined degeneration of the spinal cord caused by nitrous oxide anaesthesia–two cases. Eur J Neurol 2002;9(1):101–4.

30. Katsaros VK, Glocker FX, Hemmer B, et al. MRI of spinal cord and brain lesions in subacute combined degeneration. Neuroradiology 1998;40(11):716–9.

31. Pinnix Chelsea C, Chi Linda, Jabbour Elias J, et al. Dorsal column myelopathy after intrathecal chemotherapy for leukemia. Am J Hematol 2017;92(2): 155–60.

32. Kumar AJ, Köhler W, Kruse B, et al. MR findings in adult-onset adrenoleukodystrophy. AJNR Am J Neuroradiol 1995;16(6):1227–37.

33. Sharma Sushma, Aditya Murgai, Pankajakshan NP, et al. Teaching NeuroImages: snake eyes appearance in MRI in patient with ALS. Neurology 2013;81(5):e29.

34. Madhavan AA, Carr CM, Morris PP, et al. Imaging Review of Paraneoplastic Neurologic Syndromes. AJNR Am J Neuroradiol 2020;41(12):2176–87.

35. Samira Rabhi, Mustapha Maaroufi, Hajar Khibri, et al. Magnetic resonance imaging findings within the posterior and lateral columns of the spinal cord extended from the medulla oblongata to the thoracic spine in a woman with subacute combined degeneration without hematologic disorders: a case report and review of the literature. J Med Case Rep 2011;5:166.

36. Verdier Exequiel Patricio, Omar Konsol, Santiago Portillo. Intramedullary cervical abscess mimicking a spinal cord tumor in a 10-year-old girl: a case-based review. Childs Nerv Syst 2018; 34(11):2143–7.

37. Garg RK, Malhotra HS, Gupta R. Spinal cord involvement in tuberculous meningitis. Spinal Cord 2015;53(9):649–57.

38. Ross JS, Masaryk TJ, Modic MT, et al. MR imaging of lumbar arachnoiditis. AJR Am J Roentgenol 1987;149(5):1025–32.

39. Hiroki Morisako, Toshihiro Takami, Yamagata Toru, et al. Focal adhesive arachnoiditis of the spinal cord: Imaging diagnosis and surgical resolution. J Craniovertebr Junction Spine 2010;1(2):100–6.

40. Darouiche RO, Hamill RJ, Greenberg SB, et al. Bacterial spinal epidural abscess. Review of 43 cases and literature survey. Medicine 1992;71(6):369–85.

41. Deardre Chao, Nanda Anil. Spinal epidural abscess: a diagnostic challenge. Am Fam Physician 2002; 65(7):1341–6.

42. Olga Laur, Mandell Jacob C, Titelbaum David S, et al. Acute Nontraumatic Back Pain: Infections and Mimics. Radiographics 2019;39(1):287–8.

43. Meyers SP, Wildenhain SL, Chang JK, et al. Postoperative evaluation for disseminated medulloblastoma involving the spine: contrast-enhanced MR findings, CSF cytologic analysis, timing of disease occurrence, and patient outcomes. AJNR Am J Neuroradiol 2000;21(9):1757–65.

44. McKinney AM, Chacko Achanaril A, Knoll B, et al. Pseudo-Leptomeningeal Contrast Enhancement at 3T in Pediatric Patients Sedated by Propofol. AJNR Am J Neuroradiol 2018;39(9):1739–44.

45. Roger Chou, Fu Rongwei, Carrino John A, et al. Imaging strategies for low-back pain: systematic review and meta-analysis. Lancet 2009;373(9662): 463–72.

46. Tan Alai, Zhou Jie, Kuo Yong-Fang, et al. Variation among Primary Care Physicians in the Use of Imaging for Older Patients with Acute Low Back Pain. J Gen Intern Med 2016;31(2):156–63.

47. Modic MT, Feiglin DH, Piraino DW, et al. Vertebral osteomyelitis: assessment using MR. Radiology 1985;157(1):157–66.

48. Torda AJ, Gottlieb T, Bradbury R. Pyogenic vertebral osteomyelitis: analysis of 20 cases and review. Clin Infect Dis 1995;20(2):320–8.

49. Unkila-Kallio L, Kallio MJ, Eskola J, et al. Serum C-reactive protein, erythrocyte sedimentation rate, and white blood cell count in acute hematogenous osteomyelitis of children. Pediatrics 1994;93(1):59–62.

50. Turgut Tali E, Yusuf Oner A, Murat Koc A. Pyogenic spinal infections. Neuroimaging Clin N Am 2015; 25(2):193–208.

51. Buoncristiani AM, McCullen G, Shin AY, et al. An unusual cause of low back pain. Osteomyelitis of the spinous process. Spine 1998;23(7):839–41.

52. Satoshi Ujigo, Kazuhiko Kishi, Hideaki Imada, et al. Upper Cervical Osteomyelitis with Odontoid Process Destruction Treated with a Halo Vest in a Child: A Case Report. Spine Surg Relat Res 2020;4(3): 287–9.

53. Sans N, Faruch M, Lapègue F, et al. Infections of the spinal column–spondylodiscitis. Diagn Interv Imaging 2012;93(6):520–9.

54. Boutin Robert D, White Lawrence M, Tal Laor, et al. MRI findings of serous atrophy of bone marrow and associated complications. Eur Radiol 2015; 25(9):2771–8.

55. Nakamura Daisuke, Kondo Ryoichi, Akiko Makiuchi, et al. Empyema and pyogenic spondylitis caused by direct Streptococcus gordonii infection after a compression fracture: a case report. Surg Case Rep 2019;5(1):52.

56. Strauss SB, Gordon SR, Burns J, et al. Differentiation between Tuberculous and Pyogenic Spondylodiscitis: The Role of the Anterior Meningovertebral Ligament in Patients with Anterior Epidural Abscess. AJNR Am J Neuroradiol 2020;41(2):364–8.

57. Liu Xiaoyang, Zheng Meimei, Sun Jianmin, et al. A diagnostic model for differentiating tuberculous spondylitis from pyogenic spondylitis on computed tomography images. Eur Radiol 2021;31(10):7626–36.

58. Aysin P, Mir Ali P, Lutfu S, et al. Epidemiologic, clinical, and imaging findings in brucellosis patients with osteoarticular involvement. AJR Am J Roentgenol 2006;187(4):873–80.

59. Turgut Tali E, Murat Koc A, Yusuf Oner A. Spinal brucellosis. Neuroimaging Clin N Am 2015;25(2):233–45.

60. Solera J, Lozano E, Martínez-Alfaro E, et al. Brucellar spondylitis: review of 35 cases and literature survey. Clin Infect Dis 1999;29(6):1440–9.

61. Suzuki Tetsuya, Murai Hajime, Naohisa Miyakoshi, et al. Osteomyelitis of the spine caused by mycobacterium avium complex in an immunocompetent patient. J Orthop Sci 2013;18(3):490–5.

62. Ogawa Youichi, Ryo Hasebe, Takehiro Ohnuma, et al. Acute generalized exanthematous pustulosis associated with anti-interferon-γ neutralizing autoantibody-positive disseminated nontuberculous mycobacterial infection. Eur J Dermatol 2019;29(3):339–41.

63. Panuwat Wongkulab, Jiraprapa Wipasa, Romanee Chaiwarith, et al. Autoantibody to interferon-gamma associated with adult-onset immunodeficiency in non-HIV individuals in Northern Thailand. PLoS One 2013;8(9):e76371.

64. Colmenero Juan D, Ruiz-Mesa Juan D, Sanjuan-Jimenez Rocío, et al. Establishing the diagnosis of tuberculous vertebral osteomyelitis. Eur Spine J 2013;22(Suppl 4):579–86.

65. Choong-Hyo Kim, Hyo PJ, Chung Sang Ki, et al. Enhancing box sign : enhancement pattern of acute osteoprotic compression fracture. J Korean Neurosurg Soc 2009;46(6):528–31.

66. Patel KB, Poplawski MM, Pawha PS, et al. Diffusion-weighted MRI "claw sign" improves differentiation of infectious from degenerative modic type 1 signal changes of the spine. AJNR Am J Neuroradiol 2014;35(8):1647–52.

67. Mohammad Hossein D, Masoud P, Mohsen S, et al. Diffusion-weighted magnetic resonance imaging in differentiating acute infectious spondylitis from degenerative Modic type 1 change; the role of b-value, apparent diffusion coefficient, claw sign and amorphous increased signal. Br J Radiol 2016;89(1066):20150152.

68. Diehn Felix E, Maus Timothy P, Morris Jonathan M, et al. Uncommon Manifestations of Intervertebral Disk Pathologic Conditions. Radiographics 2016;36(3):801–23.

69. Jean-Denis L, Vuillemin-Bodaghi V, Boutry N, et al. SAPHO syndrome: MR appearance of vertebral involvement. Radiology 2007;242(3):825–31.

70. Cotten A, Flipo RM, Mentre A, et al. SAPHO syndrome. Radiographics 1995;15(5):1147–54.

Imaging of Head and Neck Infections

Joel M. Stein, MD, PhD[a],*, Junfang Xian, MD, PhD[b]

KEYWORDS

- Head and neck • Infection • Computed tomography • MR imaging • Deep spaces • Abscess
- Complications

KEY POINTS

- Imaging helps in determining the location and extent of head and neck infections, guiding abscess drainage and other interventions, and identifying important complications.
- CT is the primary imaging modality and MR imaging and ultrasound play complementary roles.
- Fat infiltration, bone erosion and diffusion restriction can be subtle signs of serious infection.
- Risk factors including immunocompromise and diabetes warrant particular attention.

IMAGING HEAD AND NECK INFECTIONS

Dating from 1760 to 1936, various eponyms associated with head and neck infections (Table 1) underscore their historical prevalence and seriousness. Although complications are much reduced with modern antibiotic use, head and neck infections remain common and imaging plays a crucial role in their management. Typical signs and symptoms often make infection apparent clinically[1] but head and neck anatomy is complex and filled with deep spaces and important structures that escape physical and visual examination (even via the otoscope, ophthalmoscope, or endoscope). Furthermore, the skin, eyes, ears, and aerodigestive tract provide multiple entry points for microorganisms. Infection can spread between spaces across fascial planes, and valveless veins and skull base foramina provide access routes to the intracranial compartment.

Thus, radiologic imaging with computed tomography (CT), ultrasound, and MR imaging becomes essential for (1) defining the location and extent of infection, (2) identifying abscesses, and (3) uncovering important complications.[1] After a few words on each modality, this review considers infections and complications by location (Table 2). Common infectious mechanisms across locations include (1) disrupted normal drainage pathways (by anatomic variation, preceding viral illness or other inflammation, stone formation, impaired clearance) and (2) underlying conditions (diabetes, immunocompromise, indwelling devices, intravenous drug use) facilitating overgrowth and spread of microorganisms.

IMAGING MODALITIES

Contrast-enhanced CT is the primary modality for imaging head and neck infection.[1] Advantages include wide availability, efficient cross-sectional coverage, rapid scans limiting motion from eye movements and swallowing, and high spatial resolution enabling multiplanar reformats. CT excels for soft tissues (including lymph nodes and vasculature) as well as osseous structures (especially maxillofacial and temporal bones), stones, calcifications, and dense foreign bodies. Both soft tissue and bone kernel reconstructions should be used and careful window leveling may be needed. Disadvantages include radiation exposure, metal artifact from dental amalgam or surgical hardware, and potential allergic reactions or renal toxicity with iodinated contrast.

[a] Department of Radiology, Hospital of the University of Pennsylvania, 1 Silverstein Pavilion, 3400 Spruce Street, Philadelphia, PA 19104, USA; [b] Department of Radiology, Capital Medical University, Beijing 100730, China
* Corresponding author.
E-mail address: Joel.Stein@pennmedicine.upenn.edu

Neuroimag Clin N Am 33 (2023) 185–206
https://doi.org/10.1016/j.nic.2022.07.016
1052-5149/23/© 2022 Elsevier Inc. All rights reserved.

neuroimaging.theclinics.com

Table 1
Eponyms in head and neck infections

Named Syndrome	Description	Primary Location	Typical Source	Complication
Bezold abscess	Osteomyelitis with muscle abscess	Sternocleidomastoid	Otomastoiditis	Deep neck or infratemporal infection, jugular vein thrombosis
Cetilli abscess	Same as above	Posterior belly of digastric	Same as above	Same as above
Gradenigo syndrome	Triad of (1) ear pain from otitis media and (2) VI nerve palsy and (3) V2/V3 nerve pain from petrous apicitis	Petrous apex	Chronic suppurative otitis media	Skull base osteomyelitis, intracranial or prevertebral abscess, meningitis
Pott puffy tumor	Osteomyelitis with subperiosteal abscess	Frontal scalp	Sinusitis	Intracranial infection
Ludwig angina	Rapidly progressive cellulitis	Floor of mouth	Dental infection	Airway compromise
Lemierre syndrome	Septic thrombophlebitis	Internal jugular vein	Pharyngitis/ tonsillitis	Pulmonary and other septic emboli
Grisel syndrome	Nontraumatic C1-2 subluxation	Cervical spine	Head and neck infection or surgery	Torticollis, pain, cervicomedullary compression

Ultrasound requires more time and local expertise but boasts similar wide availability, permits targeted dynamic examinations, facilitates biopsy and drainage, avoids ionizing radiation, and lends itself to pediatric imaging. Ultrasound readily visualizes lymph nodes, glands, superficial collections, gas, hyperemia, and calcifications, and superbly characterizes vessels and thrombosis. Cross-sectional imaging is preferred for deeper structures, surgical planning, and determining disease extent.[1]

MR imaging is less widely available, requires more expertise and longer scan times, suffers more from motion, and may not be feasible for patients with claustrophobia, agitation or implanted devices. However, MR imaging offers superior soft tissue contrast resolution and lesion characterization using multiple pulse sequences. MR imaging best assesses intracranial and spinal disease. Air-bone interfaces cause MR imaging artifact and bony margins are easier to assess on CT but MR imaging best demonstrates marrow abnormalities. Diffusion-weighted imaging (DWI) is particularly useful for abscesses.

Plain radiographs play a limited role for head and neck infections. Neck radiographs can identify epiglottitis, retropharyngeal swelling, glottitis, or swallowed radiodense foreign bodies. Dental radiographs provide detailed views of odontogenic disease in dental practice. Nuclear medicine techniques may sometimes be used for assessing osteomyelitis or response to treatment.[1]

CERVICAL LYMPH NODE INFECTIONS

Cervical adenitis (or lymphadenitis) describes inflamed infected lymph nodes. In uncomplicated cases, enlarged nodes measure greater than 1 cm but maintain normal architecture with fatty hila (hyperechoic on ultrasound and fat density on CT).[2] Complicated adenitis denotes suppuration (central liquefactive necrosis) with a loss of normal architecture and hila (anechoic/hypoechoic and avascular on ultrasound, low density on CT), often with surrounding fat inflammation or potentially rupture causing abscess.[2] Acute adenitis typically affects children, particularly due to viral upper respiratory infections (URIs) or streptococcal pharyngitis with bilateral involvement.[3] Streptococcus pyogenes and Staphylococcus aureus are the most common causes of acute unilateral disease and suppuration.[3] Subacute or chronic adenitis

Table 2
Head and neck infections organized by anatomic region

Spaces	Contents	Important Infections	Draining Lymph Nodes	Typical Sites of Secondary Spread
Temporal bone	Auditory canals, middle and inner ear, mastoid, petrous apex	Necrotizing otitis externa Otitis media Mastoiditis Petrous apicitis	Periparotid, II	Infratemporal, skull base, intracranial
Orbits	Globes, extraocular muscles, optic nerves, vessels, lacrimal ducts	Preseptal cellulitis Orbital abscess Dacrocystitis		Intracranial
Sinonasal	Paranasal sinuses	Acute and chronic bacterial sinusitis Noninvasive and invasive acute or chronic fungal sinusitis		Orbits Intracranial Periantral Scalp
Parotid	Parotid glands, lymph nodes	Parotiditis Parotid abscess	Periparotid	
Submandibular	Submandibular glands, lymph nodes	Sialadenitis	IB	
Oral cavity	Teeth, tongue, sublingual glands	Odontogenic abscess	IA, IB	Buccal, masticator, sublingual, submandibular, parapharyngeal, retropharyngeal
Pharyngeal	Tonsils	Pharyngitis Tonsilitis	II	Parapharyngeal, retropharyngeal
Parapharyngeal	Carotid sheath	Peritonsilar abscess	II	Retropharyngeal
Retropharyngeal	Retropharygneal nodes	Suppurative adenitis Retropharyngeal abscess Descending necrotizing mediastinitis	Retropharygneal	Mediastinum, prevertebral, carotid, pharyngeal
Anterior visceral	Larynx	Epiglottitis Laryngotracheobronchitis		Mediastinum, parapharyngeal

causes include *Bartonella henselae* (cat-scratch disease) and nontuberculosis mycobacteria.[3] *Tuberculous cervical lymphadenitis* (scrofula) occurs in endemic areas and immunocompromised patients with symptoms including malaise, weight loss, and nontender neck swelling.[1] Imaging features include enlarged nodes with caseation (central low density), matting (conglomerate nodes moving as a group), absent surrounding inflammation, and multiple involved sites (**Fig. 1**).[1] Adenitis can be mistaken for lymphoma or metastatic disease; clinical features, additional cross-sectional imaging, or fine needle aspiration can differentiate.[2]

TEMPORAL BONE INFECTIONS

Benign otitis externa (swimmer's ear) arises when moisture or other factors facilitate bacterial overgrowth, most commonly of *Pseudomonas aeruginosa*, or *Staphylococcus*.[4] Fungal disease caused by *Aspergillus* or *Candida* also occurs, particularly with hearing aids or altered normal flora after antibiotics.[5] Symptoms include ear pain, swelling, drainage, and pruritus. Treatment includes antibiotics or antifungals and imaging is unnecessary.

However, typically elderly diabetic or immunocompromised patients can develop *necrotizing*

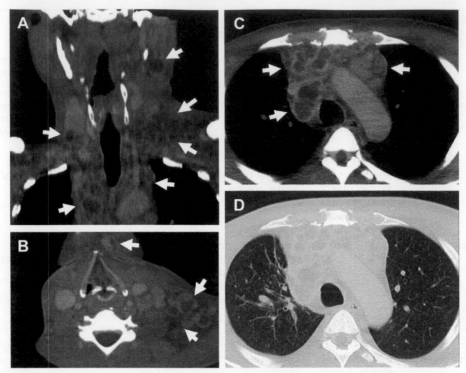

Fig. 1. Tuberculosis lymphadenitis. Coronal (*A*) and axial (*B, C*) enhanced neck CT images in a patient with newly diagnosed HIV and active tuberculosis show enlarged necrotic cervical and mediastinal lymph nodes (*arrows*). Lung window image (*D*) shows miliary nodules.

otitis externa (NOE, Fig. 2) with rapid spread of infection, almost always due to *Pseudomonas*. Otoscopy may reveal ulceration with uncovered bone along the external auditory canal (EAC).[6] Treatment includes IV antibiotics, surgical debridement, and glucose control. CT may show periauricular fat infiltration, EAC soft tissue thickening, abscess, bone erosion, or deeper neck or skull base involvement. MR imaging helps identify soft tissue infiltration, purulent collections on DWI, marrow signal abnormality, and intracranial complications including sinus thrombosis. Gaps along the cartilaginous canal (fissures of Santorini) or osseous canal (foramen of Huschke) can facilitate spread.[6,7] Masticator space[6] or retrocondylar fat pad[7] infiltration may be the only imaging features; ear pain in susceptible patients demands increased scrutiny.

NOE can be classified by direction of spread and involved structures (Table 3).[7] Medial spread is the most common cause of *skull base osteomyelitis* (SBO, Fig. 3), termed typical SBO.[8] In addition to lateral temporal bone findings, look for petrous, petroclival, or occipital bone involvement. Look for abnormal enhancing tissue in the infratemporal fossa and preclival/prevertebral region, which can mimic infiltrating neoplasm, particularly

nasopharyngeal carcinoma.[8] Atypical SBO affects the central skull base (basisphenoid and basiocciput) without preceding otologic infection. It may arise from sinusitis, deep face infections or without known local infection and more often involves bacteria other than *Pseudomonas* as well as fungus and nontuberculous mycobacteria.[8]

Otitis media (middle ear infection) occurs when Eustachian tube (ET) dysfunction permits fluid accumulation and bacterial overgrowth. This is more common in children due to shorter and more horizontal ETs and frequent URIs.[9,10] Bacteria causing *acute otitis media* (AOM) include *Streptococcus pneumoniae*, *Haemophilus influenzae*, and *Moraxella catarrhalis*.[11] AOM is the most common indication for childhood doctor visits and antibiotics in the United States, although overall incidence and pneumococcal cases have decreased with vaccination.[12] Symptoms include otalgia, otorrhea, hearing loss, fever, and headache. Otoscopic findings include a fluid-filled middle ear and bulging, thickened or ruptured tympanic membrane (TM). Adult AOM can occur from ET, immune, or ciliary dysfunction but serous effusions are more typical. *Chronic otitis media* (COM) describes TM perforation from chronic/recurrent infections, with or without serous or

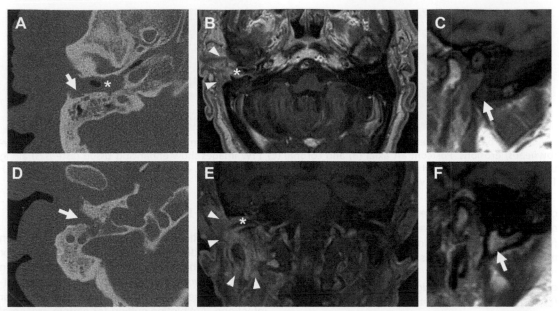

Fig. 2. Necrotizing otitis externa. Temporal bone CT images (*A, D*) show external auditory canal opacification (*asterisk*) and mastoid erosions (*arrows*). Axial (*B*) and coronal (*E*) T1W Images show enhancement (*arrowheads*) in periauricular tissues and around purulent material in the external auditory canal (*asterisk*). Sagittal T1W images show decreased signal in the right mastoid tip (*arrow* in *C*) compared with the normal left side (*arrow* in *F*).

purulent fluid. COM can cause conductive hearing loss by *tympanosclerosis* (calcification of the TM, ossicles, or ligaments) or ossicular erosion, with or without cholesteatoma formation.

Cholesteatomas (mass-like desquamated epithelium) cause conductive hearing loss by middle ear mass effect or erosion. Some are congenital, but most are acquired,[13] either from ingrown EAC epithelium in TM retraction pockets (primary acquired) or introduced by perforation (secondary acquired). Bacterial or fungal superinfection promotes bone erosion but antibiotics penetrate poorly,[14] necessitating surgery. CT shows soft tissue density, mass effect, and erosion (Fig. 4). MR imaging adds specificity, especially for recurrence

because cholesteatomas demonstrate abnormal diffusion restriction. *Labyrinthitis* (inner ear inflammation) can occur from cholestatomas, otomastoiditis, meningitis, toxins, trauma or autoimmune disease, and may cause *labyrinthitis ossificans* (Fig. 5), chronic bone deposition replacing normal fluid-filled inner ear structures. Symptoms include vertigo and profound sensorineural hearing loss.

Mastoid disease is the most common otitis media complication, often requiring mastoidectomy historically but rarely with modern prompt antibiotic treatment.[15] Benign mastoid effusions (technically mild mastoiditis) routinely accompany otitis media because these spaces communicate.[15] Effusions are common with intubation and after radiation therapy but check for nasopharyngeal carcinoma or lymphoma causing obstruction in patients with unexplained unilateral opacification. *Acute mastoiditis* (or otomastoiditis) describes symptomatic infection with postauricular pain, erythema, and swelling. Temporal bone CT is indicated to identify eroded bone around opacified air cells, signifying *coalescent mastoiditis* usually requiring intravenous antibiotics or surgery. Erosive disease can spread outward causing subperiosteal abscess (Fig. 6). Abscesses that form in the muscles attaching at the mastoid tip (Fig. 7), including the sternocleidomastoid (Bezold abscess) or posterior belly of the digastric (Citelli abscess), are difficult to palpate and can spread to

Table 3
Patterns of spread of necrotizing otitis externa

Pattern	Involved Structures
Anterior	Temporomandibular joint, masticator space, parotid gland, surrounding fat planes
Medial	Petrous segment, sphenoid, clivus, nasopharynx, cranial nerves IX–XI
Posterior	Mastoid process
Intracranial	Dura, sigmoid sinus, jugular vein

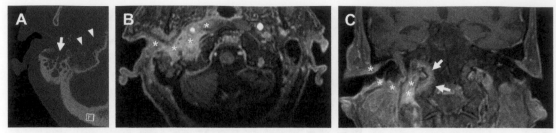

Fig. 3. Skull base osteomyelitis. Axial temporal bone CT (*A*) shows right mastoid (*arrow*) and occipital bone (*arrowheads*) erosions. Postcontrast axial (*B*) and coronal (*C*) T1W images show enhancing tissue (*asterisks*) along these sites and the carotid and prevertebral spaces, and abnormal right occipital bone enhancement (*arrows*). The right internal jugular vein was occluded.

deeper neck spaces. Medial spread into a pneumatized petrous apex can cause *petrous apicitis* (with air cell opacification, peripheral enhancement, erosion) and classic symptoms of Gradenigo syndrome (see Table 1). Intracranial complications include sigmoid sinus thrombosis (Fig. 8), meningitis, and abscess. *Chronic otomastoiditis* describes TM perforation and chronic fluid and inflammation (>4 months), typically causing mastoid sclerosis without erosion.

ORBITAL INFECTIONS

Orbital infections are common, particularly in younger children preceded by rhinosinusitis or URIs.[16,17] Other causes include trauma; foreign bodies; dacryocystitis; ophthalmic surgery or peribulbar anesthesia; and dental, facial, or middle ear infections. Antibiotics suffice for simple preseptal cellulitis and imaging is not required. However, cellulitis spreading behind the orbital septum is a

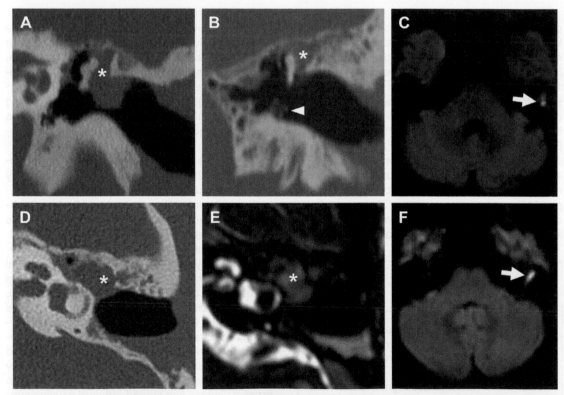

Fig. 4. Three cases of acquired cholesteatoma. Coronal temporal bone CT (*A*) shows soft tissue density pars flaccida type cholesteatoma blunting the scutum, expanding Prussak space (*asterisk*), and eroding the incus. A second case (*B*) shows a myringotomy tube (*arrowhead*) and an epitympanum cholesteatoma (*asterisk*) confirmed by MR imaging (*C*) with diffusion restriction (*arrow*). A third case after mastoidectomy shows density on CT (*D*) and heterogenous signal on T2W MR imaging (*E*) in the epitympanum (*asterisk*), a portion of which showed diffusion restriction (*arrow* in *F*).

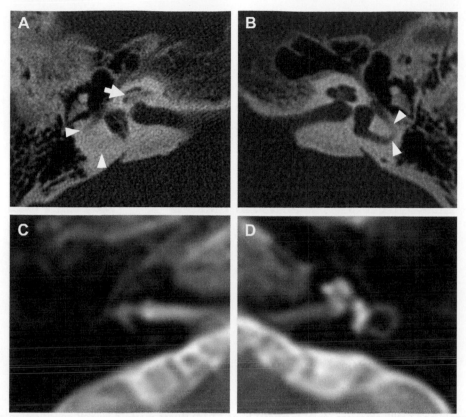

Fig. 5. Labyrinthitis ossificans following meningitis. Axial CT of the right (*A*) and left (*B*) temporal bones shows mineralization filling in the right more than left semicircular canals (*arrowheads*) and portions of the right cochlea (*arrow*). T2W MR imaging (*C, D*) shows corresponding lack of fluid signal in the right semicircular canals and cochlea.

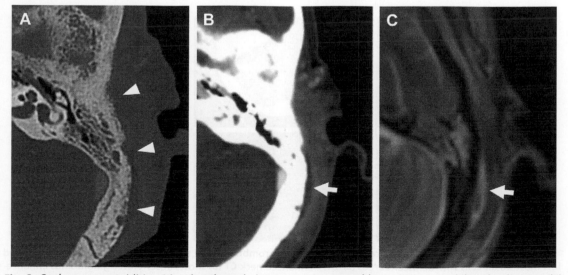

Fig. 6. Coalescent mastoiditis with subperiosteal abscess. Axial temporal bone CT in bone (*A*) and soft tissue (*B*) kernels and T2W MR imaging (*C*) show mastoid air cell opacification with cortical erosions (*arrowheads*), overlying abscess (*arrows*), and periauricular swelling.

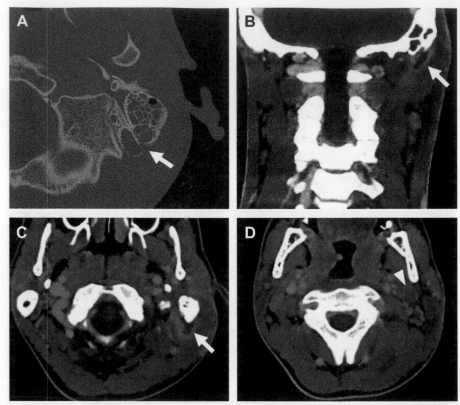

Fig. 7. Bezold and Cetilli abscesses. Axial temporal bone CT (*A*) shows mastoid air cell opacification and dehiscence (*arrow*). Coronal (*B*) and axial (*C, D*) enhanced neck CT images show an overlying abscess at the sternocleidomastoid insertion (*arrows*) and another inferiorly in the posterior belly of the digastric (*arrowhead*).

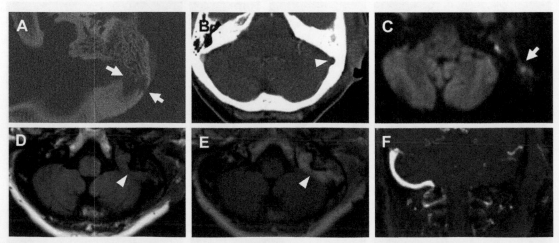

Fig. 8. Coalescent mastoiditis complicated by dural sinus thrombosis. Axial temporal bone CT (*A*) shows opacified left mastoid air cells with dehiscent areas (*arrow*). Enhanced neck CT (*B*) shows absent left sigmoid sinus enhancement (*arrowhead*) and retroauricular swelling. An underlying collection and tract extending to the skin (*arrow*) are more evident on DWI (*C*). T1W precontrast (*D*) and postcontrast (*E*) images show left sigmoid sinus enhancing clot (*arrowheads*) with a lack of flow-related enhancement on time-of-flight MR venogram (*F*).

sight-threatening and potentially life-threatening disease.[18] Focal neurologic findings, worsening symptoms, or lack of clinical improvement on antibiotics over 24 to 36 hours should prompt CT or MR imaging. Imaging detects disease extent, abscesses, intracranial complications, and sources of spread.[16,19] The modified Chandler classification stages orbital infection by location and severity (Table 4).[19,20]

Preseptal cellulitis (Chandler Group I) involves tissues anterior to the orbital septum, often due to *S aureus* or Group A *Streptococcus* and easily diagnosed by eyelid redness and swelling. Imaging to exclude higher stage disease may show periorbital fat stranding and edema. *Orbital/postseptal cellulitis* (Group II) involves tissues posterior to the septum and is more frequently associated with sinusitis, particularly ethmoiditis due to the thin lamina papyracea. Imaging demonstrates extraconal or rarely intraconal inflammation without abscess. When it occurs, abscess formation is often subperiosteal (Group III) or more rarely elsewhere in the extraconal space or in the intraconal space (Group IV). Distinguishing abscess from phlegmon is important for surgical drainage. Phlegmon describes localized enhancing inflammatory tissue, whereas abscess (Fig. 9) demonstrates peripheral enhancement around purulent fluid on CT with abnormal diffusion restriction on MR imaging.[1]

Cavernous sinus thrombosis (Group V) is a rare complication with current antibiotic therapy but critical to identify due to high morbidity and mortality. Dural venous sinuses lack valves and provide a conduit for spread of infection. Orbits protocol MR imaging scans provide the best assessment. The most useful sign is cavernous sinus expansion (see Fig. 9D) with a convex lateral margin[21] in patients with typical symptoms of ophthalmoplegia, decreased vision, chemosis, proptosis, and cranial nerve palsy. Secondary findings include superior ophthalmic vein engorgement or thrombosis,[22] extraocular muscle enlargement, and exophthalmos.

Dacryocystitis (lacrimal sac inflammation) results from lacrimal duct stenosis or obstruction, potentially congenital or acquired from surgery, trauma, or systemic diseases such as Wegener granulomatosis and sarcoidosis.[23] Clinical findings include tenderness, edema, erythema, and purulent discharge.[23] Imaging may be necessary to assess causes or complications including orbital cellulitis. CT or MR imaging will show a peripherally enhancing, circumscribed, low-density or intensity round lesion (Fig. 10) at the lacrimal fossa.[1] Antibiotics alone may be effective but many cases require surgical probing with nasolacrimal duct intubation or balloon dacryoplasty.

SINONASAL INFECTIONS

Sinusitis describes paranasal sinus mucosal inflammation, often *rhinosinusitis* with nasal cavity involvement. Symptoms include facial pain, nasal congestion, thick nasal or postnasal discharge, anosmia, halitosis, fever, and headache. Sinusitis may be viral, bacterial, or fungal, and acute (<4 weeks), subacute (4–12 weeks), or chronic (>12 weeks) in duration. Most acute cases are viral, self-limited, and not an indication for imaging or antibiotics. Symptoms that last 10 days without improvement, initially improve and subsequently worsen, or are particularly severe, suggest bacterial infection.[24] Fungal sinusitis generally manifests as chronic disease, but may be acute and progress rapidly in immunocompromised individuals.

Bacterial Sinusitis

Viral URIs often precede acute bacterial sinusitis. Sinus anatomic variants may predispose to sinus obstruction. Nasal or oral route tubes in hospitalized patients prevent proper clearance. Dental disease also contributes to maxillary sinusitis. Additional risk factors for chronic and recurrent sinusitis include cystic fibrosis with impaired clearance and allergies causing increased inflammation. Common organisms in community-acquired bacterial sinusitis include *S pneumoniae*, *H influenzae*, *M catarrhalis*, and *S pyogenes*.[25] *P aeruginosa* and other anaerobes are common in hospitalized, immunocompromised, or cystic fibrosis patients.[25]

Unenhanced CT superbly depicts sinonasal osseous anatomy and air spaces. Imaging is unnecessary for viral or uncomplicated bacterial sinusitis, and many asymptomatic individuals show incidental mucosal thickening. However, air-fluid levels (Fig. 11) suggest acute sinusitis in

Table 4		
Chandler classification and staging of orbital infection		
Group	**Involved Structures**	
I	Preseptal cellulitis	
II	Orbital cellulitis without abscess	
III	Subperiosteal abscess	
IV	Orbital abscess	
V	Cavernous sinus thrombosis	

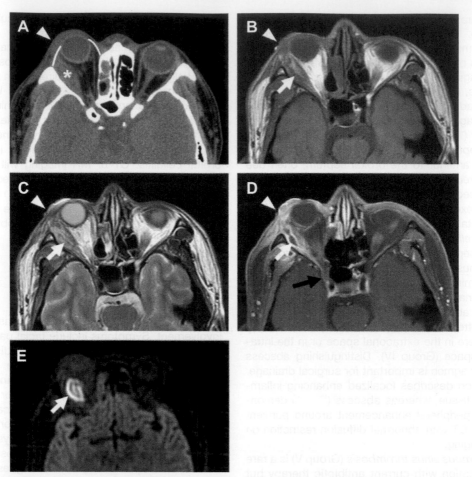

Fig. 9. Orbital cellulitis and subperiosteal abscess from rhinosinusitis. Unenhanced CT (*A*) shows periorbital swelling (*arrowhead*) anterior to the orbital septum (*white lines*) and postseptal swelling (*asterisk*) in the lateral orbit with proptosis. Corresponding T1W (*B*), T2W (*C*), postcontrast T1W (*D*), and DWI (*E*) images reveal right lateral preseptal cellulitis (*arrowheads*) and a heterogeneous subperiosteal postseptal abscess (*white arrows*), with rim enhancement and central diffusion restriction. Inflammation extends to the orbital apex. Right cavernous sinus expansion with convexity (*black arrow* in D) suggests thrombosis.

the absence of instrumentation, sinus lavage, or trauma.[26] The diagnosis is usually clinically evident but may be unexpected on scans obtained for headaches or other indications. Sinus fluid can demonstrate variable MR imaging signal intensity, most often T2-hyperintense and T1-hypointense, but becoming T2-hypointense at intermediate to higher protein concentration, and T1-hyperintense at intermediate and hypointense at higher concentrations.[27] Diffusion restricting sinus fluid suggests pyogenic bacterial sinusitis (see Fig. 11E–F).[28]

Chronic or recurrent bacterial sinusitis justifies imaging to exclude sinonasal masses and identify sites of obstruction, predisposing factors, and complications. Many otorhinolaryngology offices use low-dose cone beam CT to guide functional endoscopic surgery to improve or restore normal

drainage.[26] Chronic sinusitis CT findings include sinus mucosal thickening, variable opacification, and sclerotic wall thickening (neo-osteogenesis).[26] These features, however, overlap with those of allergic sinusitis, granulomatous inflammation, sinonasal polyposis, and prior trauma.[1]

Complications of extrasinus bacterial extension depend on the sinus involved.[1] Ethmoid disease may cause orbital infection. Sphenoid sinusitis complications tend to be intracranial, particularly cavernous sinus thrombosis. Frontal sinusitis spreading through the calvarium may cause extracranial or intracranial infection (Fig. 12). A tense subgaleal abscess in such cases is termed a "Pott puffy tumor."[29] Intracranial complications include meningitis and abscess. CT may show osseous deficiency or osteomyelitis and rim-enhancing collections. MR imaging is preferred for

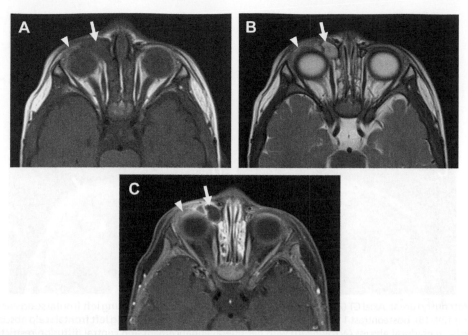

Fig. 10. Dacrocystitis. A 12-year-old boy with right-sided epiphora for 1 year, purulent for 20 days. T1W (A), T2W (B), and postcontrast T1W (C) images show eyelid edema and enhancement (arrowheads) and an enlarged circumscribed rim-enhancing lacrimal sac (arrows) centered at the lacrimal fossa. Antibiotics and drainage relieved his symptoms.

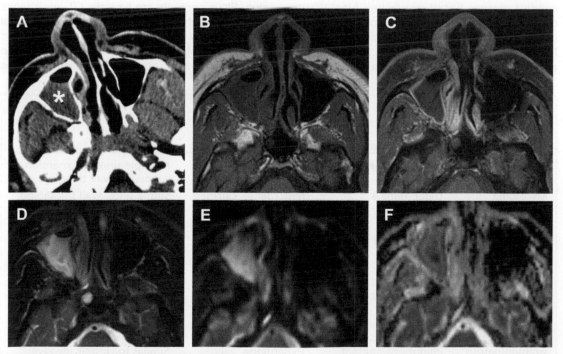

Fig. 11. Acute bacterial sinusitis. Axial unenhanced maxillofacial CT (A) shows a right maxillary sinus fluid level (asterisk). Unenhanced (B) and enhanced (C) T1W images show corresponding intermediate signal intensity fluid with peripheral mucosal enhancement. T2W (D), DWI (E), and ADC (F) images show hyperintense fluid with diffusion restriction, compatible with bacterial sinusitis.

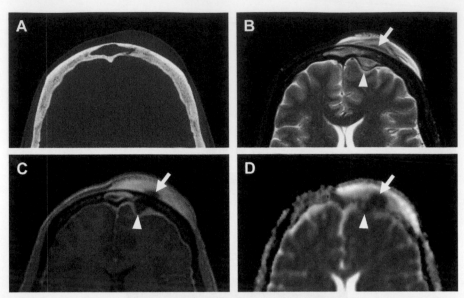

Fig. 12. Pott puffy tumor. Axial CT (*A*) shows frontal sinus opacification with overlying left frontal scalp swelling. Corresponding T2W (*B*), postcontrast T1W (*C*), and ADC map (*D*) images show overlying left frontal scalp abscess (*arrow*) and underlying epidural abscess (*arrowhead*) with peripheral enhancement and central diffusion restriction.

intracranial evaluation; look for diffusion restricting fluid and meningeal or brain enhancement.

Fungal Sinusitis

Fungal sinusitis is divided into noninvasive and invasive disease based on whether fungi remain confined to the sinus or extend into surrounding mucosa, submucosa, bone, or blood vessels.[30] Noninvasive subtypes are allergic fungal sinusitis and mycetoma. Invasive subtypes include acute,

chronic, and rare granulomatous sinusitis. Understanding their clinical and radiologic manifestations (Table 5) is important due to differing management and outcomes.[30]

Allergic fungal sinusitis is most common and usually shows multisinus opacification and expansion. Sinus contents are typically CT-hyperdense and T2-hypointense (sometimes mimicking normal aeration on MR imaging), due to paramagnetic metals, proteinaceous components, and decreased water content.[30] Clinical features

Table 5
Types of fungal sinusitis

Type	Typical Patient	Sinus Contents	Other Imaging Features
Allergic (noninvasive)	Younger, atopic	Hyperdense, T2 hypointense	Multiple sinuses, expansion, possible wall thinning
Mycetoma (noninvasive)	Older, female	Hyperdense, calcified, T2 hypointense	Single sinus, wall thickening, postobstructive opacification
Acute invasive	Immunocompromised, diabetic	Intermediate density	Bone destruction, erosion, mucosal necrosis, fat infiltration, orbital, or intracranial extension
Chronic invasive	Immunocompetent, diabetic	Hyperdense T2 hypointense	Bone destruction, sclerosis, fat infiltration, extrasinus extension may mimic tumor or orbital pseudotumor
Granulomatous invasive	Immunocompetent, rare, cases in Sudan, India, Pakistan, and the United States	Hyperdense T2 hypointense	Similar to chronic invasive

include chronic headaches and nasal congestion typically affecting younger patients. IgE-mediated allergic hypersensitivity to inhaled fungus drives the process in atopic individuals, who may also have allergic rhinitis and asthma. Treatment usually consists of surgical clearance and topical steroids to prevent recurrence.

Mycetomas (dense balls of fungal components, Fig. 13) arise due to insufficient mucocilliary clearance, leading to fungal colonization and chronic inflammation often in older individuals who may be asymptomatic. They typically involve a single sinus (usually maxillary or sphenoid) and often cause postobstructive opacification. Components are hyperdense on CT, frequently calcified, and hypointense on T2-weighted images.

Acute invasive fungal sinusitis (Fig. 14) is the most aggressive type, potentially progressing rapidly with poorly controlled diabetes (especially ketoacidosis) or immunocompromise from hematologic malignancies, transplants, chemotherapy or advanced AIDS. Clinical presentations can be dramatic with fever, facial pain, congestion, and epistaxis. Extrasinus spread can cause proptosis, vision loss, and other neurologic deficits but symptoms may be variable and unreliable. Persistent fever of unknown origin despite broad-spectrum antibiotics in immunocompromised patients should prompt sinus imaging. Common organisms include *Aspergillus* species in neutropenic patients, Mucoromycota species in diabetics, as well as *Bipolaris* and *Candida*.[30] During the COVID-19 pandemic, a surge in rhino-orbital-cerebral mucormycosis cases occurred in India,

probably exacerbated by high baseline rates, diabetes, and steroid therapy.[31] Unlike other types, acute fungal infection often lacks hyperdense CT components. Look for soft tissue density sinus opacification with subtle or extensive bone destruction. Lack of mucosal enhancement due to angioinvasion and necrosis is characteristic (see Fig. 14B). Fat stranding can be an early sign of extrasinus extension via vascular invasion, especially in orbital and periantral regions. Complications from direct extension or vascular invasion include cavernous sinus thrombosis, cavernous carotid mycotic pseudoaneurysm, orbital apex syndrome, optic nerve involvement, intracranial abscess, cerebritis, cerebral infarction or hemorrhage, and systemic dissemination. Effective therapy requires prompt recognition and aggressive surgical and medical management with debridement and systemic antifungal therapy usually with amphotericin B.

Chronic invasive fungal sinusitis (Fig. 15) also demonstrates extrasinus spread but over months to years in patients with normal or mildly suppressed immune function or diabetes. Often there are signs of chronic sinus inflammation with wall thickening and sclerosis. Mass-like components extending beyond the involved sinus may be mistaken for neoplasm. Orbital involvement can mimic idiopathic orbital inflammation (pseudotumor) and progress with steroids.[30] MR imaging again shows low signal intensity on T2-weighted images.

SALIVARY GLAND INFECTIONS

Sialadenitis (salivary gland inflammation) may be acute or chronic. In children, acute sialadenitis is typically viral, self-limited, and bilateral, most often affecting the parotid glands and due to paramyxovirus (mumps).[1,32] Adult acute sialadenitis typically arises from ascending bacteria (most commonly *S aureus*), usually associated with an obstructing calculus (sialolithiasis) and involving a single gland.[1,32,33] Submandibular glands are most often involved due to their propensity for ductal stone formation.[33] Classic symptoms are swelling and pain exacerbated by eating (salivary colic). Complications include abscess (suppurative sialadenitis), retromandibular or facial vein thrombosis, and rarely facial nerve dysfunction.[33] Treatment includes hydration, antibiotics, stone removal, and abscess drainage. Other acute causes include dehydration, immunosuppression, and certain medications including iodine administration. Chronic inflammatory sialadenitis causes include Sjogren syndrome, radiation therapy, and HIV.[34] Floor of mouth squamous cell carcinoma (SCC)

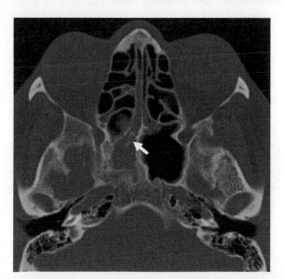

Fig. 13. Mycetoma. Axial bone kernel CT shows fungal calcification (*arrow*) at the right sphenoid sinus ostium with postobstructive opacification and sinus wall thickening indicating chronic inflammation.

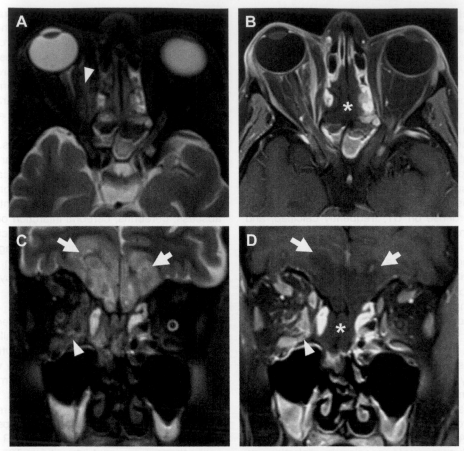

Fig. 14. Acute invasive fungal sinusitis. Lung transplant patient with headache, ophthalmoplegia, and right III–VI cranial nerve palsies. Nasal endoscopy with debridement showed necrotic mucosa with *Rhizopus* fungus. Axial and coronal fat-saturated T2W (*A, C*) and postcontrast T1W (*B, D*) images show material filling the superior nasal cavity and posterior ethmoid air cells with a notable lack of mucosal enhancement (*asterisks*) centrally indicating necrosis. Right orbital involvement results in edema and enhancement (*arrowheads*). There is intracranial extension with meningeal enhancement and brain invasion with inferior bifrontal cerebritis, hemorrhage, and infarction (*arrows*).

may cause sialadenitis by duct obstruction.[33] Ultrasound of acute sialadenitis shows enlarged, hyperechoic, and hyperemic glands. CT findings (Fig. 16) include gland enlargement, decreased density, indistinct margins, increased enhancement, and surrounding inflammation. Dilated ducts may be seen and salivary stones are most obvious on CT. Chronic inflammation may cause atrophy, fibrosis, or fatty replacement. Benign lymphoepithelial lesions (mixed cystic or solid parotid gland lesions) can be see with HIV or Sjogren syndrome.[35,36]

ORAL CAVITY INFECTIONS

Infections involving teeth (endodontal) and supporting structures (periodontal) are the most common adult head and neck infections.[37] Despite improved oral hygiene and water fluoridation

efforts, dental caries (cavities in teeth) and periodontal disease (lucencies around teeth) remain common worldwide and the major causes of tooth loss.[38] *Streptococcus viridans*, *Prevotella*, *Staphylococcus*, and *Peptostreptococcus* are common causative organisms.[39] Central pulp and root canal infections can decompress into apical bone, causing a periapical abscess.[37] Maxillary periapical infection can cause overlying odontogenic sinusitis. An oroantral fistula can develop where the site of a degenerated or extracted tooth communicates with the maxillary sinus.

BUCCAL, MASTICATOR, SUBLINGUAL, AND SUBMANDIBULAR SPACE INFECTIONS

Dental infection can also erode the lingual or buccal alveolar surface to cause a soft tissue odontogenic abscess (Fig. 17). On CT, look for

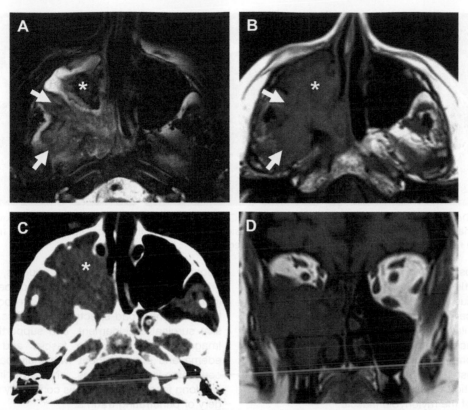

Fig. 15. Chronic invasive fungal sinusitis. Axial fat-saturated T2W (*A*), T1W (*B*), and CT (*C*) images show T2-hypointense dense fungal concretions (*asterisks*) opacifying the right maxillary sinus. There is posterior and medial sinus wall dehiscence with fungal components extending into the pterygomaxillary fissure and lateral pterygoid muscle (*arrows*). Coronal T1W image (*D*) shows additional inferior orbital involvement.

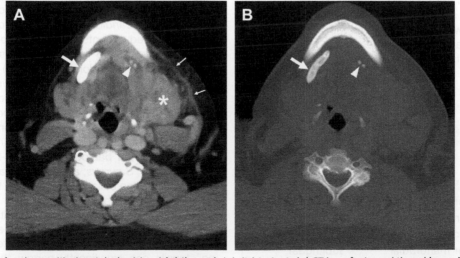

Fig. 16. Left submandibular sialadenitis with bilateral sialolithiasis. Axial CT in soft tissue (*A*) and bone kernels (*B*) shows an enlarged left submandibular gland (*asterisk*) with surrounding fat stranding and platysma thickening (*small arrows*). There is a large stone in the right submandibular duct (*arrow*) and multiple small stones (*arrowhead*) in the dilated left-sided duct.

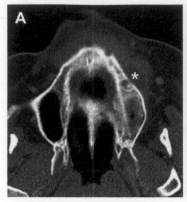
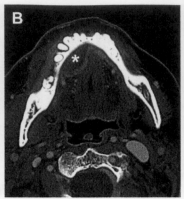
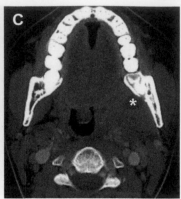

Fig. 17. Dental abscesses. Axial bone kernel-enhanced CT images show abscess formation (*asterisks*) overlying a carious maxillary tooth with buccal surface alveolar erosion (*A*), in the sublingual space (*B*), and in the masticator space (*C*) near a region of lingual surface mandibular erosion.

focal erosion with overlying asymmetric fat stranding, subtle periosteal abscess, or more extensive soft tissue collections. Affected teeth determine the space involved (Table 6). For example, anterior mandibular tooth infections spread to the sublingual space, whereas second and third molar infections spread to the submandibular space from roots posterior to the mylohyoid insertion. However, infection can spread around the free posterior border of the mylohyoid muscle.[33]

Ludwig angina (Fig. 18) describes a rapidly progressive floor of mouth cellulitis, usually from dental disease, that can cause airway compromise, requiring prompt antibiotics and airway management.[32,33] Symptoms include pain, swelling, fever, tongue elevation, and difficulty swallowing or breathing. Nonfluctuant submandibular space induration is classic. The diagnosis is clinical but imaging obtained to assess airway patency, abscess, and underlying dental disease may show multispatial edema with tongue swelling and elevation.

Necrotizing fasciitis is serious infection that can involve neck soft tissues, usually from odontogenic or oropharyngeal sources, surgery, or trauma.[1] Risk factors include diabetes and immunocompromise. Most cases are polymicrobial, requiring broad-spectrum antibiotics, aggressive surgical debridement, and supportive care. Imaging findings include fascial and muscle edema and enhancement with multispatial gas-containing fluid collections.[40] Note that incidental air along fascial planes arises commonly with surgery or penetrating trauma.

PHARYNGEAL INFECTION

Pharyngitis affects all ages. Imaging is not typically needed but may show mucosal enhancement and enlargement of Waldeyer's ring (the palatine, adenoidal, and lingual tonsils). Group A *Streptococcus* is an important cause in children. *Epstein-Barr virus* mononucleosis generates diffuse adenopathy typically in adolescents. Oropharyngeal *Candida* commonly affects immunocompromised patients. SCC should be considered with appropriate symptoms or risk factors (including human papillomavirus [HPV]) in adults with nodular mucosal thickening or evidence of metastatic (especially necrotic) lymph nodes.

Palatine tonsillitis (Fig. 19A, B) and *peritonsillar abscess* (Fig. 19C, D) are the most common deep neck infections among adolescents and young adults.[32] Common pathogens are beta-hemolytic *Streptococcus*, *S aureus*, and *H influenzae*. Symptoms include often unilateral severe sore throat, fever, tender lymphadenopathy, and tonsillar exudate. CT of uncomplicated tonsillitis shows tonsillar enlargement and edema, often a striated, "tiger stripe" appearance. Enlarged bilateral "kissing" tonsils can significantly narrow the airway. Peritonsillar abscess (quinsy) may be suspected with severe unilateral symptoms, swelling, voice changes (hot potato voice), trismus, or drooling.

Table 6	
Patterns of spread of odontogenic soft tissue infection	
Source of Infection	**Soft Tissue Space Typically Affected**
Anterior maxillary teeth	Buccal
Maxillary second molar	Masticator
Maxillary third molar	Parapharyngeal
Anterior mandibular teeth	Sublingual
Mandibular second and third molars	Submandibular

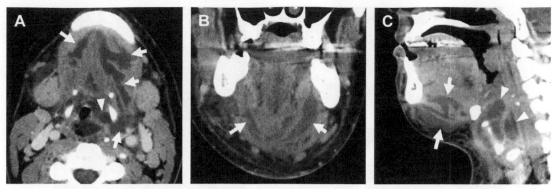

Fig. 18. Ludwig Angina. Axial (*A*), coronal (*B*), and sagittal (*C*) CT images show swelling and hypodense collections (*arrows*) involving the sublingual and submental spaces and extending to the left supraglottic larynx (*arrowhead*) with associated airway narrowing.

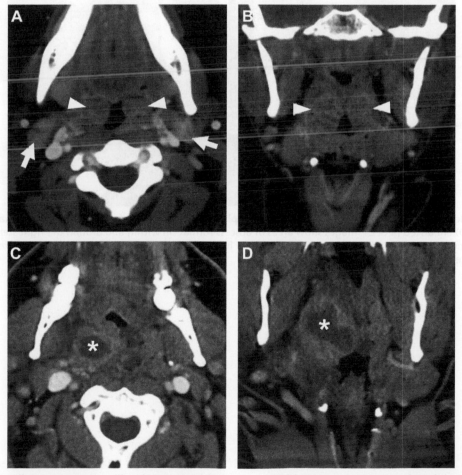

Fig. 19. Tonsillitis versus peritonsillar abscess. Axial (*A*) and coronal (*B*) enhanced CT images show bilateral tonsillitis. Enlarged palatine tonsils show characteristic striated or "tigroid" enhancement (*arrowheads*) due to alternating enhancing tonsillar septa and edema. Note reactive bilateral level II lymphadenopathy (*arrows*). Axial (*C*) and coronal (*D*) enhanced CT images in a different case show an enlarged right palatine tonsil with a lobular rim-enhancing peritonsillar abscess (*asterisk*) with surrounding edema.

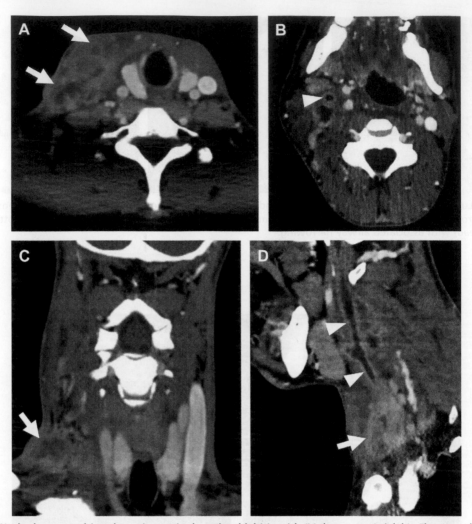

Fig. 20. Neck abscess and jugular vein septic thrombophlebitis with IV drug use. Axial (*A, B*), coronal (*C*), and sagittal (*D*) enhanced neck CT images show areas of abscess formation within and around the right sternocleido-mastoid muscle (*arrow*) and carotid space with internal jugular vein thrombosis and enhancement (*arrowheads*) and adjacent suppurative lymph nodes.

CT confirms tonsillar or peritonsilar rim-enhancing abscess collections and guides drainage.

PARAPHARYNGEAL SPACE INFECTION

Origins of parapharyngeal space infection include tonsillitis, pharyngitis, mastoiditis, parotitis, and odontogenic disease.[1] Carotid sheath involvement can cause internal jugular vein thrombosis, mycotic aneurysm, Horner syndrome, or cranial nerve IX/XII palsy.[1] *Lemierre syndrome* (postanginal septicemia) describes internal jugular vein thrombophlebitis with septic emboli particularly to the lungs. Both ultrasound and CT can depict thrombophlebitis (intraluminal filling defects with wall thickening and hyperemia) but CT is superior for showing the source or extent of infection and potential septic complications. Intravenous drug use with injection targeting neck veins can cause abscesses in the superficial and deep spaces in the neck and cause thrombophlebitis (**Fig. 20**).

RETROPHARYNGEAL SPACE, DANGER SPACE, AND PREVERTEBRAL SPACE INFECTION

Sources of retropharyngeal space (RPS) infection include retropharyngeal lymph nodes; oropharyngeal, parapharyngeal, or prevertebral infections; and trauma, foreign body, and surgery.[1,33] *Retropharyngeal abscess* is most common in children, due to an interrelated frequency of URIs and ear infections and prominence of retropharyngeal nodes, with nodal suppuration leading to abscess.[33] On enhanced CT, suppurative nodes are enlarged with hypodense centers, usually focal and unilateral.[33,41] Abscess appears as an irregular rim-enhancing fluid collection, usually extending across the midline, with surrounding mass effect (**Fig. 21**). Benign RPS edema manifests as homogeneous, symmetric, fluid mildly expanding the RPS without an enhancing rim, and may be reactive to adjacent infection, internal jugular vein thrombosis, radiation therapy, or calcific tendoinitis.[1,33] MR imaging can further distinguish among adenopathy, abscess, and edema if obtained.[33] An abscess typically warrants aggressive management and drainage to avoid airway obstruction or abscess rupture and aspiration.[33] Grisel syndrome describes rare nontraumatic atlantoaxial joint subluxation usually in children, related to ligamentous laxity after head and neck region infection including RPS abscess or surgery.[42]

Descending necrotizing mediastinitis is a rare but life-threatening acute polymicrobial infection usually arising from oral cavity, oropharyngeal or cervical infection spreading inferiorly via the retropharyngeal/danger space.[33,43] Infection may also

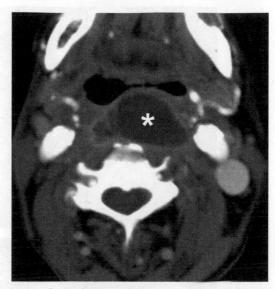

Fig. 21. Retropharyngeal abscess. A 53 year-old man with diabetes and renal transplant presenting with 1 week of sore throat, dysphagia and globus sensation. Enhanced neck CT shows a rim-enhancing fluid density abscess (*asterisk*) expanding the retropharyngeal space with mass effect.

descend laterally via the carotid space or anteriorly along a pretracheal route.[33,43] Mediastinal infection can progress rapidly to sepsis and organ failure. Delayed diagnosis due to vague symptoms (dyspnea, cough) contributes to mortality and here again diabetes and immunocompromise are common commorbidities.[43] Enhanced CT permits rapid identification of both mediastinitis and the source and route of spread (**Fig. 22**).[33] Mediastinal imaging findings include fat stranding, fluid collections, gas, and pericardial or pleural effusions.[33,43]

GLOTTIC INFECTIONS

Epiglottitis (also called supraglotitis) may require emergent intubation due to risk of airway occlusion.[33] Although traditionally affecting children aged 1 to 5 years due to *H influenzae* type B, incidence has decreased with vaccination, shifting more toward other pathogens and older children and adults.[32] Diagnosis is usually clinical (based on fever, speaking difficulty or voice changes, inspiratory stridor, and severe dysphagia) because imaging can delay intervention. The classic lateral neck radiograph finding is epiglottic and aryepiglottic fold thickening with a characteristic shape (the "thumb sign"). CT in unsuspected cases demonstrates similar thickening and surrounding inflammation.[44]

Laryngotracheobronchitis (also called subglotitis or croup) typically occurs between 6 months

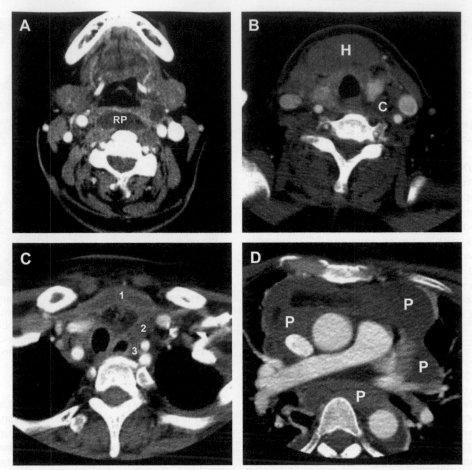

Fig. 22. Descending necrotizing mediastinitis. A 49 year-old woman with type II diabetes mellitus, HCV cirrhosis, and thrombocytopenia underwent drainage of an anterior neck abscess that grew *Klebsiella pneumonia.* Follow-up enhanced CT images from superior to inferior (*A–D*) show a ventral neck surgical site hematoma (H) and trans-spatial abscesses in the RPS (RP), left carotid space (C) and parathyroid region bilaterally. Collections track inferiorly via pretracheal (1), lateral pharyngeal (2), and retropharyngeal pathways (3) into the mediastinum with associated pericardial effusion (P). Decortication and mediastinal abscess drainage also yielded *Klebsiella.*

and 3 years of age, most often from parainfluenza virus, with a peak in fall and winter.[33] Symptoms include viral prodrome, fever, and classic "barking cough." Frontal radiographs demonstrate symmetric straightening of the normally convex appearing subglottic airway, forming the shape of a steeple (the "steeple sign").

SUMMARY

Head and neck infections are common but potentially serious, prone to spread and cause complications in susceptible patients. Diagnosis and management benefit from close coordination between care providers and radiologists. Imaging is crucial to characterize location and extent of infection, facilitate abscess drainage, and identify complications.

CLINICS CARE POINTS

- Head and neck infections are common and have the potential for serious complications, particularly in immunocompromised, diabetic, elderly, and hospitalized patients.

- Optimal management requires a multidisciplinary team including emergency medicine staff, internists or pediatricians, surgical subspecialists, and radiologists.

- Radiologists should pay close attention to the subtle signs of more aggressive infection or complications that may include fat infiltration, bone involvement, venous thrombosis, and orbital or intracranial extension.

DISCLOSURE

J.M. Stein has received support from sponsored research agreements with Hyperfine Research, Inc. and consulting income from Centaur Diagnostics, Inc. J.F. Xian has nothing to disclose.

REFERENCES

1. Hegde Amogh N, Suyash Mohan, Amit Pandya, et al. Imaging in infections of the head and neck. Neuroimaging Clin N Am 2012;22(4):727–54.

2. Białek Ewa J, Jakubowski Wiesław. Mistakes in ultrasound diagnosis of superficial lymph nodes. J Ultrason 2017;17(68):59–65.

3. Leung Alexander KC, Dele Davies H. Cervical lymphadenitis: etiology, diagnosis, and management. Curr Infect Dis Rep 2009;11(3):183–9.

4. Roland Peter S, Stroman David W. Microbiology of acute otitis externa. Laryngoscope 2002;112(7 Pt 1):1166–77.

5. Çiğdem Tepe Karaca, Seniha Şenbayrak Akçay, Sema Zer Toros, et al. External auditory canal microbiology and hearing aid use. Am J Otol 2013;34(4): 278–81.

6. van der Meer Wilhelmina L, Waterval Jérôme J, Kunst Henricus PM, et al. Diagnosing necrotizing external otitis on CT and MRI: assessment of pattern of extension. Eur Arch Otorhinolaryngol 2022;279(3): 1323–8.

7. van der Meer WL, van Tilburg M, Mitea C, et al. A Persistent Foramen of Huschke: A Small Road to Misery in Necrotizing External Otitis. AJNR Am J Neuroradiol 2019;40(9):1552–6.

8. Chapman PR, Choudhary G, Singhal A. Skull Base Osteomyelitis: A Comprehensive Imaging Review. Am J Neuroradiology 2021;42(3):404–13.

9. Harmes Kathryn M, Alexander Blackwood R, Burrows Heather L, et al. Otitis media: diagnosis and treatment. Am Fam Physician 2013;88(7):435–40.

10. Pagano Anthony S, Wang Eugene, Yuan Derek, et al. Cranial Indicators Identified for Peak Incidence of Otitis Media. Anat Rec (Hoboken) 2017;300(10): 1721–40.

11. Pichichero Michael E. Otitis media. Pediatr Clin North Am 2013;60(2):391–407.

12. Tal Marom, Tan Alai, Wilkinson Gregg S, et al. Trends in otitis media-related health care use in the United States, 2001-2011. JAMA Pediatr 2014;168(1): 68–75.

13. Semaan Maroun T, Megerian Cliff A. The pathophysiology of cholesteatoma. Otolaryngol Clin North Am 2006;39(6):1143–59.

14. Jiang Hua, Wu Chengpeng, Xu Jingjie, et al. Bacterial and Fungal Infections Promote the Bone Erosion Progression in Acquired Cholesteatoma Revealed by Metagenomic Next-Generation Sequencing. Front Microbiol 2021;12:761111.

15. McDonald Michael H, Hoffman Matthew R, Gentry Lindell R. When is fluid in the mastoid cells a worrisome finding? J Am Board Fam Med 2013;26(2): 218–20.

16. Nagaraj Usha D, Koch Bernadette L. Imaging of orbital infectious and inflammatory disease in children. Pediatr Radiol 2021;51(7):1149–61.

17. Chandler JR, Langenbrunner DJ, Stevens ER. The pathogenesis of orbital complications in acute sinusitis. Laryngoscope 1970;80(9):1414–28.

18. Theodora Tsirouki, Dastiridou Anna I, Flores Nuria Ibáñez, et al. Orbital cellulitis. Surv Ophthalmol 2018;63(4):534–53.

19. Le Tran D, Liu Eugene S, Adatia Feisal A, et al. The effect of adding orbital computed tomography findings to the Chandler criteria for classifying pediatric orbital cellulitis in predicting which patients will require surgical intervention. J AAPOS 2014;18(3): 271–7.

20. Healy G. Chandler et al.: "The pathogenesis of orbital complications in acute sinusitis." (Laryngoscope 1970;80:1414-1428). Laryngoscope 1997; 107(4).441–6.

21. Vardhan Mahalingam Harsha, Mani Sunithi E, Patel Bimal, et al. Imaging Spectrum of Cavernous Sinus Lesions with Histopathologic Correlation. Radiographics 2019;39(3):795–819.

22. Shervin Kamalian, Avery Laura, Lev Michael H, et al. Nontraumatic Head and Neck Emergencies. Radiographics 2019;39(6):1808–23.

23. Mohammad Javed Ali, Joshi Surbhi D, Naik Milind N, et al. Clinical profile and management outcome of acute dacryocystitis: two decades of experience in a tertiary eye care center. Semin Ophthalmol 2015; 30(2):118–23.

24. Rosenfeld Richard M, Piccirillo Jay F, Chandrasekhar Sujana S, et al. Clinical practice guideline (update): Adult Sinusitis Executive Summary. Otolaryngol Head Neck Surg 2015;152(4):598–609.

25. Brook Itzhak. Microbiology of sinusitis. Proc Am Thorac Soc 2011;8(1):90–100.

26. Joshi Varsha M. Sansi Rima. Imaging in Sinonasal Inflammatory Disease. Neuroimaging Clin N Am 2015;25(4):549–68.

27. Som PM, Dillon WP, Fullerton GD, et al. Chronically obstructed sinonasal secretions: observations on T1 and T2 shortening. Radiology 1989;172(2):515–20.

28. Bhatt Alok A, Donaldson Angela M, Olomu Osarenoma U, et al. Can Diffusion-Weighted Imaging Serve as an Imaging Biomarker for Acute Bacterial Rhinosinusitis? Cureus 2020;12(8):e9893.

29. Wells RG, Sty JR, Landers AD. Radiological evaluation of Pott puffy tumor. JAMA 1986;255(10):1331–3.

30. Manohar Aribandi, McCoy Victor A, Carlos Bazan. Imaging features of invasive and noninvasive fungal

sinusitis: a review. Radiographics 2007;27(5):1283–96.

31. Jesil Mathew Aranjani, Atulya Manuel, Razack Habeeb Ibrahim Abdul, et al. COVID-19–associated mucormycosis: Evidence-based critical review of an emerging infection burden during the pandemic's second wave in India. PLOS Negl Trop Dis 2021;15(11):e0009921.

32. Erin Frankie Capps, Kinsella James J, Gupta Manu, et al. Emergency Imaging Assessment of Acute, Nontraumatic Conditions of the Head and Neck. RadioGraphics 2010;30(5):1335–52.

33. Suyash Mohan, Stein Joel M, Hoeggner Ellen G, et al. The Acute Neck: Inflammation, Infections, and Trauma. Neuroimaging: The Essentials. Wolters Kluwer; 2015.

34. Bag Asim K, Curé Joel K, Chapman Philip R, et al. Imaging of Inflammatory Disorders of Salivary Glands. Neuroimaging Clin N Am 2018;28(2):255–72.

35. Kirshenbaum KJ, Nadimpalli SR, Friedman M, et al. Benign lymphoepithelial parotid tumors in AIDS patients: CT and MR findings in nine cases. AJNR Am J Neuroradiol 1991;12(2):271–4.

36. Martinoli C, Pretolesi F, Del Bono V, et al. Benign lymphoepithelial parotid lesions in HIV-positive patients: spectrum of findings at gray-scale and Doppler sonography. AJR Am J Roentgenol 1995;165(4):975–9.

37. Scheinfeld Meir H, Keivan Shifteh, Avery Laura L, et al. Teeth: What Radiologists Should Know. RadioGraphics 2012;32(7):1927–44.

38. Frencken Jo E, Sharma Praveen, Laura Stenhouse, et al. Global epidemiology of dental caries and severe periodontitis - a comprehensive review. J Clin Periodontol 2017;44(Suppl 18):S94–105.

39. Rega Anthony J, Aziz Shahid R, Ziccardi Vincent B. Microbiology and antibiotic sensitivities of head and neck space infections of odontogenic origin. J Oral Maxillofac Surg 2006;64(9):1377–80.

40. Becker M, Zbären P, Hermans R, et al. Necrotizing fasciitis of the head and neck: role of CT in diagnosis and management. Radiology 1997;202(2):471–6.

41. Hoang Jenny K, Branstetter Barton F, Eastwood James D, et al. Multiplanar CT and MRI of collections in the retropharyngeal space: is it an abscess? AJR Am J Roentgenol 2011;196(4):W426–32.

42. Stephen Osiro, Tiwari Kevin J, Petru Matusz, et al. Grisel's syndrome: a comprehensive review with focus on pathogenesis, natural history, and current treatment options. Childs Nerv Syst 2012;28(6):821–5.

43. Pinto Antonio, Mariano Scaglione, Giuseppina Scuderi Maria, et al. Infections of the neck leading to descending necrotizing mediastinitis: Role of multi-detector row computed tomography. Eur J Radiol 2008;65(3):389–94.

44. Sobol Steven E, Zapata Syboney. Epiglottitis and croup. Otolaryngol Clin North Am 2008;41(3):551–66, ix.

Imaging of Congenital/Childhood Central Nervous System Infections

TANG Phua Hwee, MBBS (Singapore), MMed (Diagnostic Radiology), FRCR (UK)[a],*,
THOON Koh Cheng, MBBS, MRCPCH, MMed (Paeds)[b]

KEYWORDS

- Congenital • Childhood • Central Nervous System Infections • TORCH • MR imaging
- Computed tomography • Ultrasound

KEY POINTS

- Cranial ultrasound remains important for diagnosis and follow-up in babies with open fontanelles.
- Patterns of infection change as countries develop, with improved sanitation, vaccines, and preventive medicine; however, characteristic "textbook" neuroimaging continues to be encountered.
- Imaging is part of the diagnostic criteria for encephalitis and can detect acute inflammation (encephalitis, meningitis, myelitis, neuritis), complications (abscess, empyema, vasculitis-induced infarcts), chronic changes (atrophy/gliosis, hydrocephalus, calcifications), as well as immune-mediated abnormalities.
- Infective epidemics and pandemics affecting children include arbovirus outbreaks, acute flaccid myelitis caused by enterovirus D68, brainstem encephalitis caused by enterovirus A71, immune-mediated acute necrotizing encephalopathy in the 2009 H1N1 pandemic, and multisystem inflammatory syndrome in the current COVID-19 pandemic.
- Hemorrhage-induced aseptic ventriculitis, genetic diseases or inborn errors of metabolism, and leptomeningeal metastasis can mimic imaging features of infection.

INTRODUCTION: EPIDEMIOLOGY OF PEDIATRIC CENTRAL NERVOUS SYSTEM INFECTION

Radiologists should be aware of the similarities as well as substantial differences among the causative organisms and risk factors in CNS infections encountered in pediatric patients; we should also pay attention to the practical challenges of transport, and requirement for anesthesia.[1] The epidemiology and pattern of central nervous system (CNS) infections in pediatric patients have changed over the years because countries developed and health services improved. Nevertheless, infections still cause significant mortality globally, with viral, bacterial, fungal, and parasitic infections giving rise to substantial neurologic, cognitive, behavioral, or mental health morbidity, especially in those in low and middle-income countries (LMIC).[2] For example, the rabies virus, a highly neuronotropic virus causing encephalomyelitis and high mortality, still accounts for thousands of deaths annually among children in LMIC,[3] although it has been eliminated from developed nations.[4] Once basic sanitation procedures are in place and effective vaccines are available, preventive medicine is the key to optimize child development.[5]

Common congenital CNS infections and their typical imaging findings have been well described in previous issues of Neuroimaging Clinics and are summarized in **Table 1**.[6] This article will focus on the main viral, bacterial, and immune-related

[a] Department of Diagnostic and Interventional Imaging, KK Women's and Children's Hospital, 100 Bukit Timah Road, Singapore 229899; [b] Department of Paediatrics, Infectious Disease, KK Women's and Children's Hospital, 100 Bukit Timah Road, Singapore 229899
* Corresponding author.
E-mail address: Tang.phua.hwee@singhealth.com.sg

Neuroimag Clin N Am 33 (2023) 207–224
https://doi.org/10.1016/j.nic.2022.07.017
1052-5149/23/© 2022 Elsevier Inc. All rights reserved.

conditions seen in children. Cranial ultrasound will be emphasized because it is less costly, radiation free, and more accessible than cross-sectional imaging; its drawback is limited to babies who still possess an open fontanelle.

ROLE OF IMAGING IN INFECTION: DIAGNOSIS AND DETECTING COMPLICATIONS

Neuroimaging contributes to confirming the diagnosis of meningitis when thickened, enhancing meninges are present (Fig. 1), encephalitis when there is swelling of the brain parenchyma (Fig. 2), and meningoencephalitis when both are detected (Fig. 3). It also can assess complications of infection such as brain abscess (Fig. 4) and empyema. The causative organism is confirmed by serology

or histopathological identification. Early antibiotic treatment can be life-saving and should not be withheld or delayed because of neuroimaging.[7]

The spread of infection can sometimes be appreciated on imaging. Contiguous spread can occur in the context of trauma when there is a breach of skull vault and dura.[8] Direct invasion from infections in the paranasal sinuses (see Fig. 3; Fig. 5) and middle ear can give rise to adjacent meningitis, encephalitis, meningoencephalitis, subdural empyemas, and brain abscesses. Hematogenous spread should be suspected when the child has bacteremia or infective endocarditis, with septic emboli giving rise to scattered microabscesses throughout the brain (Fig. 6). Abnormal neuroimaging is an important criterion for diagnosing encephalitis.[9] Neuroimaging can

Table 1
Common congenital/peripartum pediatric central nervous system infections in immunocompetent host and typical intracranial imaging findings

Infective Agent	Typical Transmission Period	Typical Intracranial Imaging Findings
Bacteria		
Group B Streptococcus	Peripartum and later	Meningitis, ventriculitis
E coli	Peripartum and later	Meningitis, ventriculitis
Listeria monocytogenes	Peripartum and later	Meningitis
Virus		
Toxoplasmosis[a]	In utero	Brain calcifications, hydrocephalus
Syphilis[a]	In utero	Meningitis, vasculitis, and arterial infarcts
Rubella[a]	In utero	Meningoencephalitis, microcephaly, brain calcifications, and delayed myelination
Cytomegalovirus[a]	In utero	Periventricular calcifications, neuronal migration disorders, and ventriculomegaly (degree inversely related to timing of infection)
Zika	In utero	Microcephaly, brain malformations, and brain calcifications
Varicella zoster virus[a]	In utero, peripartum	Microcephaly, cortical atrophy, and hydrocephalus[60] (in contrast to the encephalitis, arterial infarcts seen in infections acquired later in life)
HIV[a]	In utero, peripartum	Microcephaly, cerebral atrophy, and brain calcifications
Herpes simplex virus 2[a]	Peripartum	Widespread brain destruction. Microcephaly, multicystic encephalomalacia, dystrophic calcification, and ventriculomegaly in survivors (in contrast to the bilateral limbic encephalitis from Herpes simplex virus 1 infections acquired in infancy and beyond

[a] Common congenital CNS infections from the CHEAP TORCHES group of pathogens (chicken pox, hepatitis, enterovirus, AIDS, parvovirus, toxoplasmosis, rubella, cytomegalovirus, and herpes simplex, syphilis).

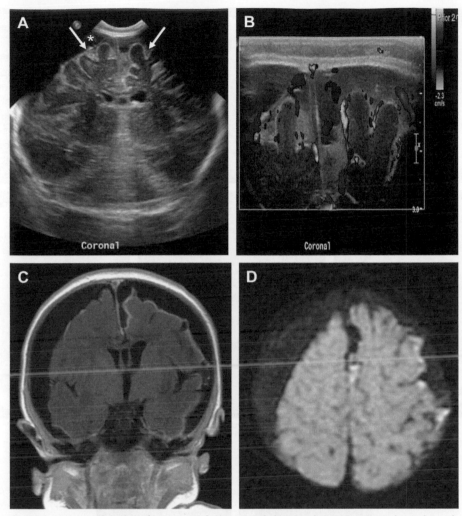

Fig. 1. *E coli* meningitis in a febrile infant. Cranial ultrasound shows echogenic material overlying both frontal lobes, extending into the depths of the sulci (*arrows*), with an anechoic right subdural fluid collection (*asterisk*, *A*). There is increased vascularity of the left frontal leptomeninges on color Doppler ultrasound (*B*). Corresponding postcontrast T1-weighted MR imaging confirms thickened enhancing leptomeninges (*C*) with foci of restricted diffusion over the cortex consistent with subarachnoid collections of pus (*D*).

also be used to monitor patient's response to treatment and guide neurosurgical interventions if required.

Role of Cranial Ultrasound

Cranial ultrasound remains the most commonly used imaging modality for neonates, being more accessible and economical than magnetic resonance (MR) imaging, and radiation-free, unlike computed tomography (CT). The typical manifestations of intrauterine infection on ultrasound depend on the gestational period during which the infection occurred. In the acute phase of intrauterine infection, cranial ultrasound may be able to detect feature of meningitis such as thickened, echogenic meninges, debris in the cortical sulci,

ventriculitis (Fig. 7), hydrocephalus (Fig. 8), parenchymal destruction, abscesses, and hemorrhages. Venous sinus thrombosis can also be identified on cranial ultrasound as the superior sagittal venous sinus is located just beneath the open fontanelle. The devastating effects of infection on brain seen in the past (Figs. 9 and 10) can be prevented when those at risk of infection are promptly investigated and treated with antibiotics.

Role of MR Imaging and CT

Unlike cranial ultrasound, MR imaging and CT can depict earlier, more subtle abnormalities because their extent of coverage are not hampered by the limited view from the anterior

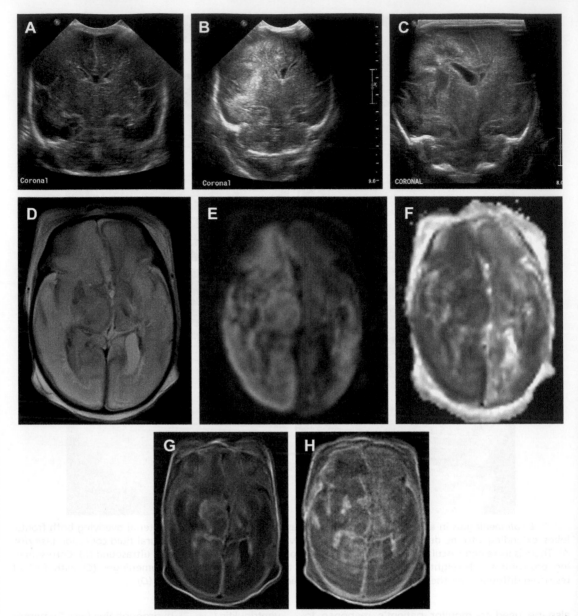

Fig. 2. Premature baby of 28-week gestation with *Enterobacter cloacae* sepsis and meningitis. Initial cranial ultrasound on day 4 of life shows only the Sylvian fissures are visible in keeping with prematurity (*A*). Ultrasound on day 11 shows increased echogenicity in a swollen right cerebral hemisphere causing midline shift to the left (*B*). Follow-up ultrasound on day 15 of life shows mixed echogenicity in a more swollen right cerebral hemisphere causing even greater midline shift (*C*). T2-weighted MR imaging on day 19 shows right cerebral hemisphere remains swollen and hyperintense with midline deviation to the left (*D*). Increased signal is seen is seen on DWI in both cerebral hemispheres, worse on the right (*E*) with corresponding low signal on apparent diffusion coefficient map (*F*). Pre (*G*) and post (*H*) contrast T1-weighted images show abnormal enhancement of the meninges and occipital lobes.

fontanelle. MR imaging gives superior soft tissue contrast compared with CT and has the advantage of multiple tissue contrasts. Diffusion-weighted imaging, for example, can be helpful to confirm cerebral abscess or empyema and to detect acute infarcts from varicella-induced angiitis (**Fig. 11**). A major drawback of MR imaging is the need for children to keep very still for each MR imaging acquisition sequence, often requiring general anesthesia because a typical MR imaging brain study with intravenous contrast exceeds half an hour, especially if

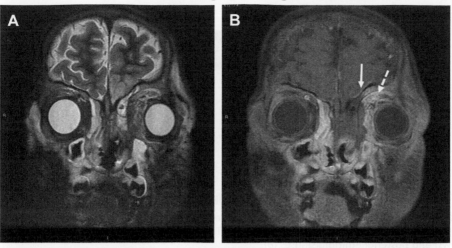

Fig. 3. Left basal frontal meningoencephalitis in a 5-year-old child with leukemia, hemifacial cellulitis, and fungal pansinusitis. Swollen and hyperintense left basal frontal lobe and with abnormal orbital and sinonasal soft tissue seen on coronal T2-weighted fat-saturated images (*A*) with enhancement of the basal frontal meninges and inflamed soft tissues in the medial left orbit and left face (*arrows, B*).

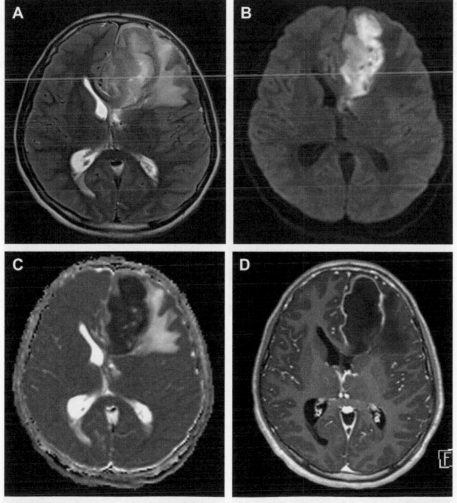

Fig. 4. Left frontal lobe abscess in a 15 year-old teenager with *Staphylococcus intermedius* bacteremia. Mass and surrounding edema result in effacement and displacement of the left frontal horn (*A*), its content showing increased signal on DWI (*B*), with corresponding low signal on apparent diffusion coefficient map (*C*). Ring-enhancing abscess seen on postcontrast MR imaging (*D*).

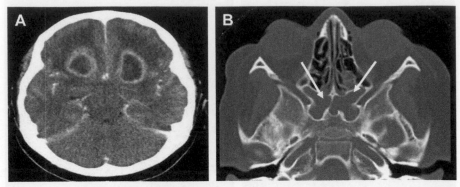

Fig. 5. Bilateral frontal lobe abscesses in an 11-year-old teenager with sinusitis, severe headache, neck pain, and torticollis. Bilateral rim-enhancing frontal abscesses on CT (*A*) with abnormal opacification of the adjacent sphenoid (*arrows*) and posterior ethmoid sinuses (*B*).

advanced pulse sequences are performed.[10,11] Carefully targeted MR imaging protocols are important for CNS infections: MR angiography is performed if vasculitic complications are suspected, the metabolite profile on MR spectroscopy can help narrow the differential diagnosis for a mass and diffusion tensor imaging can demonstrate displacement of important white matter tracts and guide biopsy trajectory. Judicious planning and preparation are crucial, and abbreviated protocols and continuous quality improvement are necessary to ensure the most appropriate and valuable use of MR imaging.[12,13]

CT remains the gold standard for the depiction of intracranial calcifications and bony anatomy, such as when the integrity of the cribriform plate

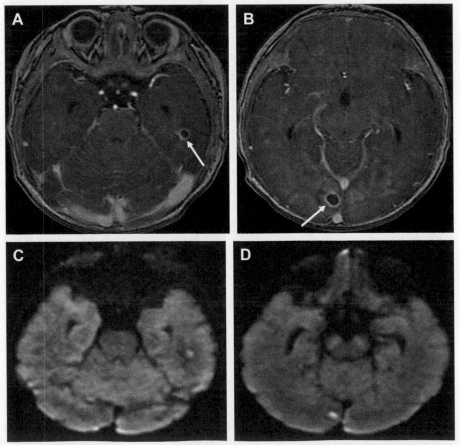

Fig. 6. Multiple abscesses in a 7-month-old septic infant. Ring-enhancing abscesses (*arrows*) are seen in the left temporal (*A*) and right occipital (*B*) lobes on postcontrast MR imaging, showing restricted diffusion (*C, D*).

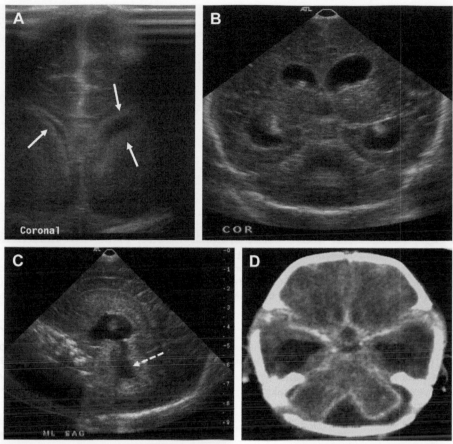

Fig. 7. *Klebsiella* meningitis and ventriculitis in a premature baby. Thickened echogenic wall of the ventricles (*arrows*) indicate inflammation (*A*). Follow-up ultrasound 5 days later shows ventriculitis has subsided but hydrocephalus has developed with dilated lateral ventricles (*B*). Sagittal midline cranial ultrasound image shows the fourth ventricle is also distended (dotted *arrow*), indicating this is communicating hydrocephalus (*C*). Corresponding CT images of the same patient confirming hydrocephalus and meningitis (*D*).

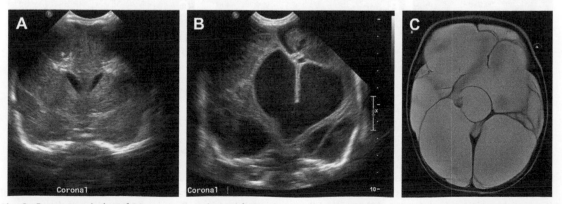

Fig. 8. Premature baby of 30-week gestation with *E coli* sepsis and meningitis. Initial ultrasound shows increased echogenicity of the bilateral white matter at 1 week of life (*A*). Dilated ventricles and cystic encephalomalacia are visible on follow-up ultrasound at 2 months of life (*B*). Only a thin layer of cerebral parenchyma is visible on MR imaging at 8 month of age (*C*).

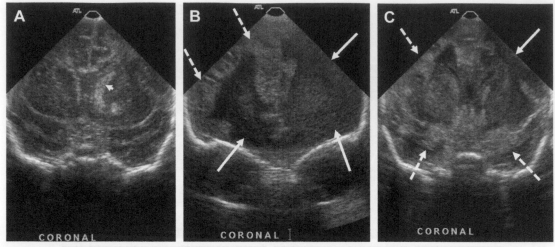

Fig. 9. Cranial ultrasound in a 1-week-old premature baby with gram-negative bacterial sepsis. Initial cranial ultrasound shows echogenic hemorrhage in the left frontal horn (*arrowhead*); the rest of the brain shows no abnormality (*A*). One day later, both cerebral hemispheres are abnormal (*B,C*) with areas of decreased (*arrows*) as well as increased (dotted *arrows*) echogenicity; brain damage can manifest as both decreased and increased echogenicity on ultrasound.

needs to be established in cases of rhinocerebral infections. CT is also faster to acquire than MR imaging, does not require as much cooperation from the child, and is often helpful when dichotomous yes/no clinical decision-making is needed, for example, if urgent neurosurgical intervention is required in suspected raised intracranial pressure.[14]

CONGENITAL AND PERIPARTUM INFECTIONS: TORCH

The acronym TORCH is often used to describe congenital infections among neonates. It stands for infections by toxoplasmosis, rubella, cytomegalovirus, herpes simplex; some authors have

recommended expanding it to CHEAP TORCHES to include chicken pox, hepatitis, enterovirus, acquired immunodeficiency syndrome (AIDS), parvovirus, and syphilis.[15] Typical CNS findings in TORCH infection include microcephaly with volume loss and intracranial calcifications (Figs. 12 and 13). Neonates with Herpes simplex virus 2 infection show widespread destructive lesions rather than the temporal lobe predisposition from Herpes simplex virus 1 infection typically seen in older children and adults.[16] Successful antenatal screening and vaccination against rubella and varicella-zoster have changed the TORCH disease pattern but this remains highly country-specific with different guidelines even among the developed countries.[17]

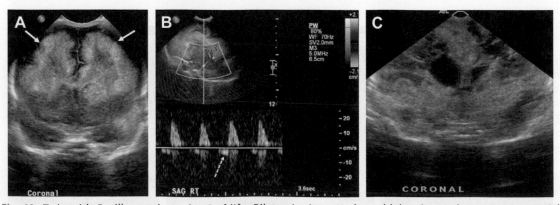

Fig. 10. Twin with *Bacillus* sepsis on day 6 of life. Bilateral echogenic frontal lobes (*arrows*) are seen on cranial ultrasound suspicious for infarction (*A*) as critical flow restriction is seen on Doppler flow study, with flow present in the middle cerebral artery only during cardiac systole, and abnormal flow reversal (dotted *arrow*) during cardiac diastole (*B*). Follow-up cranial ultrasound shows multicystic encephalomalacia has developed with ex vacuo dilatation of the right frontal horn (*C*).

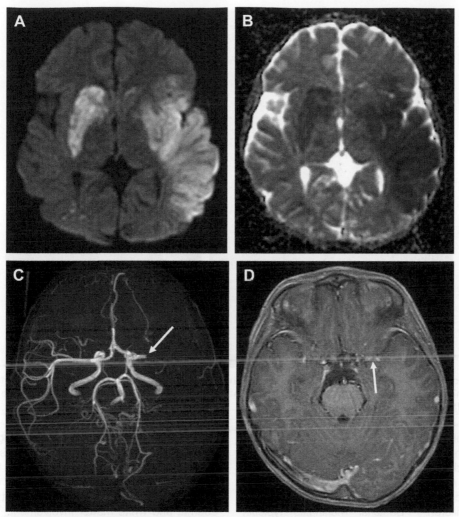

Fig. 11. Acute infarcts from vasculitis and arterial thrombosis in a 7-year-old child with primary immunodeficiency, varicella zoster virus pneumonitis, and seizures. Bilateral acute infarcts, worse on the left, are present on DWI (*A*) with corresponding low signal on apparent diffusion coefficient map (*B*). There is abrupt signal dropout from the M1 segment of the left middle cerebral artery (*arrow*) on MRA (*C*) with filling defect (*arrow*) present in the M1 segment of the left middle cerebral artery after contrast injection (*D*).

Congenital infections may be more likely when mothers are exposed to risk factors such as impaired immune systems in AIDS patients,[18] listeria from dietary intake of unpasteurized milk products,[19] and arthropod-borne viruses such as Zika, dengue, and chikungunya. The outcome of congenital infection can differ with geography, with brain abnormalities seen in 43% of Zika-infected neonates in Brazil[20] but only 11% in United States of America.[21] The different manifestations of congenital Zika infections worldwide[22] may also be attributed to the Asian strain being different from the American Zika strain,[23] with genetics of the population also playing a role (**Fig. 14**).

BACTERIAL MENINGITIS IN NEONATES AND CHILDREN

Group B Streptococcus (GBS) and *Escherichia coli* account for most of the meningitis cases in the neonatal period, typically from vertical transmission during or after birth; GBS remains a common cause of neonatal sepsis and meningitis despite intrapartum antibiotic prophylaxis.[24] Differences in clinical and neuroimaging features between common causative organisms are not specific, except for a higher percentage (up to 40%) of ischemic infarctions associated with GBS (infectious vasculitis, hypercoagulable state, septic emboli, and systemic hypotension are the proposed mechanisms of damage).[25] In contrast,

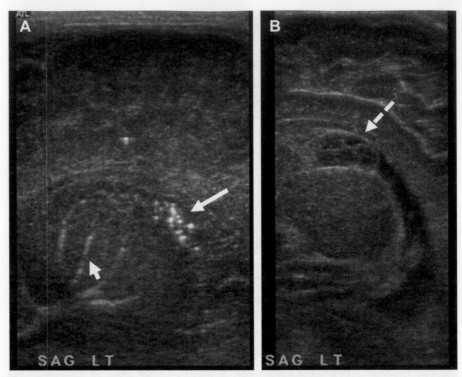

Fig. 12. Congenital rubella. Cranial ultrasound (*A, B*) shows echogenic specks of intracranial calcifications (long *arrow*), linear echogenicities suggestive of lenticulostriate vasculopathy (short *arrow*), and hemorrhage in the left caudothalamic groove (dotted *arrow*).

hydrocephalus can be seen in up to 22% of those with neonatal *E coli* infection.[26]

Beyond infancy, *Streptococcus pneumoniae*, *Neisseria meningitidis*, and *Haemophilus influenzae* type b account for most of bacterial meningitis in older children.[27] Bacterial meningitis typically carries higher risk of mortality and morbidity compared with viral meningitis if untreated but vaccination has reduced the mortality rate from more than 15% to the current rate of 5% to 10%.[28] The requirement for intensive care support is high in *S pneumoniae* meningitis, whereas neurologic morbidity 5 years postmeningitis is high in *H influenzae* type b.

CHILDHOOD OUTBREAKS OF CENTRAL NERVOUS SYSTEM INFECTIONS

In a recent epidemiologic study, most of the meningitis and encephalitis cases in healthy children in the United States were predominantly viral in origin,[29] in particular the enteroviruses.[30] Although poliovirus has been eradicated from most countries by the World Health Organization's Global Polio Eradication Initiative,[31] since 2012 multiple outbreaks caused by a nonpolio enterovirus (predominantly enterovirus D68) with polio-like symptoms have given rise to acute flaccid myelitis

with substantial disability.[32] MR imaging findings in acute flaccid myelitis typically affects the gray matter, particularly the anterior horns in the cervical cord, in a bilateral, longitudinally extensive pattern; there is minimal enhancement, variable edema, and white matter involvement.[32,33] Apart from enteroviruses, flaviviruses (such as West Nile virus) can also be responsible for damage to the spinal anterior horn cells, in contrast to other viruses such as the herpes and varicella-zoster viruses that tend to infect the brain.[34]

Hand foot and mouth disease, caused by the coxsackieviruses and enterovirus A71 (EV71), is widespread in Asia and predominantly affects preschoolers, with summer peaks in temperate regions, and spring and fall peaks in subtropical Asia.[35] The basic reproduction number of EV71 ranges from 0.5 to 5,[36,37] and the highly contagious disease often necessitates short-term closure of kindergartens and childcare centers to stem its spread.[38,39] EV71 outbreaks in Chinese, Taiwanese, Japanese, and Korean children have result in meningitis, encephalitis, brainstem encephalitis, and acute flaccid myelitis,[40,41] with characteristic pathognomonic T2 hyperintensity in the posterior brainstem described on MR imaging.[42,43] Severe brainstem encephalitis (**Fig. 15**) with damage to thalami and medulla oblongata[44]

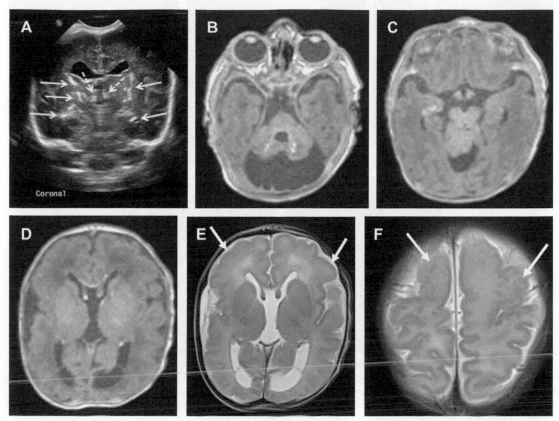

Fig. 13. Congenital cytomegalovirus infection in a term baby. Cranial ultrasound shows echogenic calcifications in the ventricular wall (dotted arrows) and in the bilateral parenchyma (arrows). (A). The calcifications are T1 hyperintense and visible in the bilateral cerebellar hemispheres (B), temporal lobes (C), and margins of the ventricles (D). Frontal cerebral gyrations seem immature (arrows) for a term infant (E) with cysts in the bilateral periventricular occipital white matter. Bilateral polymicrogyria is visible in the high frontal lobes (arrows) on T2-weighted MR imaging (F).

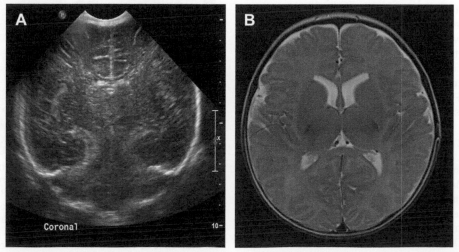

Fig. 14. Maternal Zika. Normal brain of a 1-day-old term infant born in Singapore on cranial ultrasound (A) and MR imaging (B).

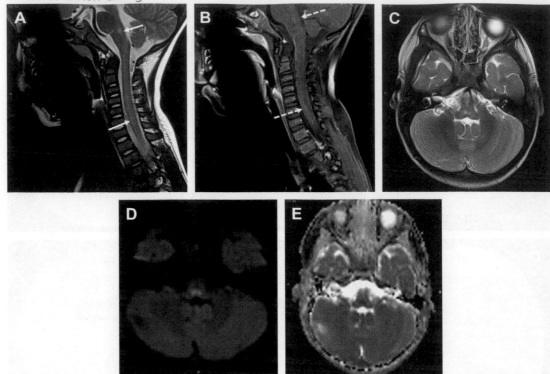

Fig. 15. Hand foot mouth disease in a 2-year-old child who presented with right upper limb lower motor neuron signs. MR imaging shows increased T2 signal in the dorsal pons and medulla with long segment of involvement of the cervical cord (arrows, A), these regions showing mild enhancement (dotted arrow) after contrast injection (B). Axial images show that the T2 hyperintensity in the dorsal medulla (C) demonstrates high signal on DWI (D) with corresponding low signal on apparent diffusion coefficient map (E).

may result in death from neurogenic pulmonary hemorrhage/edema. Prognosis is variable, and patients with mild aseptic meningitis typically recover without neurologic deficit but those with encephalitis and/or myelitis do worse.[45]

Arboviruses transmitted by the Aedes mosquito are neurotropic and include dengue, Zika, and chikungunya viruses. Although neurologic consequences have been most widely reported with Zika, vertical transmission has been described for all 3 viruses.[46,47] Dengue, which has been studied for several decades and still remains prevalent in more than 100 countries, would be a good example of the diverse effects a viral infection can have on the nervous system during cyclic outbreaks. Patients can suffer from encephalitis, meningitis, myelitis, complications such as ischemic stroke from vasculitis or hemorrhage from low platelets, and autoimmune reactions including acute disseminated encephalomyelitis (ADEM), neuromyelitis optica, optic neuritis, and Guillain-Barre syndrome. Despite the range of MR imaging findings, most patients recover well even if there was CNS involvement.[48]

Pandemics have had variable effects in children. In the 2009 influenza A (H1N1) pandemic that lasted almost a year, 90% of those affected and admitted with neurologic symptoms were children

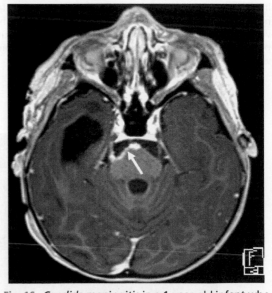

Fig. 16. Candida meningitis in a 1-year-old infant who had frontal embryonal tumor excised. Candida was isolated from the cerebrospinal fluid. MR imaging shows lepomeningeal enhancement around the brainstem (arrow). An infectious cause was favored over leptomeningeal cancer metastasis because Candida species was isolated from the cerebrospinal fluid, and MR imaging abnormalities improved after 3 weeks of antifungal treatment (not shown).

younger than 18 years, some with acute necrotizing encephalopathy (see later discussion).[49] In contrast, in the current COVID-19 pandemic, patients with neurologic manifestations have been predominantly adults[50] with a minority of children developing neurologic problems due to an immune-mediated multisystem inflammatory syndrome.[51]

OPPORTUNISTIC AND IATROGENIC INFECTIONS: IN PREMATURE INFANTS, POSTOPERATIVE AND IMMUNOCOMPROMISED CHILDREN

Multiple groups of pediatric patients are at increased risk of opportunistic infection. Premature babies are at risk of infection from immaturity of their immune system, decreased placental passage of maternal antibodies, prolonged hospitalization and use of indwelling catheters. At all ages, invasive procedures are associated with increased risk: very low birth weight neonates who require shunt implants are at the risk of developing ependymitis[52] or fungal[53] infections (Fig. 16), whereas pediatric patients with myelomeningocele are at risk for loculations and abscesses postrepair.[54] Cardiac surgery patients run the risk of developing infective endocarditis and septic emboli[55] although these have been minimized with adherence to aseptic techniques, antibiotic coverage, and careful monitoring for sepsis; the threshold to trigger neuroimaging should be low if infection is suspected in vulnerable populations.

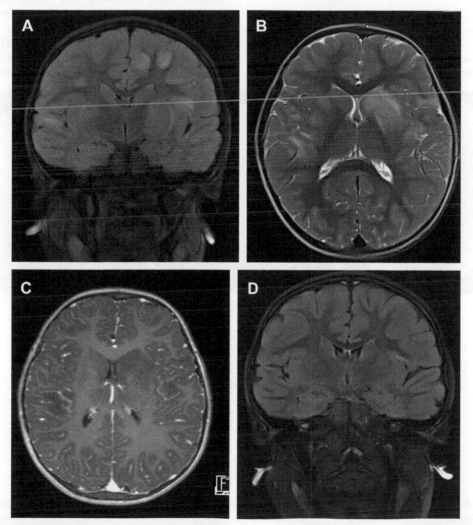

Fig. 17. Acute disseminated encephalomyelitis (ADEM) in a 3-year-old child with fever, vomiting, and seizures. Typical bilateral asymmetrical white matter T2 hyperintensities (A) with involvement of the left basal ganglia (B). There is slightly increased enhancement in the involved regions (C) with resolution of most of the white matter changes on MR imaging 2 months later (D).

Risk of opportunistic infections remains elevated for children with immune deficiency disease (congenital, acquired, or iatrogenic). Transplant patients, those on chemotherapy and those on long-term steroids have impaired immune system due to medication.[56] Sometimes, opportunistic infections are the first manifestation of unsuspected human immunodeficiency virus (HIV) infection,[57] although with optimized care, perinatal transmission of HIV can be curbed.[58] Fungal opportunistic infections in children have increased in the past decade, particularly Aspergillosis in children with hematological malignancies.[59] Organ transplantation, blood transfusion, transmission through breastfeeding have also been described as risk factors for CNS infection.[60]

IMMUNE-MEDIATED CHANGES ASSOCIATED WITH INFECTION

The human body's immune-mediated responses can also manifest in the CNS and result in tissue damage. ADEM is the most common immune-mediated encephalitis in early childhood, typically occurring 1 to 2 weeks after a nonspecific infection or vaccination, rather than directly from the infection itself.[61] Typical neuroimaging findings include asymmetric, bilateral, T2 hyperintensities in subcortical white matter and deep gray nuclei lesions in the brain, which can also be associated with long segment lesions in the spinal cord (Fig. 17). The term longitudinally extensive transverse myelitis (LETM) is used when the cord edema/inflammation spans more than 3 vertebral bodies, commonly seen in children with transverse myelitis as well as in children with ADEM with cord involvement.[62] However LETM is nonspecific because it can be seen a variety of pathologic conditions including infectious myelitis, cord infarction, and metabolic/genetic conditions.[63] Acute hemorrhagic leukoencephalopathy is thought to be an extreme form of ADEM[64] and is characterized by widespread hemorrhages in addition to the white matter changes in a rapidly deteriorating patient.[65]

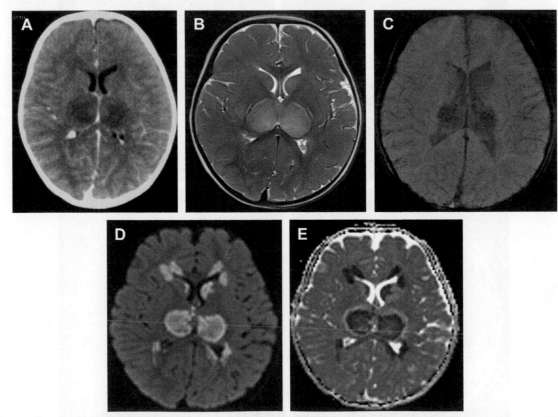

Fig. 18. Acute necrotizing encephalitis of childhood (ANEC) in a 1-year-old child with human herpes virus 6 (HHV6) infection and fluctuating consciousness. Both thalami are swollen and heterogeneously hypodense on CT (A). MR imaging shows corresponding T2 hyperintensities (B), with focal susceptibility suspicious for hemorrhage demonstrated on susceptibility-weighted images (C). DWI shows high signal in the bilateral caudate heads and bilateral periventricular white matter (D) with corresponding low signal on apparent diffusion coefficient map (E).

Acute necrotizing encephalopathy of childhood overwhelmingly affects young children in north Asia[66] with children presenting with acute encephalopathy postviral infection, including during the 2009 H1N1 influenza pandemic. Bilateral thalamic involvement is typical (Fig. 18), and these regions can be hemorrhagic or show cavitation.[67] Acute necrotizing encephalopathy score has been created and used to predict outcome in such patients.[68,69]

IMAGING MIMICS OF CENTRAL NERVOUS SYSTEM INFECTION

Neuroimaging patterns are helpful for the diagnosis of CNS infection but because similar abnormalities may be seen in a variety of other diseases, multidisciplinary collaboration is key to making a diagnosis. Multifocal intracranial calcifications in microcephalic infants (typical of TORCH infection) can also be caused by pseudo-TORCH syndrome, a rare autosomal recessive genetic disease,[70] and suspicion should be raised when TORCH screen is negative. This differential diagnosis is important because genetic counseling should be offered to the family. Intracranial calcifications can also be caused by other inborn errors of metabolism, such as basal ganglia calcification in Kearns Sayre syndrome and Aicardi Goutieres syndrome or dystrophic calcifications in the posterior cerebral hemispheres in chronic stage of X-linked adrenoleukodystrophy.[71] Hence, it is important to consider the anatomic distribution of intracranial calcifications.

Diffuse enhancement of the lumbosacral nerve roots and cauda equina mimicking infectious or malignant disease have been described in leukodystrophies such as Krabbe disease and metachromatic leukodystrophy.[72] Leptomeningeal thickening and enhancement can also be seen in neoplastic and infective causes but the presence of brain and systemic metastases may help support the former and isolation of an organism in the cerebrospinal fluid may support the latter. Ventriculitis may not always be due to infection because premature neonates are at risk of intraventricular hemorrhage and blood in the sterile cerebrospinal fluid can itself elicit ventricular inflammation (Fig. 19).

SUMMARY

Imaging has a vital role to play in the diagnosis of the extent of common pediatric CNS infection and their complications as well as in the monitoring of the patient's response to treatment. Radiologists should be aware of typical imaging features as well as the mimics of infection. Cranial ultrasound complements MR imaging and CT in babies with open fontanelles.

CLINICS CARE POINTS

- Imaging assists in localizing the sites of infection and monitoring response to treatment with cranial ultrasound able to supplement cross-sectional imaging in babies with open fontanelles.
- Infection encountered in the pediatric population is affected by endemicity of disease in the country, level of medical care available, and patient profile.

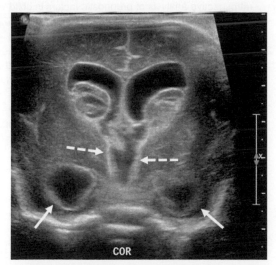

Fig. 19. Intraventricular hemorrhage-induced ventriculitis in a premature baby presenting with fever. Thickened enhancing ventricular margin of the temporal horns (arrows) and third ventricle (dotted arrows) on cranial ultrasound indicate ventriculitis. Both infection and bland, uninfected blood can cause this reaction. A helpful differentiating feature is that uninfected hemorrhage in premature babies usually occurs at the caudothalamic grooves. Ultimately, cerebrospinal fluid analysis is required to prove or exclude infection.

DISCLOSURE

The authors have nothing to disclose.

REFERENCES

1. Lim E, Rai E, Seow WT. Feasibility of anaesthetic provision for paediatric patients undergoing off-site intraoperative MRI-guided neurosurgery: the

Singapore experience from 2009 to 2012. Anaesth Intensive Care 2013;41:535–42.

2. John CC, Carabin H, Montano SM, et al. Global research priorities for infections that affect the nervous system. Nature 2015;527(7578):S178–86.

3. Banyard AC, Tordo N. Rabies pathogenesis and immunology. Rev Sci Tech 2018;37:323–30.

4. Fehlner-Gardiner C. Rabies control in North America - past, present and future. Rev Sci Tech 2018;37:421–37.

5. Anekwe TD, Newell ML, Tanser F, et al. The causal effect of childhood measles vaccination on educational attainment: A mother fixed-effects study in rural South Africa. Vaccine 2015;33:5020–6.

6. Parmar H, Ibrahim M. Pediatric Intracranial Infections. Neuroimag Clin N Am 2012;22:707–25.

7. Alamarat Z, Hasbun R. Management of Acute Bacterial Meningitis in Children. Infect Drug Resist 2020;13:4077–89.

8. Tang PH, Lim CC. Imaging of accidental paediatric head trauma. Pediatr Radiol 2009;39:438–46.

9. Messacar K, Fischer M, Dominguez SR, et al. Encephalitis in US Children. Infect Dis Clin North Am 2018;32:145–62.

10. Sum MY, Ong YZ, Low SXK, et al. Using a checklist to assess if child undergoing MRI needs general anaesthesia. Clin Radiol 2019;74:488.e17–23.

11. Ong YZ, Saffari SE, Tang PH. Prospective randomised controlled trial on the effect of videos on the cooperativeness of children undergoing MRI and their requirement for general anaesthesia. Clin Radiol 2018;73:909.e15–24.

12. Ahamed SH, Lee KJ, Tang PH. Role of a modified ultrafast MRI brain protocol in clinical paediatric neuroimaging. Clin Radiol 2020;75:914–20.

13. van Beek EJR, Kuhl C, Anzai Y, et al. Value of MRI in medicine: More than just another test? J Magn Reson Imaging 2019;49:e14–25.

14. Dorsett M, Liang SY. Diagnosis and Treatment of Central Nervous System Infections in the Emergency Department. Emerg Med Clin North Am 2016;34:917–42.

15. Ford-Jones EL. An approach to the diagnosis of congenital infections. Paediatr Child Health 1999;4:109–12.

16. Koeller KK, Shih RY. Viral and Prion Infections of the Central Nervous System: Radiologic-Pathologic Correlation: From the Radiologic Pathology Archives. RadioGraphics 2017;37:199–233.

17. Eckert N, Spicher VM. Chickenpox and shingles: one virus, two diseases and current vaccination recommendations in Switzerland. Ther Umsch 2016;73:247–52.

18. Helfgott A. TORCH testing in HIV-infected women. Clin Obstet Gynecol 1999;42:149–62.

19. Madjunkov M, Chaudhry S, Ito S. Listeriosis during pregnancy. Arch Gynecol Obstet 2017;296:143–52.

20. de Araújo TVB, Ximenes RAA, Miranda-Filho DB, et al. Association between microcephaly, Zika virus infection, and other risk factors in Brazil: final report of a case-control study. Lancet Infect Dis 2018;18:328–36.

21. Honein MA, Dawson AL, Petersen EE, et al. Birth Defects Among Fetuses and Infants of US Women With Evidence of Possible Zika Virus Infection During Pregnancy. JAMA 2017;317:59–68.

22. Baud D, Gubler DJ, Schaub B, et al. An update on Zika virus infection. Lancet 2017;390:2099–109.

23. Hu T, Li J, Carr MJ, et al. The Asian Lineage of Zika Virus: Transmission and Evolution in Asia and the America. Virol Sin 2019;34:1–8.

24. Hayes K, O'Halloran F, Cotter. A review of antibiotic resistance in Group B Streptococcus: the story so far. Crit Rev Microbio 2020;46:253–69.

25. Choi SY, Kim J, Ko JW, et al. Patterns of ischaemic injury on brain images in neonatal group B Streptococcal meningitis. Korean J Pediatr 2018;61:245–52.

26. Kralik SF, Kukreja MK, Paldino MJ, et al. Comparison of CSF and MRI Findings among Neonates and Infants with E coli or Group B Streptococcal Meningitis. AJNR Am J Neuroradiol 2019;40:1413–7.

27. Archibald LK, Quisling RG. Central Nervous System Infections. Textbook of Neurointensive Care 2013;427–517.

28. Wee LY, Tanugroho RR, Thoon KC, et al. A 15-year retrospective analysis of prognostic factors in childhood bacterial meningitis. Acta Paediatr 2016;105:e22–9.

29. Hasbun R, Wootton SH, Rosenthal N, et al. Epidemiology of Meningitis and Encephalitis in Infants and Children in the United States, 2011-2014. Pediatr Infect Dis J 2019;38:37–41.

30. Erickson TA, Munoz FM, Troisi CL, et al. The Epidemiology of Meningitis in Infants under 90 Days of Age in a Large Pediatric Hospital. Microorganisms 2021;9:526.

31. Minor P. The polio endgame. Hum Vaccin Immunother 2014;10:2106–8.

32. Murphy OC, Messacar K, Benson L, et al. Acute flaccid myelitis: cause, diagnosis, and management. Lancet 2021;397334–46.

33. Malzberg MS, Rogg JM, Tate CA, et al. Poliomyelitis: hyperintensity of the anterior horn cells on MR images of the spinal cord. AJR Am J Roentgenol 1993;161:863–5.

34. Grill MF. Infect Myelopathies. Continuum (Minneap Minn) 2018;24:441–73.

35. Koh WM, Bogich T, Siegel K, et al. The Epidemiology of Hand, Foot and Mouth Disease in Asia: A Systematic Review and Analysis. Pediatr Infect Dis J 2016;35:e285–300.

36. Xia F, Deng F, Tian H, et al. Estimation of the reproduction number and identification of periodicity for

HFMD infections in northwest China. J Theor Biol 2020;484:110027.

37. Lim CT, Jiang L, Ma S, et al. Basic reproduction number of coxsackievirus type A6 and A16 and enterovirus 71: estimates from outbreaks of hand, foot and mouth disease in Singapore, a tropical city-state. Epidemiol Infect 2016;144:1028–34.
38. Kim KH. Enterovirus 71 infection: An experience in Korea. Korean J Pediatr 2009;53:616–22.
39. Siegel K, Cook AR, La H. The impact of hand, foot and mouth disease control policies in Singapore: A qualitative analysis of public perceptions. J Public Health Policy 2017;38:271–87.
40. Li H, Su L, Zhang T, et al. MRI reveals segmental distribution of enterovirus lesions in the central nervous system: a probable clinical evidence of retrograde axonal transport of EV-A71. J Neurovirol 2019;25:354–62.
41. Wang SM, Lei HY, Su LY, et al. Cerebrospinal fluid cytokines in enterovirus 71 brain stem encephalitis and echovirus meningitis infections of varying severity. Clin Microbiol Infect 2007;13:677–82.
42. Lee KY. Enterovirus 71 infection and neurological complications. Korean J Pediatr 2016;59:395–401.
43. Lee KY, Lee MS, Kim DB. Neurologic Manifestations of Enterovirus 71 Infection in Korea. J Korean Med Sci 2016;31:561–7.
44. Gonzalez G, Carr MJ, Kobayashi M, et al. Enterovirus-Associated Hand-Foot and Mouth Disease and Neurological Complications in Japan and the Rest of the World. Int J Mol Sci 2019;20:5201.
45. Chang L, Huang L, Gau SS, et al. Neurodevelopment and cognition in children after enterovirus 71 infection. N Engl J Med 2007;356:1226–34.
46. Jones R, Kulkarni MA, Davidson TMV, RADAM-LAC Research Team, Talbot B. Arbovirus vectors of epidemiological concern in the Americas: A scoping review of entomological studies on Zika, dengue and chikungunya virus vectors. PLoS One 2020;15:e0220753.
47. Corrêa DG, Freddi TAL, Werner H, et al. Brain MR Imaging of Patients with Perinatal Chikungunya Virus Infection. AJNR Am J Neuroradiol 2020;41:174–7.
48. Li GH, Ning ZJ, Liu YM, et al. Neurological Manifestations of Dengue Infection. Front Cell Infect Microbiol 2017;7:449.
49. Prerna A, Lim JY, Tan NW, et al. Neurology of the H1N1 pandemic in Singapore: a nationwide case series of children and adults. J Neurovirol 2015;21:491–9.
50. Chougar L, Shor N, Weiss N, et al. Retrospective Observational Study of Brain MRI Findings in Patients with Acute SARS-CoV-2 Infection and Neurologic Manifestations. Radiology 2020;297:E313–23.
51. Sa M, Mirza L, Carter M, et al. Systemic Inflammation Is Associated With Neurologic Involvement in Pediatric Inflammatory Multisystem Syndrome

Associated With SARS-CoV-2. Neurol Neuroimmunol Neuroinflamm 2021;8:e999.
52. de Jesús Vargas-Lares J, Andrade-Aguilera AR, Díaz-Peña R, et al. Risk factors associated with bacterial growth in derivative systems from cerebrospinal liquid in pediatric patients. Gac Med Mex 2015;151:749–56.
53. Caceres A, Avila ML, Herrera ML. Fungal infections in pediatric neurosurgery. Childs Nerv Syst 2018;34:1973–88.
54. Anegbe AO, Shokunbi MT, Oyemolade TA, et al. Intracranial infection in patients with myelomeningocele: profile and risk factors. Childs Nerv Syst 2019;35:2205–10.
55. Krcméry V, Fedor-Freybergh PG. Neuroinfections in developed versus developing countries. Neuro Endocrinol Lett 2007;28:5–6.
56. Ren Z, Laumann AE, Silverberg JI. Association of dermatomyositis with systemic and opportunistic infections in the United States. Arch Dermatol Res 2019;311:377–87.
57. Abbasi Fard S, Khajeh A, Khosravi A, et al. Fulminant and Diffuse Cerebral Toxoplasmosis as the First Manifestation of HIV Infection: A Case Presentation and Review of the Literature. Am J Case Rep 2020;21:e919624.
58. Loh M, Thoon KC, Mathur M, et al. Management of HIV-positive pregnant women: a Singapore experience. Singapore Med J 2020 https://doi.org/10.11622/smedj.2020048.
59. Luckowitsch M, Rudolph H, Bochennek K, et al. Central Nervous System Mold Infections in Children with Hematological Malignancies: Advances in Diagnosis and Treatment. J Fungi (Basel) 2021;7:168.
60. Sampathkumar P. West Nile virus: epidemiology, clinical presentation, diagnosis, and prevention. Mayo Clin Proc 2003;78:1137–43.
61. Esposito S, Di Pietro GM, Madini B, et al. A spectrum of inflammation and demyelination in acute disseminated encephalomyelitis (ADEM) of children. Autoimmun Rev 2015;14:923–9.
62. Yiu EM, Kornberg AJ, Ryan MM, et al. Acute transverse myelitis and acute disseminated encephalomyelitis in childhood: spectrum or separate entities? J Child Neurol 2009;24:287–96.
63. Sorte DE, Poretti A, Newsome SD, et al. Longitudinally extensive myelopathy in children. Pediatr Radiol 2015;45:244–57.
64. Lann MA, Lovell MA, Kleinschmidt-DeMasters BK. Acute hemorrhagic leukoencephalitis: a critical entity for forensic pathologists to recognize. Am J Forensic Med Pathol 2010;31:7–11.
65. Varadan B, Shankar A, Rajakumar A, et al. Acute hemorrhagic leukoencephalitis in a COVID-19 patient-a case report with literature review. Neuroradiology 2021;63:653–61.

66. Ormitti F, Ventura E, Summa A, et al. Acute necrotizing encephalopathy in a child during the 2009 influenza A(H1N1) pandemia: MR imaging in diagnosis and follow-up. AJNR Am J Neuroradiol 2010; 31:396–400.

67. Wong AM, Simon EM, Zimmerman RA, et al. Acute necrotizing encephalopathy of childhood: correlation of MR findings and clinical outcome. AJNR Am J Neuroradiol 2006;27:1919–23.

68. Yamamoto H, Okumura A, Natsume J, et al. A severity score for acute necrotizing encephalopathy. Brain Dev 2015;37:322–7.

69. Lim HY, Ho VP, Lim TC, et al. Serial outcomes in acute necrotising encephalopathy of childhood: A

medium and long term study. Brain Dev 2016;38: 928–36.

70. Vivarelli R, Grosso S, Cioni M, et al. Pseudo-TORCH syndrome or Baraitser-Reardon syndrome: diagnostic criteria. Brain Dev 2001;23:18–23.

71. Biswas A, Malhotra M, Mankad K, et al. Clinico-radiological phenotyping and diagnostic pathways in childhood neurometabolic disorders-a practical introductory guide. Transl Pediatr 2021; 10:1201–30.

72. Tabarki B, Hakami W, Alkhuraish N, et al. Spinal Cord Involvement in Pediatric-Onset Metabolic Disorders With Mendelian and Mitochondrial Inheritance. Front Pediatr 2021;8:599861.

Beyond Pattern Recognition
Radiology-Pathology-Clinical Correlation

Kum Thong Wong, MBBS, MPath, FRACPath, MD[c],
Chong Tin Tan, MBBS, FRCP, MD[a], Tchoyoson Lim, MBBS, MMed[b],*

KEYWORDS

• Central nervous system • Infection • Pathogenesis • Inflammation • Immune-mediated
• Neurotropism

KEY POINTS

• Understanding the correlation between radiologic (macroscopic brain abnormalities) and pathologic (microscopic inflammatory and immunologic response) is essential for diagnoses, prognosis, and recognizing the spectrum and mechanism of central nervous system (CNS) infectious disease.
• Typically, bacteria and fungi cause acute inflammatory cellular responses, whereas viruses and immunocompromised patients tend to be associated with more diffuse or less intense response.
• Microbiological investigations of the blood and cerebrospinal fluid (CSF), including immunohistochemistry and in situ hybridization, can supplement invasive biopsy.
• Antemortem vascular complications are increasingly recognized as important contributors of CNS damage, as well as maladapted immunologic response and other secondary changes.
• Pathogenetic mechanisms and neurotropism affect anatomic predilection and pathways of spread have important effects on imaging patterns and MR imaging signal intensity; radiologists should combine clinical, pathologic data with imaging patterns to improve differential diagnoses.

INTRODUCTION TO CNS INFECTION PATHOLOGY

Radiologic pathology correlation is an important component of diagnostic radiology training: only by understanding the pathologic basis of disease, can the radiologic appearance and spectrum of disease be recognized. By combining this understanding of pathologic findings with clinical data and imaging features, clinical interpretation, differential diagnoses, and prognosis can be improved.[1] In addition to macroscopic brain abnormalities, an appreciation of the stereotypical microscopic inflammatory response to most pathogens that is common to all parts of the body, forms an important basis for understanding radiological images.

Cellular Responses to Infection Visible on Histologic Examination

In early CNS infection (first few hours or days), vascular congestion and increased permeability results in interstitial edema and parenchymal infiltration of short-lived, blood-derived neutrophils. This is followed by macrophages, lymphocytes, and plasma cells from the systemic circulation after days to 2 weeks. Thus, pathologists often regard the presence of neutrophils as suggesting an acute inflammation in CNS infections.

Perivascular cuffing represents activated leukocytes (neutrophils, macrophages, T and B lymphocytes) migrating from blood vessels as part of the systemic immune response, and is another feature characteristic of CNS infection (Fig. 1A).

[a] Department of Medicine, University of Malaya, Kuala Lumpur, Malaysia; [b] Neuroradiology, National Neuroscience Institute, Singapore; [c] Department of Pathology, Faculty of Medicine, University of Malaya, Kuala Lumpur, Malaysia
* Corresponding author.
E-mail address: tchoyoson@gmail.com

Neuroimag Clin N Am 33 (2023) 225–233
https://doi.org/10.1016/j.nic.2022.07.018
1052-5149/23/© 2022 Elsevier Inc. All rights reserved.

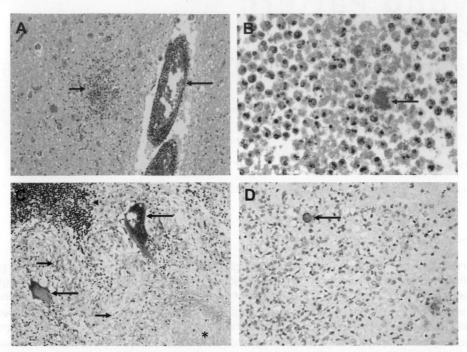

Fig. 1. *A*). Parenchymal inflammation in Enterovirus A71 encephalomyelitis showing typical features of viral encephalitis with perivascular cuffing by inflammatory cells (long *arrow*) and microglial nodule formation (short *arrow*). (*B*). In an abscess, numerous inflammatory cells consisting mainly of neutrophils and other inflammatory cells and cellular debris, often surrounding a bacterial cluster (*arrow*). (*C*) Granulomatous inflammation in tuberculosis with central necrosis (*) and surrounding multinucleated giant cells (long *arrows*), pale staining macrophages and epithelioid cells (short *arrows*) and dark staining lymphocytes at the periphery (*arrowhead*). (*D*) Cerebral toxoplasmosis with toxoplasma cyst (*arrow*) and free zoites stained brown by immunohistochemistry. Background inflammatory cells can be clearly visualized. (*A–C*): Hematoxylin and eosin stain; (*D*) Immunohistochemistry/methylene blue to detect toxoplasmal antigens.

CNS-resident microglia also proliferate, and microglial nodules are common (see Fig. 1A). Neuronophagia is a term used for phagocytosis of degenerating or necrotic neurons mainly by microglia/macrophages. It may be observed within a microglial nodule.

Encephalitis is inflammation involving the brain parenchyma, whereas leptomeningitis is inflammation of the pia–arachnoid layers. Although inflammation may be confined, often meningoencephalitis is present. Myelitis refers to spinal cord parenchymal inflammation; hence, encephalomyelitis and meningoencephalomyelitis would mean widespread inflammation of CNS parenchyma and meninges, respectively.

An abscess is a localized collection of pus cells (more neutrophils than other inflammatory cells, exudate, and cellular debris from dead cells (Fig. 1B). Older abscesses may become more circumscribed with formation of a "wall" consisting of an outer rim of fibrosis and astrogliosis. Tuberculous, fungal, or foreign body granulomata comprise circumscribed collections of mainly macrophages, epithelioid cells (spindle-shaped

macrophages resembling epithelial cells) and multinucleated giant cells (Fig. 1C). Central caseous necrosis is classically seen in mycobacterial infection but is not unique to tuberculosis; MR imaging, especially magnetization transfer imaging, may be helpful to distinguish tuberculous granuloma from pyogenic abscess, even though there is some overlap. At the periphery of granulomata, lymphocytes and plasma cells are often observed, and there is often reactive astrogliosis, part of the reparative process. In more chronic lesions or extensive parenchymal loss, astrogliosis is accompanied by new blood vessel formation (angioneogenesis). Perfusion-weighted imaging may be helpful to distinguish the walls of abscesses from necrotic brain tumor, which have significantly higher relative cerebral blood volume reflecting greater neoangiogenesis in tumors, although there is some overlap.[2,3]

Compared with bacterial and fungal infection, typical acute viral infection tends to cause more diffuse and widespread encephalitic inflammation rather than focal abscess or granuloma, especially in the late stages. Rabies encephalitis may not show much inflammation as detected by imaging studies even when the CNS is extensively involved; this correlates with the pathologic condition in rabies autopsies where inflammation is a late-stage or terminal event.[4] Inflammatory changes may be much reduced or even absent in the immunocompromised, such as AIDS or patients treated with steroids or chemotherapy, even though numerous viruses may be present; West Nile encephalitis also typically shows mild or absent inflammatory reaction.[5]

Antemortem thrombosis within a relatively intact blood vessel causes blood flow obstruction, ischemia, and tissue infarction downstream: this constitutes Virchow triad of abnormalities in vessel wall (eg, infectious vasculitis), blood flow (eg, stasis, dehydration), and blood constituents (eg, thrombophilia). In arteries, perhaps vascular wall abnormalities are commoner, whereas blood stasis probably predominates in veins.

Biopsy and CSF Microscopic Features

Compared with in-toto resection in other parts of the body, CNS biopsies by necessity yield small samples and therefore may not be representative of the pathologic lesion. Nevertheless, light microscopy may identify the likely pathogen based on the type of inflammation observed; for example, tuberculous granulomatous inflammation could suggest tuberculosis or fungal infection. This information would be lost if precious small biopsy tissues are sent to the laboratory solely for molecular testing and culture. The aim of pathogen identification is to be able to visualize bacteria, fungi, and viruses from tissue biopsy or exceptionally from even CSF and blood samples by light microscopy, immunohistochemistry, in situ hybridization (ISH), and electron microscopy. Direct CSF microscopy after staining preparations for *Cryptococcus* (combined with India ink) and *Mycobacterium tuberculosis* (Ziehl–Neelsen stain) are classic methods but suffer from low sensitivity.

Microbiological Investigations

Indirect and less invasive tests following microbial exposure take advantage of the normal antibody immune response in the body: an increasing serum IgM level as an initial response followed by increasing serum IgG levels days/weeks after that. IgM levels tend to decline after a few weeks/months, and hence, the presence of IgM is often used as a marker of recent infection. A 4-fold increase of IgG levels in paired sera, taken at the early stages of infection and about 2 weeks postinfection, is often used as an evidence of recent infection. The IgM/IgG levels

in the CSF also follow the same pattern on neuroinvasion.

Although the technology has been around for some time, immunohistochemistry (IHC) to detect pathogens has advanced identification of CNS infections tremendously. Typically, specific primary (either commercially available or produced in-house) antibodies are used to attach to the targeted microbial antigens. This antibody–antigen complex is then detected by a second antibody. An enzyme linked to this second antibody gives a color change after a substrate is added as a final step. The infected cells/tissue is then visualized with a light microscope with which is the surrounding inflammatory reaction can also be observed (Fig. 1D).

A more recent innovation that detects nucleotide sequences (present in the pathogen genome) uses a probe that can hybridize with specific genomic sequences in the tissues. This is called ISH. Similar to IHC, the presence of a pathogen is detected, and visualized with a light microscope after a series of reaction steps to provide a positive signal. The key difference between IHC and ISH is that IHC uses a specific primary antibody but ISH uses a probe that comprises specific nucleotide sequence that can complement and hybridize with part of the pathogen's genome. Similar to IHC, the advantage of ISH is being able to visualize the pathogen in the context of its targeted cell/tissue and the surrounding inflammation.

Genomic detection of pathogens in serum, CSF, or tissues represents a major advance for diagnosis. This was revolutionized by the discovery of the polymerase chain reaction (PCR) to amplify nucleotide sequences has revolutionized pathogen detection and discovery. Recently developed targeted gene panels and next-generation sequencing techniques have further improved and refined pathogen discovery samples extracted from serum, CSF, fresh and formalin-fixed biopsy tissue. In tuberculosis, molecular testing has further improved diagnostic yields in the CSF.[6] Although PCR can amplify tiny amounts of genomic material, its extreme sensitivity can sometimes lead to false-positive results.

For small biopsy samples, the other drawback is that it is not possible to know the cellular/tissue localization of the pathogen and the nature of the reactive inflammation (if any) that IHC and ISH are able to provide.[7]

Neurotropic Pathogens and Tissues of Involvement

Table 1 shows the common anatomic involvement and typical pathogens and pathogenetic mechanisms that can be inferred from neuroimaging of

Table 1
Common anatomic abnormalities and typical causes that can be inferred on neuroimaging of CNS infections

Tissue Involved on Neuroimaging	Common Inference(s)
Contiguous scalp, sinus, mastoid bone, epidural and subdural infection	Bacteria (especially Melioidosis),[35] complicating sinusitis or suppurate otitis media
Spinal vertebral body and adjacent epidural infection	Bacteria (especially tuberculosis)
Leptomeninges: base of brain	Tuberculosis, cryptococcus
Leptomeninges: over cortical surface, other than base of brain	Bacteria, fungi, viruses
Nerve root enhancement	Rabies virus, EV71 virus, Guillian-Barre disease, metastatic cancer
Olfactory bulb	Coronaviruses[36,37]
Gray matter cortex	Viruses, bacteria, autoimmune encephalitis
Gray matter cortex: temporal/frontal lobe	Herpes simplex virus
Bilateral thalamus	Japanese encephalitis, dengue, and other neurotropic flaviviruses
Cerebral white matter	JC virus (progressive multifocal leukoencephalopathy), measles virus (subacute sclerosing panencephalitis), postinfectious autoimmune demyelination
Rhombencephalus: pons & medulla	EV-A71 and other neurotropic enteroviruses, listeria monocytogenes
Large artery occlusion	Group B streptococcus in neonates, varicella virus in children, tuberculosis, SARS-CoV-1 and SARS-CoV-2 at all ages
Small artery occlusion	Aspergillus, varicella and Nipah viruses, *Rickettsia*, Group B Streptococcus
Hydrocephalus	Tuberculosis, cryptococcus

CNS infections. Aside from direct traumatic implantation or local spread, neuroinvasion is related to the ability of pathogens to travel up peripheral/cranial nerves or to cross the blood–brain barrier (BBB) hematogenously. Neurotropism refers to the ability of viruses, bacteria, fungi, and parasites to invade nervous tissue; neuronotropism is a predilection for invading neurons, especially viruses such as rabies, the herpes family, vector-borne flaviviruses, and enteroviruses.

Neurotropic anatomic predilection and preferred pathways for neuroinvasion have important effects on the topography observed on neuroimaging, with typical viral involvement of lobar cortical gray matter, deep nuclei, cerebellum, brainstem, and spinal cord. For example, herpes simplex virus enters the olfactory bulb transnasally, up the olfactory tract to involve the limbic system (including cingulate gyrus) and the temporal lobe/s. MR imaging abnormalities in fatal Enterovirus 71 infection involves the spinal cord anterior horn, dorsal brainstem, and cerebellar dentate nucleus, which correlated well with severe inflammation and viral antigens/

RNA in autopsy tissues[8] and animal models.[9] These findings support the hypothesis that viruses spread retrogradely via motor peripheral nerves (both spinal and cranial), resulting in intense inflammation/infection in spinal cord anterior horn motor neurons and brainstem motor nuclei in pontine tegmentum, often sparing the nonmotor anterior pons. A few recent MR imaging studies that demonstrated ventral root involvement where motor nerves originate have helped support this hypothesis.[10] Enterovirus D68, a recently emerging encephalitis, also showed the same CNS MR imaging findings as Enterovirus A71, involving spinal cord anterior horns in patients with acute flaccid paralysis similar to poliomyelitis.[11]

Early human Japanese encephalitis is associated with thalamic involvement on MR imaging, suggesting possible peripheral sensory nerve involvement in neuroinvasion. A recent footpad-inoculated mouse model developed to mimic mosquito bites showed early thalamic involvement giving support to this hypothesis that neuroinvasion may be via cutaneous sensory nerve endings may occur. However, peripheral nerve involvement has not been demonstrated by MR imaging so far.[12]

Viruses may alternatively invade other CNS cells such as glia (eg, JC virus, rabies) and blood vessels (eg, henipavirus, varicella zoster virus). Bacterial, fungal, and parasitic infections generally do not have a predilection for a particular neuroglial cell or endothelium. However, some fungi (eg, *Aspergillus)* have a tendency to be angioinvasive. Vascular involvement with thrombo-occlusion following henipavirus, rickettsia, tuberculosis, and varicella zoster virus infections may be associated with parenchymal infarction ranging from small infarcts to larger territorial infarcts.[13]

The Interplay Between Infective Agent and Immunologic Response

Traditionally, 3 "lines of defense" define our immunity system. The first (barrier defense eg, skin, mucous membranes) and second (neutrophil, macrophage, eosinophil, basophil, interferons, complement proteins) lines of defense are nonspecific for pathogens and are referred to as innate immunity. The third line of defense (T and B lymphocytes, antibodies) is a pathogen-specific immunity and is called acquired or adaptive immunity. Within the CNS, innate immunity comprises dendritic cells (a type of antigen-presenting cell [APC]), macrophages and neutrophils. Using pattern recognition receptors (PRR), these cells can recognize groups of pathogens by pathogen-associated molecular patterns (PAMP) and trigger a nonspecific immune response.

The various types of PRRs include toll-like receptors, nucleotide-binding oligomerization domain-like receptors, C-type lectin receptors, and RIG-1-like receptors.[14] These receptors can recognize both extracellular microorganisms (such as bacteria and fungi) and viruses within the cell cytoplasm. Examples of PAMP are bacterial flagellin and lipopolysaccharide and viral nucleic acids (upon PRR activation, neutrophil, macrophage nuclei activate genes that lead to a response cascade resulting in phagocytosis, proinflammatory cytokines, and antiviral interferon production). These responses are generally beneficial to the human host but overproduction of cytokines and other mediators may lead to a "cytokine storm" in certain infections, for example, COVID-19.

Acquired immunity as a direct response to specific pathogens generally require a longer time to be activated. In general, this response is similarly facilitated by peripheral APC (dendritic cells, macrophages) when parts of the phagocytosed microbe is presented on the cell surface as antigens. T helper (TH) or CD4-positive lymphocyte (the most important cell in acquired immunity system) interacts with the APC leading to TH1, TH2, and TH17 responses, from 3 different cell lineages. TH1 response involves the production of factors to stimulate cellular immune response, including activating cytotoxic T cells (a different subset of T lymphocytes from TH cells) to eliminate infected cells. Secreted cytokines include interferon γ, interleukin 2 and 3, tumor necrosis factor. Interleukin 12 produced by macrophages plays an important role in TH1 cell survival and growth. The TH2 response involves humoral immune response leading to specific antibody production to neutralize microbes. Secreted cytokines include interleukins 4, 5, 9, 10, and 13. Interleukin 4 is especially important for its role in antibody synthesis, whereas interleukin 10 is a key immunoregulator for infections with anti-inflammatory properties that reduce excessive TH1 responses. TH17-associated cytokines activate neutrophils and help with extracellular bacteria clearance.

Acute disseminated encephalomyelitis (ADEM) and Guillain Barre syndrome are thought to be due to molecular mimicry whereby cross-reacting antibodies that develop after an infection cause damage to myelin sheath surrounding axons resulting in abnormal axonal transmissions and so forth.

Secondary Changes after CNS Infection and other Mechanisms of Injury

In the context of care for the CNS infection patients, where there may be various surgical procedures performed, clinicians should be aware of the iatrogenic imaging changes that are commonly seen, including pneumocephalus, hemorrhage, brain shift, and diffuse pachymeningeal enhancement from intracranial hypotension caused by CSF drains. There are also several imaging changes seen in the context of infectious diseases, which are secondary to immune-mediated or unknown processes, rather than specific effects of the pathogen. Examples include reversible splenial lesions, posterior reversible encephalopathy syndrome, changes secondary to status epilepticus. These features can be difficult to distinguish from the direct effects of the primary infection.[15] However, entities such as sepsis-associated encephalopathy in severely ill patients, toxin-induced neurologic disorders, and CNS infection with minimal gross changes on postmortem brain pathologic condition are active areas of pathologic research; these are often poorly described in the imaging literature.

FROM IMAGES TO PATHOGENESIS

Inferring the pathogenesis and mechanisms of CNS injury from imaging features is important for clinical reasoning and treatment decisions; however, there exists a significant knowledge gap in the primary scientific data in radiology-pathology correlation of CNS infections. Radiologists can add value to clinical reasoning by recognizing the patterns of abnormal imaging features such as CT density, MR imaging signal intensity, combined with localizing the anatomic extent of tissue of involvement. Although this is an important first step, it would be even more helpful if the radiologist can guide the clinician's hypotheses by examining clues to the pathogenesis derived from images, and not merely recognize patterns from classic images of some specific CNS infections.

Mode of Spread

At times, the images may allow diagnosticians to infer the mode of spread, an important first step to understand the underlying pathogenesis. Classically, a new or expanding lesion located adjacent to an existing abnormality suggests direct spread, such as cerebritis or abscess from leptomeningitis, dural breach, and abscess located close to infectious sinusitis and mastoiditis (see Table 1). New CNS symptoms in patients with known associations and risk factors should increase the pretest probability (and lower the threshold for initiating CT/MR imaging studies). However, imaging abnormalities as first presentation of CNS disease often triggers a clinical and radiological search for a systemic source for infection.[16,17] These associations include preexistent hematogenous disease such as bacteremia, bacterial endocarditis, right-to-left cardiac shunt, systemic lesions such as pulmonary tuberculosis or cryptococcoma or spinal tuberculous spondylitis.

Other lesser known and less certain modes of spread include cryptococcus spreading from the basal cisterns through the Virchow-Robin spaces to affect the basal ganglia and thalamus, and cryptococcal meningitis spreading via CSF resulting in radiculopathy.[18] *Burkholderia pseudomallei* may spreading along the trigeminal nerve, over long distances along commissural and projection white matter tracts, including the corpus callosum, corticospinal tract, and cerebellar peduncle.[19,20] Longitudinal studies such as these, with the benefit of multiple imaging abnormalities detected at different time points, often help establish increasing involvement and modes of spread; nevertheless, even cross-sectional studies may help suggest possible mechanisms based on CNS infection radiologic-pathology knowledge.

Pathogenesis, Complications, and Refining Differential Diagnoses

Modern MR imaging, with its multiple acquisitions of different tissue contrast, can often help to elucidate the pathogenesis or complication of the CNS abnormalities associated with infection, refining the likelihood of diagnosis and infer causative organisms. The followings are some specific examples.

First, imaging may help to confirm the relatively benign uncomplicated aseptic (viral) meningitis. In aseptic meningitis, there is little or minimal leptomeningeal enhancement and no signal abnormalities in the brain. However, in septic meningoencephalitis from bacterial or fungal infection, there is both leptomeningeal enhancement and adjacent brain abnormalities. In encephalitis, the imaging changes are primarily in the brain substance.[21]

Second, imaging is able to detect and often differentiate the various process of inflammation, including blood–brain barrier breakdown, cerebral edema, necrosis and formation of brain abscess capsules, and hemorrhagic complications.

Third, the imaging may detect vascular complications. A well-known example would be cerebral infarction of the basal ganglia or thalamus caused by basal leptomeningeal inflammation and occlusion of penetrating arteries associated with in tuberculous meningitis.[22] In Nipah encephalitis, the disseminated small discrete lesions detected on diffusion-weighted MR imaging, probably resulted from infarction following vasculitis-induced thrombosis and occlusion of arterioles.[23,24] This pattern is likely different from the larger contiguous "geographic" lesion seen in relapsed Nipah encephalitis with focal cerebritis.[25] In cerebral malaria, MR imaging lesions may be the result of ischemia from parasitized red blood cell sequestration in brain capillaries, leading to impaired perfusion.[26] Finally, severe acute respiratory caused by the SARS-CoV-1 virus was associated with fatal large artery territory cerebral infarction, some with hemorrhagic conversion.[27] The rich literature on infectious vasculitis and ischemia associated with CNS infection is one of the reasons for the interest in large vessel infarction and other complications in the current COVID-19 pandemic.[28]

Fourth, hydrocephalus complicating meningitis implies tuberculous or cryptococcal infection (and rarely metastatic brain tumor), usually indicating obstruction to the foramina of Magendie and Luschka. However, obstructive hydrocephalus is unusual in viral meningoencephalitis or autoimmune encephalitis.[21,29]

Fifth, disseminated multifocal discrete lesions suggests systemic involvement at some point in the pathogenesis, for instance multiple abscesses from disseminated bacterial endocarditis. However, a single abscess may still be from systemic involvement but localized infection should be sought such as adjacent paranasal sinusitis or mastoiditis.

Sixth, the appearance of cerebral cyst with intracystic nodule, different stages of the enhancing wall and adjacent cerebral edema, allow inference of the different stages of acute inflammation induced by antigens released from the dying neurocysticercosis, based on characteristic imaging patterns.[30]

Normal Imaging or Near-normal Imaging in encephalitis

In practice, it is common to find severe clinical encephalitic illness, with grossly abnormal electroencephalogram (EEG) indicating diffuse brain abnormality, yet neuroimaging may be normal or show minimal changes only. How does one understand this enormous clinical-radiology corelation gap, and the underlying pathogenesis?

First, when the pathologic condition is limited to the brainstem (especially the medulla oblongata) rather than the cerebral hemispheres, brain imaging may be relatively normal. In acute Nipah virus encephalitis, the multifocal disseminated, small, infarcts caused by infectious arteritis do not correspond with high mortality, and direct neuronal infection and viral cytolysis in the brainstem could not be detected on brain imaging.[31] Second, the imaging changes tend to be more easily visible when there is more intense localized inflammation; such as breakdown of BBB, necrosis, infarction, vasculitis, edema, hemorrhage, or abscess formation. However, if widespread but mild encephalitis is confined to the cellular microstructural level, the stereotypical inflammatory changes widely described in this article and elsewhere may not be detected on MR imaging. Examples include sepsis-associated encephalopathy, wherein damage caused by proinflammatory cytokines and glutamate secreted by the microglia, would be invisible on neuroimaging.[32] Thus, in viral encephalitis, it is the variable intensity of inflammatory response by the host to the virus, rather than the virus itself, that is the core of pathophysiological change in CNS viral infections. Neuroimaging assists in documenting the extent of this inflammation but still cannot predict or prognosticate final neurologic deficit that can be caused by MR imaging-invisible cellular damage.[33]

We may also compare with other pathologic conditions that are also known to have significant clinical-radiology gap. These include metabolic diseases such as hypoglycemia and hyperglycemia,

some autoimmune encephalitidis, degenerative and psychiatric diseases, where late-stage neuronal loss is reflected only as nonspecific cerebral atrophy on imaging.[34] In CNS infection, normal or near-normal neuroimaging in the presence of severe clinical disease suggests that the pathologic condition is probably at the microstructural and cellular level, with relative lack of intense inflammation, blood–brain barrier breakdown, edema, infarction, or hemorrhage. Although MR imaging is sensitive to detect inflammation, it is still limited, and there are other noninflammatory processes that imaging cannot yet detect.

SUMMARY

Although CNS infection has varied etiology, radiologic pathology correlation can help understanding of the imaging features, especially when inflammatory processes are well developed. Despite the high sensitivity of multiparametric MR imaging, there are instances where there is disconnect between the clinical and radiological images. Although clinician radiologists should be familiar with the classic imaging patterns of infection, we should also ask how the images may help in the understanding of the underlying pathogenesis. By combining pathologic and clinical data with imaging features, clinical interpretation, differential diagnoses, and prognosis can be improved.

CLINICS CARE POINTS

- Understanding cellular and immune-mediated response to pathogens, vascular and other complications are essential for radiologic pathology correlation.
- Imaging patterns can sometimes inform pathogenetic mechanisms and pathways of spread.
- Multidisciplinary collaboration is essential to aggregate clinical, pathologic data with imaging patterns because there is substantial overlap.

DISCLOSURE

The authors have nothing to disclose.

REFERENCES

1. Murphey Mark D, Madewell John E, Olmsted William W, et al. A History of Radiologic Pathology Correlation at the Armed Forces Institute of Pathology and

Its Evolution into the American Institute for Radiologic Pathology. Radiology 2012;262(2):623–34.

2. Holmes TM, Petrella JR, Provenzale JM. Distinction between cerebral abscesses and high-grade neoplasms by dynamic susceptibility contrast perfusion MRI. AJR Am J Roentgenol 2004;183(5):1247–52.

3. Chiang IC, Hsieh TJ, Chiu ML, et al. Distinction between pyogenic brain abscess and necrotic brain tumour using 3-tesla MR spectroscopy, diffusion and perfusion imaging. Br J Radiol 2009;82(982): 813–20.

4. Melo GDD, Parize P, Jouvion G, et al. In: Chretien F, Wong KT, Sharer LR, et al, editors. Rabies. Infections of the central nervous system: pathology and Genetics. 1st Edition. John Wiley & sons Ltd; 2020. p. 121–9.

5. Kleinschmidt-DeMasters BK, Beckham DJ. West Nile virus encephalitis 16 years later. Brain Pathol 2015;25:625–33.

6. Cresswell FV, Nathan LT, Bahr NC, et al. on behalf of ASTRO-CM team. Xpert MTB/RIF Ultra for the diagnosis of HIV-associated tuberculous meningitis: a prospective validation study. Lancet Inf Dis 2020; 20:208–17.

7. Wong KT, Ng KY, Ong KC, et al. Enterovirus 71 encephalomyelitis and Japanese encephalitis can be distinguished by topographic distribution of inflammation and specific intraneuronal detection of viral antigen and RNA. Neuropathol Appl Neurobiol 2012;38:443–53.

8. Wong KT, Munisamy B, Ong KC, et al. The distribution of inflammation and virus in human enterovirus 71 encephalomyelitis suggests possible viral spread by neural pathways. J Neuropathol Exp Neurol 2008; 67:162–9.

9. Ong KC, Badmanathan M, Devi S, et al. Pathologic characterisation of a murine model of human Enterovirus 71 encepalomyelitis. J Neuropathol Exp Neurol 2008;67:532–42.

10. Cheng Hua, Zeng Jinjin, Hongjun, et al. Review: Neuroimaging of HFMD infected by EV71. Radiol Infect Dis 2015;1:103e108.

11. Messacar Kevin, Asturias Edwin J, Hixon Alison M, et al. Enterovirus D68 and acute flaccid myelitis-evaluating the evidence for causality. Lancet Infect Dis 2018;18(8):e239–47.

12. Fu TL, Ong KC, Tan SH, et al. Japanese encephalitis virus infects the thalamus early followed by sensory-associated cortex and other parts of the central and peripheral nervous system. J Neuropathol Exp Neurol 2019;78:1160–70.

13. Ong KC, Wong KT. Henipavirus Encephalitis: Recent Developments and Advances. Brain Pathol 2015; 25(5):605–13.

14. British Soc for Immunology. Available at: https://www.immunology.org/public-information/bitesized-immunology/receptors-and-molecules/pattern-recognition-receptor-prrs. Accessed December 2021.

15. Goh GX, Tan K, Ang BSP, et al. Neuroimaging in Zoonotic Outbreaks Affecting the Central Nervous System: Are We Fighting the Last War? Am J Neuroradiology 2020. https://doi.org/10.3174/ajnr.A6727.

16. Tan K, Wijaya L, Chiew HJ, et al. Diffusion-Weighted MRI Abnormalities in an Outbreak of Streptococcus agalactiae Serotype III, Multilocus Sequence Type 283 Meningitis. J Magn Reson Imag 2017;45: 507–14.

17. Lim MCK, Ahmad ZA, Low SC, et al. Non-bacterial thrombotic endocarditis: A rare manifestation of cervical adenocarcinoma. Neurol Asia 2018;23(1): 97–9.

18. Ng WK, Tan CT. Peripheral nerve involvement in immunocompetent hosts with cryptococcal meningitis: a clinical and electrophysiological study. Neurol J Southeast Asia 1996;1:33–7.

19. Currie Bart J, Fisher Dale A, Howard Diane M, et al. Neurological melioidosis. Acta Tropica 2000;74: 145–51, Issues 2–3.

20. Hsu CCT, Singh D, Kwan G, et al. Neuromelioidosis: Craniospinal MRI Findings in Burkholderia pseudomallei Infection. J Neuroimaging 2016;26:75–82.

21. Bhoi SK, Naik S, Kumar S, et al. Cranial imaging findings in dengue virus infection. J Neurol Sci 2014;342:36–41.

22. Tai SML, Viswanathan S, Rahmat K, et al. Cerebral infarction pattern in tuberculous meningitis. Scientific Rep 2016;6:38802.

23. Lim CCT, Lee KE, Lee WL, et al. Nipah Virus Encephalitis: Serial MR Study of an Emerging Disease. Radiology 2002;222(1):219–26.

24. Wong KT, Shieh WJ, Kumar S, et al. Nipah virus infection: pathology and pathogenesis of an emerging paramyxoviral zoonosis. Am J Pathol 2002;161:2153–67.

25. Sarji SA, Abdullah BJJ, Goh KJ, et al. MR Imaging Features of Nipah Encephalitis. Am J Roentgenol 2000;175:437–42.

26. Potchen MJ, Kampondeni SD, Seydel KB, et al. Acute Brain MRI Findings in 120 Malawian Children with Cerebral Malaria: New Insights into an Ancient Disease. Am J Neuroradiology 2012;33(9):1740–6.

27. Umapathi T, Kor AC, Venketasubramanian N, et al. Large artery ischaemic stroke in severe acute respiratory syndrome (SARS). J Neurol 2004;251: 1227–31.

28. Yaghi S, Ishida K, Torres J, et al. SARS-CoV-2 and Stroke in a New York Healthcare System. Stroke 2020;51(7):2002–11.

29. Zhang T, Duan Y, Ye J. Brain MRI Characteristics of Patients with Anti-N-Methyl-D-Aspartate Receptor Encephalitis and Their Associations with 2-Year Clinical Outcome. Am J Neuroradiol 2018;39(5):824–9.

30. Kimura-Hayama E, Higuera JA, Corrona-Sedillo R, et al. Neurocysticercosis: Radiologic-Pathologic Correlation. RadioGraphics 2010;30(6).

31. Goh KJ, Tan CT, Chew NK, et al. Clinical features of Nipah virus encephalitis among pig farmers in Malaysia. N Engl J Med 2000;342(17):1229–35.

32. Verdonk F, Mazeraud A, Chretian F, et al. Sepsis-Associated Encephalopathy. In: Chetrian F, Wong KT, Sharer LR, editors. Infections of the central nervous system: pathology and Genetics. Willey Blackwell; 2020. p. 11–20.

33. Koeller Kelly K, Shih Robert Y. Viral and Prion Infections of the Central Nervous System: Radiologic-Pathologic Correlation: From the Radiologic Pathology Archives. RadioGraphics 2017;37(1):199–233.

34. Shenton ME, Dickey CC, Frumin M, et al. A review of MRI findings in schizophrenia. Schizophr Res 2001; 49(1–2):1–52.

35. Fong SL, Wong SJ, Tan AH, et al. Neurological melioidosis in East Malaysia: Case series and review of the literature. Neurol Asia 2017;22(1): 25–32.

36. Politi LS, Salsano E, Grimaldi M. Magnetic Resonance Imaging Alteration of the Brain in a Patient With Coronavirus Disease 2019 (COVID-19) and Anosmia. JAMA Neurol 2020; 77(8):1028–9.

37. Hwang C. Olfactory neuropathy in severe acute respiratory syndrome: report of a case. Acta Neurol Taiwanica 2006;15(1):26.

Moving?

Make sure your subscription moves with you!

To notify us of your new address, find your **Clinics Account Number** (located on your mailing label above your name), and contact customer service at:

Email: Journalscustomerservice-usa@elsevier.com

800-654-2452 (subscribers in the U.S. & Canada)
314-447-8871 (subscribers outside of the U.S. & Canada)

Fax number: 314-447-8029

**Elsevier Health Sciences Division
Subscription Customer Service
3251 Riverport Lane
Maryland Heights, MO 63043**

*To ensure uninterrupted delivery of your subscription, please notify us at least 4 weeks in advance of move.

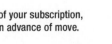

Printed and bound by CPI Group (UK) Ltd, Croydon, CR0 4YY

Printed and bound by CPI Group (UK) Ltd, Croydon, CR0 4YY

03/10/2024

01040308-0005